Metatheory and Interviewing

Metatheory and Interviewing

Harm Reduction and Motorcycle Safety in Practice

Emily J. Haas and Marifran Mattson

LEXINGTON BOOKS
Lanham • Boulder • New York • London

Published by Lexington Books
An imprint of The Rowman & Littlefield Publishing Group, Inc.
4501 Forbes Boulevard, Suite 200, Lanham, Maryland 20706
www.rowman.com

Unit A, Whitacre Mews, 26-34 Stannary Street, London SE11 4AB

British Library Cataloguing in Publication Information Available

Library of Congress Cataloging-in-Publication Data Is Available

ISBN 978-0-7391-8056-3 (cloth : alk. paper)
ISBN 978-0-7391-8057-0 (electronic)

♾™ The paper used in this publication meets the minimum requirements of American National Standard for Information Sciences—Permanence of Paper for Printed Library Materials, ANSI/NISO Z39.48-1992.

Printed in the United States of America

To my mom, Joyce, and dad, Bob, for your continuous encouragement, faith, and love. —EJH

To Jim and Simon (woof!) for your unconditional love and support. —MM

To the motorcyclists who participated in this research project. Their time and willingness to share their experiences and opinions made this research project possible and contributed to making the roads safer for everyone.

Contents

Preface ix

Acknowledgments xiii

1 The Origins and Iterations of Harm Reduction Theory 1

2 Setting the Stage for Harm Reduction Metatheory 35

3 Improving the Theoretical Utility of Harm Reduction: A Motorcycle Safety Exemplar 73

4 A Qualitative Approach to Applying Harm Reduction Metatheory 97

5 Qualitative Analysis Informed by Harm Reduction Metatheory: Implications for Motorcycle Safety 121

6 Validity and Reflexivity in Harm Reduction Qualitative Research 175

7 Harm Reduction Championing Research Ethics 201

Summary: Future Directions for Harm Reduction Metatheory 239

Appendices 243

Index 277

About the Authors 279

Preface

We believe this book fills a void in current harm reduction research methodology offerings by discussing a new, applied use for harm reduction as a metatheory and connecting this metatheory to qualitative methodology in an effort to enhance harm reduction research and theory. This book explains and demonstrates a unique approach and provides a practical tool for conducting harm reduction, qualitative research interviews with at-risk individuals. Specifically, we argue that using harm reduction as a metatheory to guide qualitative interviews strengthens (1) the use and acceptance of harm reduction and (2) constructs within health theories, resulting in more effective application of those theories.

To demonstrate how harm reduction metatheory can guide and inform health theory while conducting research, we provide *Research in Practice Illustrations* throughout the book that focus on the development, implementation, and analysis of in-depth interviews with at-risk motorcyclists as a qualitative approach to research methodology. The *Research in Practice Illustrations* applies Harm Reduction Theory (HRT) as a metatheory (Haas, 2012) to the Reconceptualized Health Belief Model (RHBM; Mattson, 1999) in targeting motorcyclists to practice safety behaviors on the road.

AUTHORS' UNIQUE EXPERIENCES IN HARM REDUCTION THEORY AND MOTORCYCLE SAFETY

As you read this book you may wonder why we chose motorcycle safety as the case study illustration. Both I and my co-author, Marifran Mattson, have unique experiences that eventually led us to become interested in motorcycle safety independently and then together, with an end goal of making the roads safer for motorcyclists. Our experiences bring different perspectives to this health and safety issue that allows for a rich discourse and analysis surrounding motorcycle safety. Our stories are presented in turn.

When I arrived home after my first year of college in Summer 2004, I found out that my cousin, Ryan, bought a new Harley-Davidson Sportster motorcycle. Although some people in my family had positive or negative reactions to Ryan's purchase, I had not thought about motorcycle safety as an important health issue that warranted attention. However, later that summer, Ryan was in a motorcycle accident. After striking a curb, Ryan was thrown from his motorcycle and his head struck the base of the crossing arm of a railroad signal device. He died eight hours later due to a closed head injury. Ryan was not wearing a helmet and his blood alcohol content (BAC) level was 0.26.

After Ryan's death I wondered what role I could have had in preventing his tragic accident. But, even if I wanted to communicate with Ryan about motorcycle safety, I did not know what to say. After I realized that I did not know how to appropriately and accurately communicate safety concerns to my cousin, I wanted to learn how to communicate with other people who were engaging in risky driving behaviors. This experience ultimately led me to start studying health communication, with a specific interest in motorcycle safety.

Much like my desire to learn about motorcycle safety, a Motorcycle Safety Campaign came about literally by accident. About three months after my cousin died my colleague, Marifran Mattson, who I had not yet met, was involved in a motorcycle accident. While motorcycle riding with a small group of friends in Fall 2004, she collided with a semitruck. The accident resulted in severe injuries, including a severed leg. After a life-saving emergency helicopter transport, a month-long stay in a trauma unit, and several months in recovery and rehabilitation, she returned to campus scheduled to teach a graduate course on evaluating health campaign messages. Students, however, encouraged the development of a two-course graduate-level sequence on health campaigns culminating in the design, implementation, and evaluation of a motorcycle safety campaign, known today as the Motorcycle Safety at Purdue (MS@P) campaign.

This ongoing campaign targets motorcyclists, friends and family of motorcyclists, and drivers of cars and trucks. Although I was not in the original classes that conceived the campaign, I became involved in the campaign soon after arriving on campus as a PhD student in 2008. Around the same time, Marifran introduced me to Harm Reduction Theory. I immediately gravitated toward the nonjudgmental and realistic tenets of this theory, realizing how difficult abstinence from risky behaviors can be for different target audiences. Marifran agreed to work with me in further assessing the use of HRT in health campaign research, and we began focusing on motorcycle safety as a case study approach for how HRT could be used to gradually guide behavior change.

While working together both on expanding the use of HRT and new motorcycle safety initiatives, the combination of our experiences and dedication to this issue helped us conceptualize harm reduction as a metatheory, apply the proposed metatheory to theory, and observe how motorcyclists' responses were more open and honest in comparison to previous research studies. Because of our previous research experience with motorcycle safety, we could see how using harm reduction as a metatheory was enhancing the quality of the in-depth interviews being conducted.

We sincerely hope both our personal experiences and research experiences revolving around motorcycle safety help us better communicate how harm reduction metatheory enhanced our research methodology, and helps provide you with an opening to insert your own health and research interests.

ORGANIZATION

The book begins by discussing the history and definitions of Harm Reduction Theory and how this has been applied in health and safety research. The subsequent chapters conceptualize harm reduction as a metatheory and address how harm reduction metatheory can reinforce the application of theory in interview research including the development of interview protocols, conducting interviews, analyzing data, and utilizing the results to address target audiences. These chapters are organized around motorcycle safety research in practice illustrations to provide in-depth examples of how this unique approach to interviewing can be used to link metatheory, theory, methodology, and ultimately application and translation of research results. The book culminates with a discussion of how applying harm reduction from a metatheoretical perspective to conduct and analyze interviews can enhance the use of theory in research and practice while facilitating a deeper, more intimate conversation with research participants by encouraging them to incorporate the same, overarching harm reduction framework to provide pragmatic feedback about changing specific health behaviors.

We encourage you to utilize this book as a tool to learn more about how to integrate harm reduction as an overarching framework in your future research projects and hope offering our approach to the research methodology of interviewing can serve as a reference to assist you in adapting your own research projects.

Acknowledgments

We would like to acknowledge the support provided throughout different phases of this research project:

Tamara Loew, Nancy Maylath, and Stephanie Orstad for their contributions to the harm reduction approach to address high-risk drinking among college students. Their tireless work to address high-risk drinking behaviors at Purdue University via a harm reduction approach has served as a model for other universities.

Adam Barry for his contribution to the high-risk drinking literature. His research focus helped further support reasons for a harm reduction approach to address high-risk behaviors.

College of Liberal Arts at Purdue University for supporting the funding of a portion of the typesetting costs.

The Motorcycle Safety at Purdue (MS@P) campaign for providing an outlet to study harm reduction motorcycle safety initiatives.

Stacey Connaughton, Robin Jensen, and William McInerney, for their constructive comments in the early phases of this research project.

I also would like to thank those who helped instigate and then support this book throughout the writing process:

Marifran Mattson, for introducing me to Harm Reduction Theory, being an instigator to keep this project going, and sharing qualitative research insights and expertise, which I apply every day to help keep other individuals as healthy and safe as possible.

Thomas, for calling just to "check-in," Cassie, for providing constant humor in our research life, and Joe, for always having a positive and patient attitude throughout the weekends of writing and celebrating every accomplishment along the way.

Safe and Healthy Regards,
Emily J. Haas, PhD

Chapter 1

The Origins and Iterations of Harm Reduction Theory

This book is primarily dedicated to expanding the theoretical utility of harm reduction in health and safety research and practice. Harm Reduction Theory (HRT) has informed various research projects and applications in the fields of public health, health promotion, health communication, psychology, and public policy. If you have reviewed HRT in any of these disciplines or domains, you probably noticed that HRT is defined and used in various ways. Because varying definitions and uses of HRT are discussed in the literature, it is important to establish a common lexicon as you continue reading this book. This chapter provides an introduction to HRT and is guided by the following objectives:

- Provide a brief history of HRT
- Discuss barriers that prevent consistent use of HRT in health and safety research and practice
- Discuss other terms that are associated with HRT
- Highlight varying definitions of HRT and propose a comprehensive definition of HRT
- Present and define five consistent tenets of HRT

This chapter begins by discussing the origins of HRT. HRT is a longstanding concept with modest beginnings (Einstein, 2007; Stimson & O'Hare, 2010). Initially, HRT was considered a model that transcended traditional boundaries and bridged gaps between medicine and public health (Marlatt, 1998). The primary roots of HRT are in "the scientific public health model, with deeper roots in humanitarianism and libertarianism" (Newcombe, 1992, p. 1) HRT "contrasts with abstentionism, which is rooted more in the punitive law enforcement model, and in medical and religious paternalism" (p. 1).

Since its application in the field of public health, a main focus of harm reduction is to initiate and encourage healthy behavior change (Wintstock, Wolff, & Ramsey, 2004). According to Marlatt (1998), HRT is an umbrella term for interventions aiming to reduce the problematic effects of negative health behaviors. Essentially, HRT supports any steps toward positive behavior change.

Although the general concepts of HRT have been applied in practice for decades (see examples in Table 1.1), the term "harm reduction" was not adopted until approximately the mid-1980s during the initial years of the HIV/AIDS epidemic (Springer, 1991; Stimson, 2007). Around the same time, John Ashton in the Department of Health at the University of Liverpool, and later the Mersey Regional Director of Public Health, in addition to Howard Seymour, head of the Health Promotion of the Mersey Regional Health Authority (MRHA), began working on ideas for the *New Model for Public Health* (O'Hare, 2007). They used tenets of HRT to describe their public health goals for the new model, which was designed to recognize the social aspects of health problems that impact individual lifestyles. Their approach emphasized primary care, multi-agency interaction, and public engagement (Ashton & Seymour, 2010). Conceptualizing a new model for public health that incorporated harm reduction strategies helped avoid victim blaming during health interventions (Ashton & Seymour, 1988). In addition, the foundational tenets of HRT began to reorient health practitioners toward aiding prevention efforts rather than solely responding to and treating an existing disease and/or addiction (O'Hare, 2007).

By the mid-1980s, harm reduction facilities were established at the new Mersey Region Drug Treatment Centre in the United Kingdom (UK), including three needle exchange programs (NEPs). Other countries quickly followed this example, as displayed in Table 1.2. These early HIV/AIDS projects paved the way for harm reduction developments around the world (Stimson & O'Hare, 2010) with interventions operating in a wide range of social, cultural, and religious settings (Kamarulzaman & Saifuddeens, 2010).

Table 1.1 Early Examples of Harm Reduction Practices

1912–1923	Narcotic maintenance clinics in the US
1926	Report of the *UK Departmental Committee on Morphine and Heroin Addiction* supported opiate prescriptions to help maintain normality for heroin-dependent patients
1960s	Emergence of "controlled drinking" as an alternative to abstinence-based treatments for some alcohol users
1960s+	Grassroots work on reducing harms connected to the use of LSD, cannabis, amphetamines, and glue sniffing

Source: Cook, Bridge, & Stimson, 2010, p. 38.

Table 1.2 Early Timeline of Harm Reduction Needle Exchange Programs

1984	Junkie-Bond in the Netherlands started a needle exchange program in response to the hepatitis B epidemic (Stimson & O'Hare, 2010)
1984	Switzerland began developing harm reduction centers (Stimson & O'Hare, 2010)
1986	Grassroots community approaches began in Sydney, Australia, and many European cities when additional needle exchange programs formed (Cook, Bridge, & Stimson, 2010)
1988	The United States formed a needle exchange program in New York and adopted the term "harm reduction" (Newcombe, 1987)

So far this review indicates that HRT is most frequently associated with substance misuse and abuse. Other than reducing the risk of HIV transmission by supporting NEPs, HRT also can function to help encourage less risky alcohol consumption for underage individuals; safer sex; mindful eating skills; and minimal exercise each day (Logan & Marlatt, 2010). These harm reduction efforts occur in a variety of settings including individual counseling centers and school-based interventions (e.g., McBride et al., 2004; Poulin & Nicholson, 2005), college-based interventions (e.g., Dimeff, Baer, Kvlahan, & Marlatt, 1999; Larimer & Cronce, 2007; Little & Franskoviak, 2010), worksite interventions with older adults (e.g., Cook, Back, & Trudeau, 1996; Matano et al., 2000), trauma center interventions (e.g., Gentilello et al., 1999; Schermer, Moyers, Miller, & Bloomfield, 2006), interventions in areas where the homeless congregate (e.g., Tsemberis, Gulcur, & Nakae, 2004), and community intervention sites such as nicotine replacement centers, opioid substitution, needle exchange programs, and safe injection sites (Little & Franskoviak, 2010; Logan & Marlatt, 2010).

In some cases abstinence may be the ultimate goal of these interventions, but more often HRT focuses on accepting and reducing individuals' risky health behaviors (Heather, 2006). So, the general goal of HRT interventions is not necessarily to eliminate the behavior but to manage the negative effects of the behavior. In managing risky health and safety behaviors, Marlatt (1998) stated that HRT approaches help address "the power differential between those who administer and deliver health services and those who receive them, to give a voice in the decisions of how, where, and in what manner people are treated" (p. xii).

HRT interventions are based on several tenets, including humanistic value (Mattson & Basnyat, 2008; Riley & O'Hare, 2000), pragmatism (Des Jarlais, 1995; Lenton & Single, 2004), immediacy and goal setting (Marlatt & Witkiewitz, 2010; Mattson & Basnyat, 2008), empowering individuals through choice (Reid, 2002; Shepard, 2007), and community collaboration (Little & Franskoviak, 2010), to facilitate healthier and safer behaviors.

In general, guidelines from these tenets help practitioners communicate with risky individuals including accepting where individuals' attitudes are regarding their ability and motivation to change behaviors. These tenets are defined, discussed, and applied in detail in subsequent sections of the book. Now that a brief background of HRT is established, the next section discusses some reasons why HRT has not been regularly integrated into health and safety research and practice.

BARRIERS TO INTEGRATING HARM REDUCTION THEORY INTO RESEARCH AND PRACTICE

Throughout the iterative refinement of HRT interventions from the 1960s to current applications, HRT continues to encounter barriers to consistent use in health and safety research and practice. In reference to these barriers, Sweanor (2007) argued during an interview with *Eudoxa*, an independent research foundation, that policymakers often forget that HRT is a key aspect of public policy regarding a wide range of health issues. However, it is apparent that the regulative history of several health and safety areas such as medical services and devices, pharmaceuticals, processed foods, automobiles, building standards, municipal water supplies, etc. and their subsequent policies were based in part on HRT tenets (Sweanor, 2007, p. 2).

This oversight regarding the influence of HRT on public policy exists because HRT most often is associated with health concerns such as nicotine addiction, alcohol abuse, illicit drug use, sexual activity, and other issues that arouse strong moral debates within society (Sweanor, Alcabes, & Drucker, 2007). Although research shows that HRT is effective in reducing risky health behaviors and the consequences of those behaviors, the tenets of HRT still are very controversial. However, the positive health outcomes of HRT approaches suggest that health and safety researchers and practitioners need to reconsider how HRT is framed and articulated. This chapter initiates that dialogue by discussing barriers to HRT application relative to the discourse surrounding this topic and how to move beyond those barriers.

Negative Discourse Surrounding Harm Reduction Theory

According to Nadelmann (1993), the "wonderfully neutral" language of harm reduction has made significant contributions in Europe, Australia, and Canada but the same language have failed to take hold in the US. The challenges that face HRT in the US are partly political and partly technical

(Hathaway, 2001). HRT serves as an alternative to prohibition or legalization, both of which may be difficult to accept when referring to illegal behaviors (DuPont & Ford, 2000). After revealing some of the discourse and rhetorical limits of HRT, and later including more empowering discourse into its definition, the health-promoting meaning of HRT may be more apparent and positively valenced. First, HRT is associated with negative and/or inaccurate metaphors that socially construct HRT approaches as promoting the legalization of illicit drugs rendering HRT a very controversial subject. These metaphors allow individuals to imagine the negative effects of HRT approaches in a more emotional tone than via a literal description of the term HRT. The most common metaphor that continues to disempower HRT initiatives is "Trojan horse."

Harm Reduction as a Trojan Horse

HRT often is described as a *Trojan horse*. For example, Hall (2007) argued that HRT is pejorative in the US primarily because it is considered a Trojan Horse for drug legalization (p. 338). Because HRT accepts that people use drugs, individuals argue that HRT interventions may make it easier for people to continue using illegal drugs. In response, when health practitioners use the term HRT to discuss the reduction of negative health outcomes due to risky health behaviors such as drug use, the public may perceive this language as support for legalizing drugs. In this regard, some researchers argue that HRT interventions that facilitate easier drug use are considered a Trojan horse because they seem positive but actually are detrimental to the society (DuPont & Ford, 2000). Specifically, DuPont (2013) argues that those who are in favor of harm reduction strategies have limited firsthand experience with addicts and do not realize that HRT tactics may negatively affect highly vulnerable populations including the homeless, young, and poor.

One of the primary problems with the Trojan horse metaphor is the implication that harm reduction only applies to drug use (Marlatt, 1998). Initially some national and international health organizations (e.g., National Institutes of Health [NIH], Centers for Disease Control and Prevention [CDC], and the World Health Organization [WHO]) supported more general HRT interventions, but political initiatives, such as the US declaration of a "war on drugs," kept HRT interventions from proliferating. The war on drugs was socially constructed by the Nixon administration in 1971 and largely shaped how the United States perceived the tenets of HRT (Dobbs, 2007). Since the declaration of the war on drugs and subsequent development of the Trojan horse metaphor, administrations continually denied national efforts to include harm reduction language in national drug policy

(Lillis, 2010). The US government continued to argue that harm reduction language is ambiguous and may support controversial interventions, such as drug legalization. Instead, the government continued to initiate policy proposals trying to reduce legal restrictions against the use and sale of illegal drugs (DuPont & Voth, 1995). Rather than calling for more emphasis on personal choice and safer habits for drug use, they recommended stronger national policies to reduce the harm of drug use through harm elimination, or abstinence.

Because of its association as a Trojan horse, HRT is criticized for sending the wrong message to the public. However, if benefits of HRT interventions become more apparent and are applied to a variety of other health behaviors, more positive perspectives about HRT may emerge and initiate more optimistic discourse about HRT. Besides utilizing Trojan horse as a metaphor to improperly describe HRT, another barrier to implementing HRT interventions is confusion about HRT terminology. The next section discusses the terms harm minimization and risk reduction and their relationships with harm reduction efforts.

Clarifying the Terms of Harm Reduction

Two terms are used interchangeably with harm reduction: harm minimization and risk reduction. In addition to being used interchangeably, these terms often are used simultaneously within the same research project, causing confusion and inaccurate portrayals of the goals of HRT (Inciardi & Harrison, 2000). Like the Trojan horse metaphor used to describe HRT, the use of harm minimization and risk reduction affects how individuals view the goals and implementation of HRT, creating an inaccurate frame of reference (Lakoff, 2005; Schon, 1993). Although the terms harm minimization and risk reduction may seem similar, Roche, Evans, and Staton (2001) argued that it is difficult to identify what harm reduction *is not* due to the lack of clarity among these terms. This causes ambiguity because HRT is used in place of and/or is compared to other concepts such as harm minimization and risk reduction (Reid, 2002; Roche et al., 2001). This confusion creates a discourse that limits the use of HRT. Consequently, the differences among "harm" terms need to be deciphered and simplified before HRT research can progress (Weatherburn, 2008). To address this, we discuss both terms, harm minimization and risk reduction, and emphasize the distinctions from but connections with HRT.

Harm Reduction and Harm Minimization

Harm minimization is a common goal of drug and alcohol policy, which is to minimize all harm related with drug and alcohol abuse behavior

(Weatherburn, 2008). According to Rumbold and Hamilton (1998), *harm minimization* attempts to "assess the actual harm associated with any particular drug and then asks how these harmful effects may be minimized within an amoral framework" (p. 135). Kellehear, Rumbold, and Hamilton (1998) described harm minimization as a continuous approach to reducing drug use. Although several studies discuss implementing "harm minimization" strategies, harm minimization is seldom defined (McBride et al., 2004; Vogl et al., 2009) or researchers include harm minimization in the title of the study and then use the term harm reduction throughout the study (Winstock, Wolff, & Ramsey, 2001).

As defined above, harm minimization may seem similar to HRT. However, harm minimization more often is used as an umbrella term for harm reduction strategies (Miller, 1999). In addition, internationally (e.g., Australia), harm minimization is used as a metaphor to indicate abstinence-based goals and strategies by reducing the demand for illicit drug use (Bessant, 2008; Blewett, 2004). Therefore, the term harm minimization was used interchangeably with harm reduction to frame HRT efforts within higher moral standards, creating a more powerful rhetorical tool for prohibitionists (Lakoff, 2005). However, while HRT aims to reduce the negative health-related outcomes of engaging in risky behaviors, harm minimization seeks to reduce the supply and demand of the source of the behavior. As Table 1.3 indicates, the goals of harm minimization and HRT are clearly different; harm minimization has abstinence as an end goal whereas HRT does not necessarily strive for abstinence.

Researchers have noted that harm minimization efforts have simply been used to strategically help implement HRT tenets (Kellehear et al., 1998; Rumbold & Hamilton, 1998) and are not effective apart from HRT. Particularly, harm minimization does not emphasize immediacy and goal setting in regards to behavior change, or consistent collaboration with others as important tenets of HRT interventions (Kellehear et al., 1998).

The few, ambiguous, unevaluated uses of harm minimization in combination with HRT have blurred the boundaries of abstinence-based and harm minimization dialogue over time (Miller, 2001). Since harm minimization "failed to adequately consider the role of discourse within its theoretical conceptualizations" (Miller, 2001, p. 169), its contribution to date, especially

Table 1.3 Harm Minimization vs. Harm Reduction

Harm Minimization	*Harm Reduction*
• Aims to reduce supply and demand of the source of the behavior. • Abstinence is more often an end goal.	• Aims to reduce the negative health outcomes of a risky behavior. • Abstinence is less often an end goal.

in the arena of drug use, is minimal. As a result, the use of the term harm minimization failed to influence health behaviors and should not be used in combination with harm reduction. Although the framing of HRT may shift and initially be more difficult to understand for those familiar with harm minimization terminology, the reframing of HRT to its original intention eventually will benefit its acceptance (Lakoff, 1999). Now that harm minimization was discussed as a term confusing to the definition and application of HRT, we address another term confusing the HRT landscape in the next section.

Harm Reduction and Risk Reduction

Another term often associated with HRT is risk reduction (Inciardi & Harrison, 2000). According to Herring et al. (2010), the distinction between harm reduction and risk reduction is that, whereas "harm reduction aims to reduce harm once it has actually been caused, *risk reduction* aims to prevent harm from being caused in the first place" (p. 280). Therefore, as Table 1.4 indicates, risk reduction initiatives operate more on a primary prevention level, since they try to prevent the initial onset of occurrences. HRT clearly is different from this concept, as it strives to reduce harm that, to some extent, already exists in society or in a situation (i.e., secondary prevention).

Much like harm minimization, generally the concept of risk reduction is included in studies and either not defined or researchers begin using harm reduction midway through the study report (DiClemente & Wingood, 1995; Kamb et al., 1998), which can be very confusing to researchers and practitioners trying to utilize harm reduction tenets. In addition, the use of the term risk reduction may serve as a metaphor to conceptualize a less controversial version of HRT for skeptics. Although interchanging these terms may not be negative for HRT, it is confusing, creating a barrier to the advancement of HRT research.

Besides harm minimization and risk reduction, even lesser used terms associated with HRT include responsible drug use, problem prevention, secondary prevention, and risk management (Inciardi & Harrison, 2000). Although these terms are used sparingly and not often confused with HRT, discontinuing use of these terms in conjunction with HRT would be

Table 1.4 Risk Reduction vs. Harm Reduction

Risk Reduction	*Harm Reduction*
• Aims to prevent harm from being caused in the first place. • Primary prevention strategies.	• Aims to reduce harm once it has actually been caused or is in its onset. • Secondary prevention strategies.

beneficial. For example, if the term secondary prevention is used to describe the positive outcome of a HRT intervention, using harm reduction instead of secondary prevention may support a more positive dialogue surrounding HRT. The next section further discusses strategies to help surpass communication barriers surrounding HRT.

Other Disempowering Discourse Surrounding Harm Reduction Theory

So far this review has discussed some reasons that HRT is misunderstood and criticized as encouraging illegal activities or spreading the wrong message to individuals and society (Sweanor, 2007). We highlighted that this misunderstanding is due, in part, to the negative and inaccurate discourse used to represent HRT. In addition, the noncritical and realistic approaches of HRT in practice further position harm reduction as an immoral and irrational approach to drug policy, in particular (Hathaway, 2001). Further, negative discourse surrounding HRT has been perpetuated because of political agendas (Bessant, 2008; Schon, 1993). Rhodes and Hedrich (2010) argued that it is naïve to think that HRT would not be linked to political debate, as is the case with any new public health policy or intervention.

The political debate makes evidence-based arguments and evaluations even more necessary to advancing HRT application. Reid (2002) agreed arguing that the absence of effective and evaluated HRT counseling and health education limits the ability of HRT to achieve and quantify behavior change. Hathaway (2001) also contended that additional empirical resources are needed to pursue a more critical line of HRT research. Although several pro harm reduction researchers agree that additional empirical studies involving harm reduction would be helpful for health and safety research, these researchers also acknowledge that, due to the types of barriers and resistant discourse we have discussed, HRT interventions lack the necessary resources to be rigorously implemented (Stevenson, 1994). These barriers are further exacerbated by current economic conditions, which create a critical need for community organizations and individuals to work together and share resources (Alter & Hage, 1993).

Instead of continuing to participate in political debates over HRT, conceptualizing a less controversial definition and forwarding an empirical method to study HRT initiatives may be most needed to reposition HRT philosophy, and subsequently utility in health and safety research and practice. In the next section we review several definitions of HRT, followed by relevant concepts that can be incorporated into the definition of HRT to facilitate adoption and use. A long-term commitment to this comprehensive conceptualization of HRT may eventually extend the reach and quality of HRT research and interventions (Inciardi & Harrison, 2000) and perhaps even reposition HRT as a viable framework that has more practical utility in health and safety research and practice.

THE VARYING DEFINITIONS OF HARM REDUCTION THEORY

Harm Reduction Theory does not have a consistent, agreed-upon definition (Bigler, 2005; Castro & Foy, 2002; Hilton, Thompson, Moore-Dempsey, & Janzen, 2001; Hunt et al., 2003; Rehm et al., 2010; Riley & O'Hare, 2000; Single, 2000). The lack of an objectively-defined concept of HRT often is blamed for halting the progression of harm reduction research and limiting its empirical basis for implementation and evaluation (Hall, 2007; Leshner, 2008; Rehm & Fisher, 1997). Not only is there not an agreed-upon definition of HRT, but also many meanings and definitions exist, which provoke a variety of reactions, some of which are quite critical (Hall, 2007).

In an effort to forward a consistent definition of HRT, we provide a review of current definitions. Based on the origins of HRT, a majority of the definitions of HRT emphasize the topics of drug-related harm and HIV/AIDS (Burke & Clapp, 1997; Castro & Foy, 2002; Erickson, 1997; Farrell, Gowing, Marsin, Ling, & Ali, 2005; Kimber et al., 2010; Marlatt, 1998; Mattson & Basnyat, 2008; McNeece, 2003; Wiessing et al., 2009; Wodak & Cooney, 2005). More recently, HRT has been applied to other health-related behaviors and services (Castro & Foy, 2000; Eshrati et al., 2008; Nichter et al., 2008; Riley & O'Hare, 2000). To advance the utility of harm reduction, a definition that encompasses a variety of risky health and safety behaviors is necessary. Table 1.5 contains some common definitions used to describe HRT.

Although the substance abuse definitions are inclusive of a spectrum of behaviors that can be addressed in HRT interventions, due to their emphasis on illicit drug use, they are limited in terms of expansion into other health issues. Over time some researchers attempted to forward a more general definition by applying HRT to broader areas of health. For example, Single (1995) described HRT as a health-centered approach seeking to reduce the health and social harms associated with risky behaviors. Another broader definition (Reid, 2002) described HRT as an intervention and/or policy strategy that is used to improve health, social, or economic consequences associated with negative behaviors. The "behavior" can refer to a variety of behaviors including but not limited to decreasing risky alcohol consumption of underage college students, encouraging safer sex, providing clean

Table 1.5 Definitions of Harm Reduction

Examples that Focus on Substance Abuse
• "A set of interventions which seek to reduce the negative consequences of drug use, incorporating a spectrum of strategies from safer use, to managed use to abstinence. HRT is not making drug use solely acceptable but it's accepting that people use drugs" (Harm Reduction Coalition, 2004, p. 26). • "An attempt to ameliorate adverse health, social or economic, consequences of mood-altering substances without necessarily requiring a reduction in the consumption of these substances" (Heather, Wodak, Nadelmann, & O'Hare, 1993, p. vi). • "An attempt to ameliorate health, social, or economic consequences associated with the use, misuse, and abuse of legal, illegal, or psychoactive substances without necessarily requiring a reduction in their consumption" (Einstein, 2007, p. 257). • "A framework for addressing substance use and other potentially risky behaviors, aims to reduce the harmful consequences of these behaviors without requiring abstinence as a goal or a prerequisite of treatment. It is an alternative to traditional treatments that require abstinence and extends the reach of treatment to substance users who are unwilling or unable to embrace abstinence" (Tatarsky & Marlatt, 2010, p. 117).
Examples that Focus on Broader Health Behavior
• "An approach acknowledging that people engage in unhealthy behaviors and seeks to reduce harm that results from that behavior" (Brown, Luna, Ramirez, Vail, & Williams, 2005, p. 318). • A framework "not intended to completely eliminate behavioral risk, but instead, it aims to help minimize possible adverse consequences of the behavior" (Odets, 1998, p. 5). • HRT aims to "reduce the problematic effects of unhealthy behaviors and can include techniques ranging from prevention to intervention to maintenance" (Logan & Marlatt, 2010, p. 203).

razors for those who participate in self-cutting, and supporting minimal exercise each day (Logan & Marlatt, 2010). It is not uncommon to read HRT definitions that are written in research projects to include entire communities (Little & Franskoviak, 2010) and several racial/ethnic minorities (Blume & Lovata, 2010).

Although definitionally HRT has varied widely across settings, some concepts are consistently applied across definitions. For example, most definitions of HRT primarily emphasize the outcome of a behavior rather than the behavior itself. And, a major goal of HRT that is illustrated within most definitions is to reduce negative health outcomes (Rehm et al., 2010). A harm reduction approach differs from typical prevention measures because it emphasizes a pragmatic, nonjudgmental approach and supports any steps taken in the direction toward healthy behavior change (Logan & Marlatt, 2010; Marlatt, 1998). The consistencies in these definitions indicate that although the purpose of HRT is broad, its role in reducing risky health behaviors is quite simple (Bigler, 2005).

However, in order for HRT to move beyond the barriers previously discussed and be broadly accepted and applied, this rather simple concept needs a consistent, noncontroversial definition to highlight the practical tenets that HRT promotes. Although a common goal inherent in these definitions is to improve health outcomes, these definitions do not communicate the unique attributes of HRT that address this goal and advance health research and practice. To address this definitional challenge three concepts are introduced along with what these concepts contribute to a reconceptualization of HRT including what may be missing from current discussions surrounding harm reduction: health promotion, motivational interviewing, and goal setting.

Harm Reduction Theory and Health Promotion

The first concept that may be explicitly missing from HRT is health promotion, sometimes referred to as health protection. Several researchers argue that HRT is closely intertwined with health promotion because HRT tenets and health promotion were initiated during the "new public health" (Ashton & Seymour, 1988; Peterson & Lupton, 1996; Rhodes & Hedrich, 2010). Ashton and Seymour (1988) suggested that health promotion is a broad-based approach to achieving the highest level of health possible for each individual. They defined *health promotion* as, "the means to health is seen as a process of enabling people to increase control over and improve their health" (p. 25). Health promotion emphasizes an individual-level approach and the individual unit of analysis when enabling healthier behaviors. Therefore, health promotion practice encompasses HRT because it focuses on individual control and increasing self-efficacy.

In 1986 the *Ottawa Conference on Health Promotion* developed principles that could strengthen the applicability of health promotion to advance positive health behaviors. When comparing these health promotions principles with the tenets of HRT, there is consistency in the terminology and goals. Table 1.6 shows this comparison.

Table 1.6 Health Promotion Principles vs. Harm Reduction Theory Tenets

Health Promotion Principles	*Harm Reduction Theory Tenets*
• Create public policies that support health	• Implement policy changes
• Create supportive environments	• Strengthen community outreach
• Strengthen community action	• Empower individuals
• Develop personal skills	• Modify the relationship between individuals and their environment
• Reorient health services	• Strengthen personal skills such as goal setting

Source: WHO, 1986; Marlatt, 1998

The similarities between health promotion and HRT indicate that incorporating principles from health promotion (i.e., strengthen community action, environmental support, and personal skills) into the definition of HRT may increase positive connotations associated with this approach to health and safety. For example, in emphasizing the community collaboration aspect of health promotion, Ashton and Seymour (1988) discussed the importance of recognizing that most causes of poor health are due to influences outside of the medical context. In response, health practitioners must be willing to work beyond the boundaries of their institutional offices to investigate and influence the causes of risky health behaviors. This notion of community outreach also is evident in HRT interventions because community collaboration and meeting the client in the appropriate setting is crucial to success (Little & Franskoviak, 2010; Mattson & Basnyat, 2008). Thus the concept of community outreach provides a useful intersection between health promotion and HRT.

In addition, health promotion supports change at the individual level through empowerment. Both HRT and health promotion emphasize the importance of respecting and empowering individuals to increase opportunities to maximize health, regardless of circumstances. This overlap implicates HRT into the conceptual framework of health promotion with "the reduction of risks and harms forming one part of the broader continuum of strategies to promote health and avoid disease" (Downie, Fyfe, & Tannahill, 1990; Marlatt, 1998, p. 9).

It is possible that by integrating health promotion elements within the reconceptualization of HRT, negative connotations associated with HRT may decrease. Although typical health interventions often excessively emphasize the negative aspects of individual health and health behaviors (Downie et al., 1990), health promotion and harm reduction both stress positive efforts individuals make to change health behaviors. For example, the principles of health promotion and tenets of harm reduction recognize that individual behavior change may have positive effects on and strengthen the organization, community, and societal levels (Ashton & Seymour, 1988). In general, both areas stress that any positive change is a healthy change (Logan & Marlatt, 2010).

Because the ecology of the new public health that began in Liverpool focused on the principles of health promotion, HRT tenets emerged from this model of health. However, over the years, the health promotion aspect became separated from HRT. We encourage researchers and practitioners to intentionally link these two areas of research back together in an effort to more accurately depict the goals of HRT. In the next section we consider MI as another health concept to integrate into a new definition of HRT.

Harm Reduction Theory and Motivational Interviewing

Motivational interviewing (MI) often is implicitly integrated within HRT research that focuses on the individual and is consistently recommended as a concept to incorporate into the definition of HRT. MI is designed to activate an individual's own motivation to change and adhere to recommended health behaviors. Generally, *motivational interviewing* is defined as ". . . a collaborative, person-centered form of guiding to elicit and strengthen motivation for change" (Miller & Rollnick, 2009, p. 137). An earlier definition offered by the same researchers was a "A client-centered method for enhancing intrinsic motivation to change by exploring and resolving ambivalence" (Miller & Rollnick, 2005, p. 25). Arkowitz, Westra, Miller, and Rollnick (2008) also described MI as strongly client (individual) centered as it is rooted in Carl Rogers's (1959) therapy.

Not surprisingly, the emphasis of MI is to understand the individual's frame of mind, concerns, and inconsistencies between their behaviors and values (Arkowitz et al., 2008). The three skills necessary for effective MI are asking, informing, and listening. The guiding principles of MI are provided in Table 1.7. The principles illustrate that MI promotes guiding rather than directing and emphasizes listening as much as telling (Rollnick, Miller, & Butler, 2008).

MI posits that people go through stages during the process of changing behaviors (Shernoff, 2006). Shepard (2007) described MI as participants identifying and considering the pros, cons, and contradictory feelings about their behaviors throughout their process of changing behaviors. Research demonstrated that patients exposed to MI versus other treatments were more likely to enter, stay, and complete treatment, including follow-up visits. Shernoff (2006) argued that MI is an appropriate approach to HRT because it enables therapy that targets where the client is, instead of where the therapist wishes the client would be in their progression toward change. Table 1.8 further depicts some similarities and connections between MI and HRT.

These guiding principles of MI are parallel to the tenets of HRT such as empowering, providing choices for the individual, and being nonjudgmental about the past and current decisions of the individual. In light of the similarities between HRT and MI, it is not uncommon to see MI principles

Table 1.7 Guiding Principles of Motivational Interviewing

- Resist the righting reflex
- Understand and explore the individual's own motivations
- Listen with empathy
- Empower the individual encouraging hope and optimism

Source: Miller & Rollnick, 2012

Table 1.8 Motivational Interviewing Principles vs. Harm Reduction Theory Tenets

Motivational Interviewing Principles	*Harm Reduction Theory Tenets*
• Collaborative, evocative, and honors patient autonomy • The partnership between the client and healthcare practitioner is emphasized as a crucial aspect of effective dialogue and health outcomes (Keefe, 1978; Mattson, 2000) • Expresses empathy and building rapport with clients (Logan & Marlatt, 2010) • Commonly used method to empower individuals (Shernoff, 2006)	• Works with individuals as they make their own choices for change and respects these choices without judgment • Recognizes the importance of relationship building and helping clients develop self-efficacy to facilitate behavior change (Brown et al., 2005; Little & Franskoviak, 2010; Mattson, 1999; Shepard, 2007). • Empowerment and the notion of choice is a central focus of HRT interventions (Marlatt, 1998; Mattson & Basnyat, 2008; Shepard, 2007)

incorporated into interventions that focus on harm reduction. For example, Shernoff (2006) applied the principles of MI to influence harm reduction techniques used by gay men. When using these two approaches together throughout the intervention, he found that many men engaged in harm reduction practices such as communicating with their partner and practicing safer sex to reduce risk of HIV transmission.

In addition, one of the areas lacking in current HRT research and practice is the inclusion of consistent communication skills into interventions. Because MI offers three core communication skills to utilize when communicating with individuals, asking, informing, and listening, we believe MI can enhance the communication strategies included in HRT interventions. Specifically, previous studies (Arkowitz et al., 2008; Little & Franskoviak, 2010; Miller & Rollnick, 2002; Whiteside et al., 2010) indicated that the most successful interventions with young adults utilized these three core communication skills, and personal feedback, within the context of MI. As a result, it is possible that using MI techniques during conversations with individuals throughout HRT interventions may strengthen the client-practitioner relationship. To show support for this integration, later in this book we showcase an example of how principles from MI and tenets of HRT came together to influence interviews with at-risk motorcyclists. The final area we highlight as an area to explicitly include into the definition of HRT is goal setting.

Harm Reduction Theory and Goal Setting

Finally, goal setting is another concept we consider beneficial to incorporate into the definition of HRT. Mainly, explicitly discussing the importance of goal setting in HRT practice makes sense, given that aspects of goal setting have been referenced as a tenet of HRT through adhering to a hierarchy of goals (Brocato & Wagner, 2003; Mattson & Basnyat, 2008; O'Hare, 2007; Reid, 2002). Like the previous two concepts we discussed, clearly including goal setting terminology also may help reorient HRT toward more positive connotations. For example, some HRT interventions referred to *goal setting* in which setting realistic goals was consistently correlated with retention and success among the at-risk audience being engaged to modify a behavior (Mattson & Basnyat, 2008; Rogers & Ruefli, 2004). In addition, counselors and other health practitioners often help clients reach goals by working interactively with them to discover connections between their complex attitudes, behaviors, and the changes that they try to pursue (Brocato & Wagner, 2003).

According to research by Locke and Latham (2002), goal setting helps elevate performance, facilitate development, and enhance overall effectiveness of interventions. Likewise, if an individual or organization has poorly developed goals, change likely is hampered or setbacks in progress occur. Consequently, incorporating the concept of small-scale, individualized goals into the definition of HRT is worthwhile. Later in this chapter you will notice the concept of goal setting integrated with an existing HRT tenet, immediacy.

Now that some positive connections between the intentions of HRT have been made with other health-related initiatives in public health promotion research and practice, the next section begins to discuss the conceptualization of a more universal and practitioner-friendly definition of Harm Reduction Theory.

A Comprehensive Definition of Harm Reduction Theory

Erickson (1995) indicated that our interpretations of terms, such as HRT, transform over time and that this change is healthy and essential in the full articulation of an "emerging public health perspective" (p. 238). However, in order for HRT application to expand, a definition with more positive connotations must emerge, since the negative discourse surrounding HRT continues to stifle its use and integration into health and safety research and practice. Based on the variety of definitions and associated concepts reviewed, the following comprehensive, communication-oriented definition of *Harm Reduction Theory* was proposed by Haas (2012):

> Harm reduction theory is a concept and a practical model that seeks to ask, listen, and inform individuals and groups in an effort to understand why and how they engage in risky behaviors. Subsequently, HRT provides guidance for reducing the health risks associated with those behaviors by communicating with individuals to develop a hierarchy of goals that, over time helps protect the health of individuals and of those in their sphere of influence.

We utilize this definition throughout this book to refer to how we envision HRT in health and safety research and practice. This definition highlights that HRT is a concept and a model that seeks to reduce the risks associated with risky health behaviors. Part of what was missing from previous definitions is how HRT can communicate about and inform behavior change in practical applications. To accommodate for this absence, aspects of MI were incorporated into the proposed definition, including asking, listening, and informing individuals. In addition, the concept of goal setting was added into the proposed definition to address the notion of a time frame into HRT interventions. Health promotion also is indicated toward the end of the definition, by emphasizing the well-being of the individual and eventually their society. This definition also is broad enough to be applied to any health or safety intervention as a conceptual starting point to assess the reduction of the negative effects associated with the risky health behaviors practiced by individuals.

In addition, this definition is attempting to move away from past associations with harm minimization and risk reduction that influenced the negative connotations associated with HRT or caused confusion about the general goals of HRT. Instead, this reconceptualization allows HRT to move in a more positive direction by accounting for and addressing the reasons for risky health behaviors in hopes of shifting those behaviors toward more healthy behaviors among individuals. Now that a comprehensive definition of HRT is established for you to reference throughout this book, it is necessary to outline the central tenets of HRT stemming from the definition, which form a framework to guide health and safety research and practice.

CENTRAL TENETS FROM COMPREHENSIVE DEFINITION OF HARM REDUCTION THEORY

Similar to the lack of a consistent and comprehensive definition of HRT, a model to design, implement, and evaluate HRT interventions also does not exist. It is common to encounter several tenets of HRT when reviewing previous HRT applications. However, HRT tenets vary widely across interventions. Establishing consistent tenets to complement the reconceptualization of HRT and to associate with HRT design, implementation, and evaluation is important to expand the use of HRT and subsequently consistently apply harm reduction interventions.

It is common for HRT interventions to be tailored to the specific needs of an individual or community. For this reason, a universal intervention for implementing harm reduction tenets is not possible or practical (Marlatt & Witkiewitz, 2010). Since it is not realistic to create a one-size-fits-all behavior change intervention, it is important for HRT to contain consistent tenets that can be adapted to individuals and communities. For example, upon receiving a cue to action, such as reading a persuasive health message about motorcycle safety, to initiate health behavior change, individuals likely have different situations and may need to change their environment or reassess their personal risks. It is possible that among the varying circumstances and resources individuals experience when deciding how to respond to a particular cue to action, tenets of HRT can be utilized to fit individual situations.

Haas (2012) conducted a review and analysis of HRT tenets to determine which tenets should be proposed as adaptable across HRT applications. From this review, five tenets emerged: humanistic value; pragmatism; immediacy and setting/balancing goals; empowering the individual through an egalitarian relationship of choice; and evidence of collaboration with the community. In the following sections, each tenet is presented and discussed in turn. Later, these tenets are further discussed using motorcycle safety as the health and safety issue to illustrate their application in research and practice, and in tandem with other health behavior theories. For now, we emphasize the definition and utility of each tenet.

Humanistic Value

The first central tenet of HRT is humanistic value. Overall, humanistic value as a tenet in HRT practice emphasizes respect of individuals. To practice this tenet means to acknowledge that risky health behaviors exist in society but also ensure that individuals who participate in these risky behaviors are treated in a nonjudgmental way because all humans have value (Non-Prescription Needle Use Consortium [NPNUC], 2000). Riley and O'Hare (2000) defined *humanistic value* as respecting the dignity and rights of individuals, regardless of the behavior in which they are engaging. In an extensive review of HRT tenets to introduce a study of HIV-test counseling, Mattson and Basnyat (2008) also discussed the importance of humanistic value. They discussed humanistic value as the recognition of individuals' decisions about their health and respecting individuals' right to make their own choices. According to Marlatt (1998), the concept of humanistic value recognizes that people use drugs and engage in other risky health behaviors, and that idealistic visions of a drug-free and completely healthy society are unlikely to become reality.

Recognizing this reality, HRT encourages a less coercive approach to helping people with problems and works to reduce the stigma associated with risky health behaviors (Marlatt, 1998; Tucker, Donovan, & Marlatt, 1999). It is crucial to adopt a humanistic perspective in HRT interventions so dignity and respect are accorded to drug users and others who participate in risky behaviors, and they are not judged because of these behaviors (Brocato & Wagner, 2003). If health and safety practitioners acknowledge and accept individuals' behavior choices, it may help reduce barriers that impede at-risk individuals from seeking and responding to assistance. A harm reduction philosophy allows health practitioners to provide practical service without discrimination toward those who are engaging in risky health behaviors (NPNUC, 2000; Race, 2007). Once humanistic value occurs in HRT interventions, pragmatism often is incorporated as a complementary tenet.

Pragmatism

A related core tenet of HRT is the creation of pragmatic responses to individuals who participate in risky health behaviors (Des Jarlais, 1995; Lenton & Single, 2004). Basically, *pragmatism* emphasizes understanding as the main, cognitive goal of decision-making (Boersema, 2009). Pragmatism developed as a movement in the late nineteenth century and appealed to Americans because "it places human destiny in the hands of users" (Sharpes, 2009, p. 113). Riley and O'Hare (2000) classified pragmatism simply as doing what works. Rorty (1999) summarized the concept of pragmatism by stating that for those who practice pragmatism, "There is no sharp break between natural science and social science, nor between social science and politics, nor between politics, philosophy and literature. All areas of culture are parts of the same endeavor to make life better" (p. xxv). Similarly, Habermas noted that the greatest strength of pragmatism is its combination of anti-skepticism and naturalistic approaches to the human mind (as quoted in Aboulafia, Bookman, & Kemp, 2002). Along these same lines, Sharpes (2009) described the epistemology of pragmatism as acting on sensory experience and creating one's own knowledge through interacting with the surrounding environment.

In HRT, pragmatism refers to the principle of compassionate pragmatism versus moralistic idealism (Marlatt, 1998). In other words, practicing pragmatism means being realistic about the behaviors of individuals and communities and focusing on harm-reducing actions instead of abstinence from a risky behavior (Heather, 2006). Pragmatism in HRT interventions can help ensure that policies and/or strategies that are impossible to achieve or that create more harm than good are not pursued (Stronach, 2003). HRT accepts individuals' participation in risky health behaviors as reality and focuses on reducing the harms or risks associated with those behaviors (Reid, 2002). Acceptance of risky health behaviors may guide the development of more productive methods to reduce potentially harmful consequences. Working with an individual to develop realistic intervention goals and focus on consistent efforts toward reducing the harms of a continued risky health behavior is one way to incorporate pragmatism into HRT (Des Jarlais, 1995; Lenton & Single, 2004).

Generally, pragmatism is described as being realistic and accepting of individuals' health behaviors and providing realistic goals in response to those behaviors. For example, in an HIV-test-counseling session, a counselor would employ pragmatism by "accepting unconditionally that individuals engage in risky behaviors and rather than eliminating the cause (i.e., unsafe sex), they would focus on reducing the negative effects of the risk such as negotiating relevant skills to employ in the future, increase general knowledge, and provide access to condoms" (Mattson & Basnyat, 2008, p. 151). Pragmatism has been emphasized as a central tenet to modify individuals' behaviors to reduce risks to their health and safety (Brocato & Wagner, 2003).

Health practitioners cannot be pragmatic about health behavior change until attention to humanistic value (i.e., acceptance of an individual's risky health behavior) occurs. However, once recognition and acceptance of risky behaviors occurs it is possible to help individuals engage in goal setting until they gradually achieve a healthier goal, which eventually may be abstinence. Pragmatism is a value or attitude that should be considered by health practitioners to help engage others in leading healthier lives. Complementing the accepting and realistic approaches previously discussed as important tenets of HRT, developing a hierarchy of goals is an important way to effectively reduce immediate harm to individuals and is considered another tenet of HRT.

Immediacy/Goal Setting

HRT also emphasizes the consequences of immediate harms rather than focusing on a long-term goal. *Immediacy*, essentially described as prioritizing, does not mean that HRT excludes long-term treatment or abstinence as an ultimate goal (Marlatt, 1998; Mattson & Basnyat, 2008; NPNUC, 2000; Reid, 2002). Rather, a goal is to aid the individual in developing specific coping strategies, often in the form of a hierarchy of goals, to begin reducing the negative behaviors and subsequently the consequences of those behaviors (Riley & O'Hare, 2000). Often, this occurs by understanding the risky health behaviors and how those behaviors impact the community (Mattson & Basnyat, 2008). Immediacy and the concept of goal setting also is highlighted by Brocato and Wagner (2003) who argued for the importance of prioritizing the amelioration of physical, social, and economic harms associated with drug use, rather than prioritizing the elimination of drug use.

The concepts of immediacy/goal setting created some controversy about HRT. Some behaviors, such as reducing the amount of alcohol an individual consumes, are less controversial than providing clean needles for drug users. Marlatt and Witkiewitz (2010) recognized this when they suggested that a main purpose of HRT is to identify, measure, and assess the importance of harms while balancing the costs and benefits of trying to reduce harms. Based on the severity of an individual's behaviors, a spectrum of short-term and long-term goals may be negotiated, addressing realistic goals that may quickly reduce immediate harm.

Since HRT prefers a nonjudgmental, pragmatic approach, its methods aim for any positive progress over no progress in achieving an ultimate health goal. Despite criticism from those who value abstinence-only models, supporters of HRT remind us that HRT recognizes abstinence as an ideal outcome but accepts alternatives that reduce harm (Marlatt, 1998; Reid, 2002). In other words, harmful effects of risky behaviors including unsafe drug use or sexual activity can be placed along a continuum that ranges from less to more harmful (Prochaska & Velicer, 1997).

Since one of the overarching concepts in the definition of HRT is to reduce harm associated with risky health behaviors, it is imperative that immediacy and goal setting are included and assessed during HRT interventions. Within this tenet, health practitioners can apply different strategies, such as messaging or MI, to decrease risky health behaviors and the negative effects of those risky behaviors on the individual and society. Addressing these immediate goals with the individual may help increase self-efficacy (Bandura, 1991), motivating the individual to continue setting goals toward better health. This tenet is an important aspect of HRT implementation and evaluation because the majority of communication with an individual likely occurs during goal setting, when an individual is motivated to alter current behavior.

Much like the previous three tenets, the fourth proposed tenet of HRT emphasizes the individual as the agent of change. However, this tenet specifically focuses on empowering individuals by allowing them to make their own choices when deciding what behaviors to change and to what extent.

Empowerment of the Individual

In order to reduce the negative outcomes associated with risky health behaviors, empowerment is another fundamental emphasis of HRT. Traditionally, public health practice places healthy decision-making as the responsibility of the individual (Peterson & Lupton, 1996). However, it is also recognized that the social environment plays a role in shaping the risks individuals are surrounded by on a daily basis (Rhodes, 2002). Health practitioners can help empower individuals by encouraging implementation of short-term pragmatic goals over long-term idealistic goals (Reid, 2002). *Empowerment* involves communicating choices with individuals, a key aspect of effective HRT interventions (NPNUC, 2000; Shepard, 2007). Shepard (2007) stated, "When clients are given the choice of treatment, they do better than if they are assigned a treatment by someone else" (p. 26). Practicing empowerment and providing choices are themes that should be emphasized in HRT interventions. When provided with choices, individuals gain a sense of control over their own lives, often leading to increased health and well-being (NPNUC, 2000).

The importance of empowering individuals has been emphasized consistently in HRT research, but has not regularly been assessed in the implementation and outcomes of HRT interventions. Although empowerment can be facilitated by short-term goal setting, working with at-risk populations to create choices for each individual also needs to be emphasized separately. In addition to providing choices, health practitioners must listen to individuals' responses to their choices, which are consistent with the MI principles of asking, listening, and informing (Rollnick & Miller, 2002).

HRT promotes low-threshold access to services as an alternative to traditional, high-threshold approaches (Marlatt, 1998). Low-threshold interventions reach out and achieve community partnerships within target populations in order to help more accurately develop new interventions and services (Marlatt, 1998). Counseling is an example of a low-threshold program and is a method used to empower individuals who are trying to change their risky health behaviors. In addition, empowering the individual also increases individuals' self-efficacy, or self-confidence, which are integral to initiating and maintaining behavior change (Denning, 2000).

For example, Mattson (2000) indicated that HRT has the "theoretical and practical vitality to reduce the relevant harms of HIV/AIDS through HIV-test-counseling discourse that empowers and promotes clients' agency" (p. 339). Consistent with HRT Mattson (2000) suggested that the HIV-test-counseling protocol needed to shift from being test driven to more client-centered (Centers for Disease Control and Prevention [CDC], 1993). Like HIV-test-counseling protocols, messages for other health issues may need to be altered to be more client-centered and empowering. Therefore, harm reduction is an applicable fit for HIV-test-counseling because it promotes that individuals have choices about their health behaviors.

Keefe (1978) also argued that harm reduction practitioners need to promote an egalitarian spirit of partnership between practitioner and client. Because discussing a harm-reducing lifestyle is a main goal of HRT interventions, the opinions of clients about what methods would best reduce the risks in their lives should be considered. For example, developing a guiding script, such as the protocol suggested by Mattson (2000), using HRT tenets may empower individuals to make healthier choices. The final tenet of HRT emphasizes the importance of community collaboration during interventions in order to initiate healthy behavior change.

Community Collaboration

HRT emerged primarily as a bottom-up approach based on advocacy for drug addicts, rather than a top-down policy promoted by drug policymakers (Marlatt, 1998). Therefore, it is not surprising that community-based efforts are used to implement effective HRT interventions. Harm reduction enhances the community as a whole, via *community collaboration*, by focusing on the interests of the individual that also impact the interests of the surrounding community (Mattson & Basnyat, 2008). Current approaches to health recognize the need to create more "enabling environments" to facilitate harm reduction and behavior change (WHO, 1986). In order to create these more enabling environments, communicating action and cooperation is necessary (WHO, 1986). As a result, HRT interventions "recognize and reduce the harmful costs of risky behaviors while maximizing the benefits of healthy behaviors for everyone" (Mattson & Basnyat, 2008, p. 151). HRT aims to accomplish community interventions by brainstorming and balancing the costs and benefits of the interventions (Mattson & Basnyat, 2008), demonstrating the importance of conceptualizing treatment as collaboration (Brocato & Wagner, 2003), and maximizing healthy behaviors for the individual.

In some situations, collaboration is considered the missing link in creating more effective HRT interventions. Community-based research is necessary for the development and evaluation of an effective HRT intervention (Brown et al., 2005). According to Little and Franskoviak (2010), a community-based setting is where "people congregate that is not designated as a formal therapy office, mental health clinic, or drug or alcohol treatment program" (p. 177). These community settings can vary from public health settings to outreach interventions such as needle exchange programs (NEPs), sexually transmitted disease (STD) prevention interventions, food pantries, community centers, individual housing, and employment research centers (Little & Franskoviak, 2010).

Many HRT studies include collaboration between individuals trying to change their behavior and other people within their communities whom they affect or are affected by in terms of health decisions (e.g., Dhand, 2006; Cooper et al., 2005; Nichter et al., 2008; Rogers & Ruefli, 2004; Ruefli & Rogers, 2004). However, research also indicates that initially sustaining community collaborations often is a greater challenge than establishing positive links with people in the community (Brocato & Wagner, 2003; Brown et al., 2005). Brown et al. (2005) contended that one of the most effective ways to improve collaboration may be through more tailored communication.

Little and Franskoviak (2010) stated, "A fundamental characteristic of community-based treatment is that the frame of the treatment is informed by the needs of the members of the community in which the program is located" (p. 179). In other words, HRT interventions cannot neglect the environmental factors that promote or hinder success in reducing risky health behaviors. For example, previous research (Carey, Scott-Schelden, Carey, & DeMartini, 2007; Larimer & Cronce, 2007) suggested that HRT techniques strongly impact self-efficacy among adolescents. Therefore, HRT interventions, in addition to the necessary formative research, may be particularly germane in high school and college settings, targeting adolescents engaging in risky health behaviors.

Once formative research is conducted and applicable community collaborations are established, the next step is to devise a strategic plan to work with the particular target audience. Sheon (2004) offered suggestions specific to harm reduction to apply when collaborating with the community. These suggestions include: recognizing and removing judgments of others; acknowledging that any reduction in harm is a step in a positive direction; developing and practicing pragmatic policies; creating an exchange of ideas with intervention participants; understanding that change is not always linear; and incorporating each participant in the planning and evaluation of interventions. These suggestions are consistent with the five tenets of HRT proposed in this book indicating the importance of community collaboration within an overall framework of HRT.

Brown et al. (2005) made a similar observation, noting that it is important for community collaboration to occur during the planning, design, implementation, and evaluation of a project. Community collaboration helps sustain interventions. As Bazzoli et al. (1997) stated, "public-private partnerships form to help develop an infrastructure for assessment, planning, and evaluation of community health needs and to integrate health and human services into collaborative service networks" (p. 533). Including this concept into the tenets of HRT may motivate organizations and individuals to partner when establishing an HRT intervention and may assist health practitioners in consistently assessing if additional collaborations are necessary.

Although the literature shows that community-research collaboration is necessary for both the development and evaluation of HRT interventions (Brown et al., 2005), a major barrier to collaboration is that capacity building often takes time. Therefore, it may take an extensive amount of time before an HRT intervention is implemented and its collaborative efforts evaluated.

Summary of HRT Tenets

This discussion of HRT interventions supports that harm reduction approaches tend to share common characteristics and goals, such as providing a range of services that are responsive to the needs and preferences of individuals, rather than continuing the "one size fits all" approach of most traditional treatment interventions (Tucker et al., 1999). We also discovered that, although most HRT interventions communicate similar ideas, different vocabularies are used to describe those ideas. We argue that it is necessary to have a consistent approach to help guide researchers and practitioners as they consider, design, implement, and evaluate HRT interventions. Ideally, this consistency needs to encompass all tenets of HRT and include consistent phrasing so that the outcomes of interventions can be compared across health and safety issues. Incorporating these five tenets into an overarching framework may encourage consistent interventions and comparable data for analysis and feedback.

SUMMARY

This chapter provided an overview of HRT showing that, initially, the objectives of HRT were simple and focused on drug abuse. The main goals of HRT were to reduce the negative health outcomes that may occur as a result of sharing drug injection equipment, injecting drug use, and street drug use, and if possible increase abstinence. These concepts were presented as a hierarchy of objectives (O'Hare, 2007). Since its inception, HRT was known for its radical and revolutionary approach to dealing with risky health behaviors (O'Hare, 2007) and recently expanded beyond drug prevention and abuse to the reduction of a variety of risky health behaviors including addiction, overdose prevention, safer sex, sexual health education, nutrition, gambling, and motor vehicle safety.

Recently, literature has expressed doubts about whether HRT can be systematically applied and replicated in micro projects (Stimson & O'Hare, 2010). Islam, Day, and Conigrave (2010) argued, "The next generation of HRT needs to occur through the integration of harm reduction into general health systems" (p. 132), moving harm reduction from the "exceptional to the mainstream" (Stimson & O'Hare, 2010, p. 92). This book and the highlighted motorcycle safety research study begin addressing this gap by advancing the systematic and theoretical application of HRT.

The next chapter continues to provide a more in-depth overview of HRT by discussing specific studies that have incorporated harm reduction tenets and the results of these studies. Then, we move on to highlight two short case examples that show how harm reduction tenets have been incorporated to guide other theories in health and safety research. After presenting how HRT has worked in research and practice, we propose that harm reduction may function as a metatheory in health and safety research and begin framing a motorcycle safety research case study designed to empirically test the metatheoretical utility of HRT.

REFERENCES

Aboulafia, M., Bookman, M., & Kemp, C. (2002). *Habermas and pragmatism* (Eds.), New York: Routledge.

Alter, C., & Hage, J. (1993). *Organizations working together.* Newbury Park, CA: Sage.

Arkowitz, H., Westra, H. A., Miller, W. R., Rollnick, S. (2008). *Motivational interviewing in the treatment of psychological problems.* New York, NY: The Guilford Press.

Ashton, J. R., & Seymour, H. (2010). Public health and the origins of the Mersey model of harm reduction. *International Journal of Drug Policy, 21*, 94–96.

Ashton, J. R., & Seymour, H. (1988). *The new public health.* Milton Keynes: Open University Press.

Bandura, A. (1991). Social cognitive theory of self-regulation. *Organizational Behavior and Human Decision Processes, 50,* 248–287.

Bazzoli, G. J., Stein, R., Alexander, J. A., Conrad, D. A., Sofaer, S., & Shortell, S. M. (1997). Public-private collaboration in health and human service delivery: Evidence from community partnerships. *The Milbank Quarterly, 75,* 533–561.

Bessant, J. (2008). From 'harm minimization' to 'zero tolerance' drugs policy in Australia: How the Howard government changed its mind. *Policy Studies, 29,* 197–214.

Bigler, M. O. (2005). Harm reduction as a practice and prevention model for social work. *The Journal of Baccalaureate Social Work, 10*(2), 69–86.

Blewett, N. (2004). *Harm minimization and Australia's national drug strategies'.* Presented at the 15th International Conference on the Reduction of Drug-Related Harm, Melbourne, Australia.

Blume, A., & Lovato, L. (2010). Empowering the disempowered: Harm reduction with racial/ethnic minority clients. *Journal of Clinical Psychology: In Session, 66*(2), 189–200.

Boersema, D. (2009). *Pragmatism and reference.* Cambridge, MA: The MIT Press.

Brocato, J., & Wagner, E. F. (2003). Harm reduction: A social work practice model and social justice agenda. *Health & Social Work, 28*(2), 117–125.

Brown, N. L., Luna, V., Ramirez, H., Vail, K. A., & Williams, C. A. (2005). Developing an effective intervention for IDU women: A harm reduction approach to collaboration. *AIDS Education and Prevention, 17*(4), 317–333.

Burke, A. C., & Clapp, J. D. (1997). Ideology and social work practice in substance abuse settings. *Social Work, 42*(6), 552–562.

Carey, K. B., Scott-Sheldon, L. A. J., Carey, M. P., DeMartini, K. S. (2007). Individual level interventions to reduce college student drinking: A meta-analytic review. *Addictive Behaviors, 32*, 2469–2494.

Castro, R. J., & Foy, B. D. (2002). Harm reduction: A promising approach for college health. *Journal of American College Health, 51*(2), 89–91.

Centers for Disease Control and Prevention (CDC). (1993). Technical guidance on HIV counseling. *Morbidity and Mortality Weekly Report, 42*(RR-2), 11È17.

Cook, C., Bridge, J., & Stimson, G. V. (2010). The diffusion of harm reduction in Europe and beyond. In T. Rhodes & D. Hedrich (10th Ed.), *European Monitoring Centre for Drugs and Drug Addiction Monographs: Harm reduction evidence, impacts, and challenges* (pp. 37–56). Luxembourg: Publications Office of the European Union.

Cook, R., Back, A., & Trudeau, J. (1996). Preventing alcohol use problems among blue-collar workers: A field test of the Working People program. *Substance Use and Misuse, 31,* 255–275.

Cooper, H., Moore, L., Gruskin, S., Krieger, N. (2005). The impact of a police drug crackdown on drug injectors' ability to practice harm reduction: A qualitative study. *Social Science & Medicine, 61*, 673–684.

Denning, P. (2000). *Practicing harm reduction psychotherapy: An alternative approach to addictions.* New York, NY: The Guilford Press.

Des Jarlais, D. C. (1995). Harm reduction: A framework for incorporating sciences into drug policy. *American Journal of Public Health, 85,* 10–12.

Dhand, A. (2006). The roles performed by peer educators during outreach among heroin addicts in India: Ethnographic insights. *Social Science & Medicine, 63,* 2674–2685.

DiClemente, R. J., & Wingood, G. M. (1995). A randomized controlled trial of an HIV sexual risk-reduction intervention for young African-American women. *JAMA, 27*, 1271–1276.

Dimeff, L. A., Baer, J. S., Kivlahan, D. R., & Marlatt, G. A. (1999). *Brief alcohol screening and intervention for college students (BASICS): A harm reduction approach.* New York: Guilford.

Dobbs, L. (2007, February 13). The war within, killing ourselves. Retrieved on December 6, 2010, from http://articles.cnn.com/2007-02-13/us/Dobbs.Feb14_1_drug-overdoses-drug-abuse-illegal-drugs/2?_s=PM:US.

Downie, R. S., Fyfe, C., & Tannahill, A. (1990). *Health promotion models and values.* Oxford: Oxford University Press.

DuPont, R. L. (2013). *The selfish brain: Learning from addiction.* Center City, MN: Hazeldon.

DuPont, R. L., & Ford, B. (2000). *The selfish brain: Learning from addiction.* Center City, MN: Hazeldon Publishing.

DuPont, R. L., & Voth, E. A. (1995). Drug legalization, harm reduction, and drug policy. *Annals of Internal Medicine, 123,* 461–465.

Einstein, S. (2007). Harm and risk reduction: History, theories, issues, and implications. *Substance Use & Misuse, 42,* 257–265.

Erickson, P. G. (1995). Harm reduction: What it is and is not. *Drug and Alcohol Review, 14,* 283–285.

Eshrati, B., Asl, R. T., Dell, C. A., Afshar, P., Millson, P. M., Kamali, M., Weekes, J. (2008). Preventing HIV transmission among Iranian prisoners: Initial support for providing education on the benefits of harm reduction practices. *Harm Reduction Journal, 5*(21). Published online 2008 June 9. doi: 10.1186/1477-7517-5-21.

Farrell, M., Gowing, L., Marsen, J., Ling, W., & Ali, R. (2005). Effectiveness of drug dependence treatment in HIV prevention. *International Journal of Drug Policy, 16* (Supplement 1), S67–S75.

Gentilello, L. M., Rivara, F. P., Donovan, D. M., Jurkovich, G. J., Daranciang, E., Dunn, C. W., et al. (1999). Alcohol interventions in a trauma center as a means of reducing the risk of injury reoccurrence. *Annals of Surgery, 230,* 473–480.

Haas, E. J. (2012). *Toward harm reduction as a metatheory for health communication campaigns: An empirical study of harm reduction metatheory and the reconceptualized health belief model addressing motorcycle safety. Unpublished doctoral dissertation.* West Lafayette, IN: Purdue University.

Hall, W. (2007). What's in a name: *Addiction, 102*, 691–692.

Harm Reduction Coalition (2004). *Principles of harm reduction.* Retrieved March 31, 2014, from http://harmreduction.org/about-us/principles-of-harm-reduction/.

Harris, R. A. (2010). *A handbook of rhetorical devices.* Retrieved on February 5, 2011, from http://www.virtualsalt.com/rhetoric5.htm#Metaphor.

Hathaway, A. D. (2001). Shortcomings of harm reduction: Toward a morally invested drug reform strategy. *International Journal of Drug Policy, 12,* 125–137.

Heather, N. (2006). Controlled drinking, harm reduction and their roles in the response to alcohol-related problems. *Addiction research and theory, 14,* 7–18.

Heather, N., Wodak, A., Nadelmann, E. A., & O'Hare, P. (1993). *Psychoactive drugs and harm reduction: From faith to science* (Eds.), London: Whurr Publishers.

Herring, R., Thom, B., Beccaria, F., Kolind, T., & Moskalewicz, J. (2010). Alcohol harm reduction in Europe. In T. Rhodes & D. Hedrich (Eds.), European Monitoring Centre for Drugs and Drug Addiction (EMCDDA), *Harm reduction: evidence, impacts, and challenges* (pp. 275–301). Scientific Monographs Series No. 10, Luxembourg: Publications Office of the European Union.

Hilton, B. A., Thompson, R., Moore-Dempsey, L., & Janzen, R. G. (2001). Harm reduction theories and strategies for control of human immunodeficiency virus: A review of the literature. *Journal of Advanced Nursing, 33*(3), 357–371.

Hunt, N., Ashton, M., Lenton, S., Mitchseon, L., Nelles, B., & Stimson, G. (2003). *A review of the evidence-base for harm reduction approaches to drug use.* Forward Thinking on Drugs. Retrieved on March 31, 2014 from http://www.neilhunt.org/pdf/2003-evidence-base-for-hr-hunt-et-al.pdf.

Inciardi, J. A., & Harrison, L. D. (2000). *Harm reduction: National and international perspectives.* California: Thousand Oaks Press.

Islam, M. M., Day, C. A., & Conigrave, K. M. (2010). Harm reduction healthcare: From an alternative to the mainstream platform? *International Journal of Drug Policy, 21*(2), 131–133.

Kamarulzaman, A., & Saifuddeens, S. M. (2010). Islam and harm reduction. *International Journal of Drug Policy, 21*(2), 115–118.

Kamb, M. L., Fishbein, M., Douglas, J. M., Rhodes, F., Rogers, J., Bolan, G., Zenilman, J., Hoxworth, T., Malotte, K., Iatesta, M., Kent, C., Lentz, A., Graziano, S., Byers, R. H., & Peterman, T. A. (1998). Efficacy of risk-reduction counseling to prevent human immunodeficiency virus and sexually transmitted diseases. *JAMA, 280*(13), 1161–1167.

Keefe, T. (1978). The economic context of empathy. *Social Work, 11,* 460–465.

Kellehear, A., Rumbold, G. R., & Hamilton, M. A. (1998). *Drug use in Australia: A harm minimization approach.* Melbourne: Oxford University Press.

Kimber, J., Palmateer, N., Hutchinson, S., Hickman, M., Goldberg, D., & Rhodes, T. (2010). Harm reduction among injecting drug users: Evidence of effectiveness. In T. Rhodes & D. Hedrich (Eds.), European Monitoring Centre for Drugs and Drug Addiction (EMCDDA), *Harm reduction: evidence, impacts, and challenges* (pp. 115–162). Scientific Monographs Series No. 10, Luxembourg: Publications Office of the European Union.

Lakoff, G. (2005). *Don't think of an elephant.* Melbourne: Scribe.

Lakoff, G. (1999). *Moral politics: how conservatives and liberals think.* Chicago, IL: University of Chicago Press.

Larimer, M. E., & Cronce, J. M. (2007). Identification, prevention, and treatment revisited: Individual-focused college drinking prevention strategies: 1999–2006. *Addictive Behaviors, 32*, 2439–2468.

Lenton, S., & Single, E. (2004). The definition of harm reduction. *Drug Alcohol Review, 17,* 213–220.

Leshner, A. (2008). By now, "harm reduction" harms both science and the public health. *Clinical Pharmacology and Therapeutics, 83,* 513–514.

Lillis, M. (2010, March 18). White house shifts away from 'war on drugs' rhetoric: Government moves more toward treating addiction as illness. *The Washington Independent*, (np).

Little, J., & Franskoviak, P. (2010). So glad you came! Harm reduction therapy in community settings. *Journal of Clinical Psychology, 66*(2), 175–188.

Locke, E. A., & Latham, G. P. (2002). Building a practically useful theory of goal setting and task motivation. *American Psychologist, 57*(9), 705–715.

Logan, D. E., & Marlatt, A. G. (2010). Harm reduction therapy: A practice-friendly review of research. *Journal of Clinical Psychology, 66*(2), 201–214.

Marlatt, G. A. (1998). *Harm reduction: Pragmatic strategies for managing high-risk behaviors.* New York: The Guilford Press.

Marlatt, G. A., & Witkiewitz, K. (2010). Update on harm-reduction policy and intervention research. *Annual Review of Clinical Psychology, 6,* 591–606.

Matano, R. A., Futa, K. T., Wanat, S. F., Mussman, L. M., & Leung, C. W. (2000). The employee stress and alcohol project: The development of a computer-based alcohol abuse prevention program for employees. *Journal of Behavioral Health Services and Research, 27,* 152–165.

Mattson, M. (2000). Empowerment through agency-promoting dialogue: An explicit application of harm reduction theory to reframe HIV test counseling. *Journal of Health Communication, 5,* 333–347.

Mattson, M. (1999). Toward a reconcepualization of communication cues to action in the Health Belief Model: HIV testing counseling. *Communication Monographs, 66,* 240–263.

Mattson, M., & Basnyat, I. (2008). Infusing HIV test counseling practice with harm reduction theory: An integrated model for voluntary counseling and testing. In T. Edgar, S. Noar, & V. Freimuth (Eds.). *Communication perspectives*

for HIV/AIDS in the 21st century (pp. 137–167). New York: Lawrence Erlbaum Associates.
McBride, N., Farrington, F., Midford, R., Meuleners, L., & Phillips, M. (2004). Harm minimization in school drug education: Final results of the School Health and Alcohol Harm Reduction Project (SHAHRP). *Addiction, 99,* 278–291.
McNeece, C. A. (2003). After the war on drugs in over: Implications for social work education. *Journal of Social Work Education, 39,* 193–212.
Miller, P. G. (2001). A critical review of the harm minimization ideology in Australia. *Critical Public Health, 11*(2), 168–178.
Miller, P. G. (1999). *What factors led to the rejection of the proposed A.C.T. heroin trials by the Federal Government in 1997?: A discourse analysis.* Unpublished thesis, School of Social Inquiry, Faculty of Arts, Deakin University, Greelong.
Miller, W. R., & Rollnick, S. (2012). *Motivational interviewing: Helping people change* (3rd Ed.), New York, NY: Guilford Press.
Miller, W. R., & Rollnick, S. (2002). *Motivational interviewing: Preparing people for change* (2nd Ed.), New York, NY: The Guilford Press.
Miller, W. R., & Rollnick, S. (1991). *Motivational interviewing: Preparing people to change addictive behavior.* New York, NY: The Guilford Press.
Nadelmann, E. A. (1993). Progressive legalizers, progressive prohibitionists and the reduction of drug-related harm. In N. Heather, A. Wodak, E. Nadelmann, & P. O'Hare (Eds.), *Psychoactive drugs and harm reduction: From faith to science.* London: Whurr Publishers Ltd.
Newcombe, R. (1992). The reduction of drug-related harm: A conceptual framework for theory, practice, and research. In P. O'Hare, R. Newcombe, A. Matthews, E.C. Buning, & E. Drucker, (Eds.), *The reduction of drug-related harm* (pp. 1–15). New York, NY: Routledge.
Newcombe, R. (1987). High time for harm reduction. *Druglink, 2*(1), 10–11.
Nichter, M., Nichter, M., Adrian, S., Goldade, K., Tesler, L., Muramoto, M. (2008). Smoking and harm-reduction efforts among postpartum women. *Qualitative Health Research, 18(*9), 1184–1194.
Non-Prescription Needle Use (NPNU) Consortium (2000). *Harm reduction information kit: For professionals working with at-risk populations.* The Government and Public Awareness Task Group of NPNU Consortium.
Odets, W. (1998). HIV test site counseling for gay men: Harm reduction and a client-centered approach. In J.W. Dilley & R. Marks, *The UCSF AIDS health project guide to counseling: Perspectives on psychotherapy, prevention, and therapeutic practice.* San Francisco: Jossey-Bass Publishers.
O'Hare, P. (2007). Merseyside, the first harm reduction conferences, and the early history of harm reduction. *International Journal of Drug Policy, 18,* 141–144.
Parsons, T. (1991). *The social system.* New York, NY: The Free Press.
Peterson, A., & Lupton, D. (1996). *The new public health and self in the age of risk.* Newbury Park, CA: Sage Publications.
Poulin, C., & Nicholson, J. (2005). Should harm minimization as an approach to adolescent substance use be embraced by junior and senior high schools? Empirical evidence from an integrated school and community-based demonstration

intervention addressing drug use among adolscents. *International Journal of Drug Policy, 16*, 403–414.
Prochaska, J. O., & Velicer, W . F. (1997). The transtheoretical model of health behavior change. *American Journal of Health Promotion, 12*, 38–48.
Race, K. (2008). The use of pleasure in harm reduction: Perspectives from the history of sexuality. *International Journal of Drug Policy, 19,* 417–423.
Rehm, J., Fischer, B., Hickman, M., Ball, A., Atun, R., Kazatchkine, M., Southwell, M., Fry, C., & Room, R. (2010). Perspectives on harm reduction- what experts have to say. In T. Rhodes & D. Hedrich (Eds.), European Monitoring Centre for Drugs and Drug Addiction (EMCDDA), *Harm reduction: evidence, impacts, and challenges* (pp. 79–108). Scientific Monographs Series No. 10, Luxembourg: Publications Office of the European Union.
Reid, R. J. (2002). Harm reduction and injection drug use: Pragmatic lessons from a public health model. *Health and Social Work, 27*(3), 223–226.
Rhodes, T. (2002). The "risk environment": A framework for understanding and reducing drug-related harm. *International Journal of Drug Policy, 13,* 85–94.
Rhodes, T., & Hedrich, D. (2010). Harm reduction and the mainstream. In T. Rhodes & D. Hedrich (10th Ed.), *European Monitoring Centre for Drugs and Drug Addiction Monographs: Harm reduction evidence, impacts, and challenges* (pp. 19–33). Luxembourg: Publications Office of the European Union.
Riley, D., & O'Hare, P. (2000). Harm reduction: History, definition, and practice. In J.A. Inciardi & L.D. Harrison (Eds.), *Harm reduction: National and international perspectives* (pp. 1–26). Thousand Oaks, CA: Sage.
Roche, A., Evans, K., & Staton, W. (2001). Harm reduction: Road less traveled to the Holy Grail. *Addiction, 92,* 1207–1212.
Rogers, C. R. (1959). A theory of therapy, personality, and interpersonal relationships as developed in the client-centered framework. In S. Koch (Ed.), *Psychology: The study of a science: Vol. 3. Formulations of the person and the social contexts* (pp. 184–256). New York: McGraw Hill.
Rogers, S. J., & Ruefli, T. (2004). Does harm reduction programming make a difference in the lives of highly marginalized, at-risk drug users? *Harm Reduction Journal, 1*(7). Published online 2004 June 1. doi: 10.1186/1477-7517-1-7.
Rollnick, S., Miller, W. R., Butler, C. C. (2008). *Motivational interviewing in healthcare: Helping patients change behavior*. New York, NY: The Guilford Press.
Rorty, R. (1999). *Philosophy and social hope*. New York: Penguin.
Ruefli, T., & Rogers, S. J. (2004). How do drug users define their progress in harm reduction interventions? Qualitative research to develop user-generated outcomes. *Harm Reduction Journal, 1*: 8. Published online 2004 August 26. doi: 10.1186/1477-7517-1-8.
Rumbold, G., & Hamilton, M. (1998). Addressing drug problems: the case for harm minimisation. In M. Hamilton, A. Kellehear, & G. Rumbold (Eds.), *Drugs in Australia: A harm minimization approach* (pp. 130–145). Singapore: Oxford University Press.
Schermer, C. R., Moyers, T. B., Miller, W. R., & Bloomfield, L. A. (2006). Trauma center brief interventions for alcohol disorders decrease subsequent driving under the influence arrests. *Journal of Trauma, 60,* 29–34.

Schon, D. (1993). Generative metaphor: A perspective on problem setting in social policy. In A. Ortony, *Metaphor and thought* (2nd Ed.), (pp. 137–164.) Cambridge: Cambridge University Press.

Sharpes, D. K. (2009). *The evolution of the social sciences.* Lanham, MD: Rowman & Littlefield Publishing Group, Inc.

Shepard, B. (2007). Harm reduction outreach services and engagement of chemically dependent homeless people living with HIV/AIDS: An analysis of service utilization data to evaluation program theory. *Einstein Journal of Biology and Medicine, 23,* 26–32.

Shernoff, M. (2006). Condomless sex: Gay men, barebacking, and harm reduction. *Social Work, 51,* 106–113.

Single, E. (2000). *The effectiveness of harm reduction and its role in a new framework for drug policy in British Columbia.* Paper presented to the National Federal/Provincial/Territorial Meeting on Injection Use, Vancouver, BC, Canada.

Single, E. (1995). Defining harm reduction. *Drug and Alcohol Review, 14,* 287–290.

Springer, E. (1991). Effective AIDS prevention with active drug users: The harm reduction model. *Journal of Chemical Dependency Treatment, 4*(2), 141–157.

Stevenson, R. (1994). Harm reduction, rational addiction, and the optimal prescribing of illegal drugs. *Contemporary Economic Policy, 12,* 101–108.

Stimson, G. V., & O'Hare, P. (2010). Harm reduction: Moving through the third decade. *International Journal of Drug Policy, 21,* 91–93.

Stimson, G. V. (2007). Harm reduction-coming of age: A local movement with global impact. *International Journal of Drug Policy, 18,* 67–69.

Stronach, B. (2003), 'Alcohol and harm reduction'. In E. Buning, M. Gorgullo, A. G. Melcop, & P. O'Hare, (Eds.), *Alcohol and harm education: an innovative approach for countries in transition,* Amsterdam, ICAHRE, pp. 27–34.

Sweanor, D. (2007). Harm reduction with David Sweanor. Retrieved January 30, 2010, from http://www.eudoxa.se/content/archives/2007/06/harm_reduction_7.html.

Sweanor, D., Alcabes, P., & Drucker, E. (2007). Tobacco harm reduction: How rational public policy could transform a pandemic. *International Journal of Drug Policy, 18*(2), 70–74.

Tatarsky, A., & Marlatt, G. A. (2010). State of the art in harm reduction psychotherapy: An emerging treatment for substance misuse. *Journal of Clinical Psychology: In session, 66*(2), 117–122.

Tsemberis, S., Gulcur, L., & Nakae, M. (2004). Housing first, consumer choice, and harm reduction for homeless individuals with dual diagnosis. *American Journal of Public Health , 94*(4), 651–656.

Tucker, J. A., Donovan, D. M., & Marlatt, G. A. (1999). *Changing addictive behavior: Bridging clinical and public health strategies.* New York: The Guilford Press.

Vogl, L., Teesson, M., Andrews, G., Bird, K., Steadman, B., & Dillon, P. (2009). A computerized harm minimization prevention program for alcohol misuse and related harms: Randomized controlled trial. *Addiction, 104,* 564–573.

Weatherburn, D. (2008). Dilemmas in harm minimization. *Addiction, 104,* 335–339.

Whiteside, U., Cronce, I. M., Pedersen, E. R., & Larimer, M. E. (2010). Brief motivational feedback for college students and adolescents: A harm reduction approach. *Journal of Clinical Psychology: In Session, 66,* 150–163.

Wiessing, L., Likatavicius, G., & Klempova, D. (2009). Associations between availability and coverage of HIV-prevention measures and subsequent incidence of diagnosed HIV infections among injection users. *American Journal of Public Health, 99,* 1049–1052.

Winstock, A. R., Wolff, K., & Ramsey, J. (2001). Ecstasy pill testing: harm minimization gone too far? *Addiction, 96,* 1139–1148.

Wodak, A., & Cooney, A. (2005). Effectiveness of sterile needle and syringe interventions. *International Journal of Drug Policy, 16,* S1, S31-S44.

World Health Organization, Health and Welfare Canada, Canadian Public Health Association (1986). Ottawa Charter for Health Promotion, WHO, Copenhagen.

Chapter 2

Setting the Stage for Harm Reduction Metatheory

In the previous chapter you read about the historical roots of HRT. Throughout the process of discussing and reconceptualizing the definition and tenets of HRT, we referenced broad uses and examples of HRT in research and practice. This chapter gives more attention to those applications of HRT within certain health and safety issues. After focusing on ways that HRT is typically utilized as a theory throughout health interventions, we begin considering harm reduction as a metatheory in health and safety research. This chapter is guided by the following objectives:

- Discuss common applications of HRT in health and safety research and practice
- Highlight gaps in the evaluation of previous HRT applications
- Provide two research-in-practice examples that demonstrate how HRT can be applied concurrently with other theories to guide social science research and inform application and evaluation
- Propose harm reduction as a metatheory in health and safety research
- Discuss why motorcycle safety is an appropriate health and safety issue for which harm reduction may have metatheoretical utility

THE ROLE OF HARM REDUCTION THEORY IN HEALTH AND SAFETY RESEARCH

HRT has a rich application history mainly in the fields of public health and counseling. These HRT applications include interventions and policies involving a variety of health issues including needle exchange, tobacco and other drugs, gambling, and alcohol abuse. A main goal of these HRT interventions is to reduce the health and social harms of these risky behaviors for those individuals who engage in the behaviors and their surrounding communities and societies (Rhodes & Hedrich, 2010). In doing so, these interventions focus on personal responsibility of the individuals and individual choices rather than choosing methods that emphasize punishing their behaviors (Marlatt, 1998). This harm reduction approach to interventions addresses already affected people and high-risk groups through its pragmatic, nonjudgmental, and humane philosophy (Marlatt, 1998).

HRT interventions also are termed "combination interventions" by some practitioners because of their tailored design to individual needs and local settings (Rhodes & Hedrich, 2010). As a part of targeting and adapting to needs of at-risk individuals, harm reduction interventions include a variety of treatments and options such as allowing individuals to make their own choices when contemplating behavior change (Tucker, Donovan, & Marlatt, 1999). This section begins by discussing needle exchange programs, which were *the* first programs that were labeled as harm reduction initiatives in the field of public health.

Harm Reduction and Needle Exchange Programs

In the first chapter we discussed the relatively neutral stance of harm reduction. This neutral stance worked as a public health strategy to initially promote needle and syringe distribution services on a national and international level (Stafford, 2007). These distribution services are known as needle exchange programs. *Needle exchange programs* (NEPs) provide a way for injection drug users (IDUs) to safely dispose used needles and then obtain sterile needles at no cost (Centers for Disease Control & Prevention [CDC], 2005). Obtaining sterile needles helps minimize the transmission of HIV and other infections. In addition to receiving sterile needles, these sites also function as an education and outreach facility in which IDUs receive sex education and prevention materials, referrals to medical care, legal services, or social services, if desired (Drucker, Lurie, Wodak, & Alcabes, 1998).

When offering these services the intention is that IDUs are communicated with in a way that is absent of discrimination or negative stigma and rather, treated as individuals who are taking positive steps to regain control over their lives. A comprehensive harm reduction strategy should include education about the risk of contracting HIV from sharing injection materials, providing needle syringe programs, providing access to drug treatment, and community development (Wodak & McLeod, 2008). For example, at needle exchange centers, nurses may communicate and work closely with IDUs to show them safer ways to inject needles (Inciardi & Harrison, 2000).

NEPs are most often labeled as an HRT intervention (Ksobiech, 2004a, 2004b; Springer, 1991). Prior research shows that full participation in harm reduction interventions, in the form of NEPs, are associated with a lower risk of HIV and hepatitis C viral (HCV) infections in IDUs, compared to IDUs who do not participate in such programs (Van Den Berg et al., 2007). Nationally and internationally, harm reduction efforts in the form of NEPs, also termed as "substitution treatment" continue to progress and become more prevalent in society.

For example, according to the Central Eastern European Harm Reduction Network (CEEHRN), in 2004, 76 harm reduction NEPs existed in the regional area and approximately 6,565 individuals in central eastern European and central Asian countries were receiving methadone or buprenorphine treatments. In 2006, this number increased to more than 15,000 individuals (Subata & Stuikyte, 2006). Based on the increased number of individuals utilizing such services, it is apparent that there is a need for additional harm reduction programming. Challenges that exist to maintaining harm reduction interventions, in the form of NEPs, include vaccination, prevention in prisons, issues of quality control, sustaining services, and reaching adequate coverage in certain areas (Sarang, Stuikyte, & Bykov, 2007).

The inclusion of the HRT tenet community collaboration is an important component for NEPs to be effective in reducing individuals' risky behaviors as well. For example, Cooper, Moore, Gruskin, and Krieger (2005) found that heightened surveillance and arrests in response to drug crackdowns endangered individuals' capacity to practice harm reduction through NEPs. Specifically, where more surveillance was present, drug users were likely to inject more quickly, skip steps in cleaning their needles, not clean their injection site, or exchange dirty needles with other IDUs (Cooper et al., 2005). These riskier methods were used by IDUs to avoid encounters with law enforcement officers but at the same time, heightened IDUs' risk for negative health outcomes. In contrast, where NEPs are present and individuals are not lawfully reprimanded when exchanging their needles, this harm reduction strategy is more likely to facilitate less harmful injections (Reid, 2002). These results indicate the importance of community officials being on-board with harm reduction methods, such as NEPs. Even if such services facilitate continued drug use, the likelihood of transmitting disease could decrease.

Due to their locations nationally and internationally, more quantitative evaluation data exists about NEPs than any other type of harm reduction oriented intervention. One analysis of eight NEPs found that these programs typically reduce the amount of time dirty needles are in circulation (Ksobiech, 2004a). Another meta-analysis of 26 NEPs also showed a decreased time that used needles were in circulation in addition to an increase in HIV/AIDS education outreach efforts and saturation (Ksobiech, 2004b). In addition, an earlier analysis of 12 NEPs that examined the risky injection behaviors of IDUs found that 11 of the programs showed improvement in safety behaviors among IDUs including a decrease in syringe sharing (Drucker et al., 1998). Although debate is likely to continue about the efficacy of these programs, several analyses indicate the effectiveness of NEPs. However, the results of these programs to date do present the need for more specific evaluation procedures to further their support and use, which are discussed in a later section of this chapter.

Applications of HRT in other health interventions are more limited. However, some studies also demonstrate effectiveness in reducing negative health consequences, including those focused on tobacco consumption.

Harm Reduction and Tobacco Abuse

Despite the evidence known about tobacco's harmful health effects, smoking continues to be a major public health issue. The remaining quarter of the population that still smokes is a target audience for the development of tobacco harm reduction replacement products that claim to preserve tobacco pleasure while reducing its negative health consequences and perhaps eventual consumption of tobacco products (Stratton et al., 2001). A common harm reduction strategy includes the substitution of products that contain less nicotine than cigarettes, such as e-cigarettes. *E-cigarettes* are battery-powered nicotine devices that, when smoked, convert liquid that contains nicotine into aerosol vapor (US Food and Drug Administration [FDA], 2009). When inhaled, this vapor delivers nicotine into the smoker's lung (FDA, 2009). It is common for advertising around e-cigarettes to utilize a harm reduction messaging approach. For example, one commercial that first aired during Super Bowl Sunday 2013, for the NJOY brand e-cigarette was, "Finally, smokers have a real alternative. Cigarettes, you've met your match" (Fairchild, Bayer, & Colgrove, 2013, p. 2).

Research about the health effects of e-cigarettes is not complete and many opponents exist for these types of health products. Like many harm reduction strategies, e-cigarettes have become a focal point of public health disputes, with opponents and supporters of these harm reduction alternatives to aid behavior change. Besides the research being inconclusive about the side effects of e-cigarettes, opponents discuss e-cigarettes as a product that has the potential to minimize long time efforts to de-normalize smoking (Fairchild et al., 2013) which could halt attempts at smoking cessation. As an example, data collected by the CDC (2013) showed that twice as many young people experimented with e-cigarettes in 2012 as in 2011. Also, because of the many efforts at policy implementation to eliminate tobacco on a global level, tobacco control advocates or officials are more likely to be against any device that aids the continued use of tobacco products. These individuals continue to express concern that e-cigarettes could threaten bans on public smoking currently in place.

However, there also are many public health researchers and advocates who argue that e-cigarettes are an effective harm reduction strategy for smokers. For instance, research has shown that e-cigarettes can aid smoking reduction and eventually smoking cessation by serving as an alternative to tobacco (Etter, 2010; Siegel, Tanwar, & Wood, 2011). Also, some research supports that the ingredients in e-cigarettes are less harmful than those in traditional cigarettes (Bullen et al., 2010). Regardless of whether e-cigarettes continue to be allowed on the market or are publically banned, it has been suggested to avoid using the term "safer cigarette" to evade the connotation that e-cigarettes are safe because they can still pose health risks to some individuals (Stratton, Shetty, Wallace, & Bondurant, 2001). The example of e-cigarettes demonstrates why harm reduction methods remain controversial in public health promotion research and practice.

Other tobacco substitution products besides e-cigarettes also are on the global market. Specifically, in 2003 harm reduction strategies were heavily initiated in Sweden as new messages persuaded smokers to consume less harmful tobacco products such as snus. *Snus* is a powder tobacco that is consumed by placing it under the lip for an extended period of time. It has been used as a healthier replacement for smoking and chewing tobacco. One of the reasons for the encouragement to choose snus instead of trying to be abstinent from tobacco is the years of limited success of antismoking campaigns (Harrison, 2011). The limited cessation success of antismoking campaigns is more than likely due to unrealistic messaging in an effort to completely eliminate tobacco use in society. The snus-based campaign that originated in Sweden, however, promoted harm reduction messages that focused on individuals' ability to change tobacco behaviors and supported other options to become healthier, including other smoking alternatives that could offer some small health gains (Gartner et al., 2007). Now, snus is heavily sold and is offered in a variety of flavors to attract smokers to this smoking alternative (Swedish Match, 2013).

Separate from e-cigarettes and other tobacco substitution options, harm reduction interventions also are developed and implemented to simply reduce the amount of nicotine, or number of cigarettes that smokers consume. These interventions, which often target a specific audience, such as pregnant women or adolescents, have experienced varying levels of success. However, effective tobacco harm reduction interventions have consistently included positive communication between peer supporters and/or nonsmokers. This positive, nonjudgmental communication has been a contributing factor that influences smokers' determination not to smoke (Audrey et al., 2006). To further illustrate, another intervention that targeted pregnant women who smoked found that, more often after these pregnant smokers deliver their babies, support networks such as their personal healthcare practitioner, friends, and family gradually stopped asking about the new mothers' smoking status (Nichter et al., 2008). The lack of positive communication or even peer pressure that others placed on these new mothers made harm reduction smoking efforts more difficult. Instead of stopping the dialogue about smoking reduction or cessation after a pregnancy, Nichter and colleagues concluded that these new mothers preferred that their support networks continue to acknowledge and encourage their smoking reduction efforts. Not surprisingly, the smoking mothers desired a nonjudgmental approach as they tried to reduce smoking, similar to the communication emphasized throughout the humanistic value tenet of HRT.

In addition, some HRT interventions utilize properly trained peer educators to raise awareness and promote positive communication about minimizing or maintaining abstinence from tobacco and other drugs. Specifically, Dhand (2006) integrated the tenets of HRT into the development of narrative role plays between peer educators and students to help address the broad issues of preventing and reducing drug use among minors in India. The peer educators conducted daily community outreach to raise awareness about negative health outcomes of drug use. The peer outreach, in the form of creating and rereading narratives with students, positively influenced and altered the at-risk students' norms toward drug misuse. HRT narratives, through role playing, helped reduce threats among at-risk individuals and opened a nonjudgmental space to communicate about these behaviors.

Besides NEPs and tobacco interventions, alcohol abuse is a primary focus in HRT research, with interventions focusing on at-risk groups from adolescent drinkers to alcoholics. An overview of this research area is provided in the next section. We also discuss alcohol abuse in more detail during the research to practice illustration presented in this chapter.

Harm Reduction and Alcohol Abuse

Alcohol interventions, like other health behavior interventions that incorporate HRT, do not strive for abstinence but aim to reduce negative consequences of drinking alcohol (Robson & Marlatt, 2006). In the discussion of harm reduction strategies for alcohol-related problems throughout this chapter we utilize historical and prominent resources to provide a broad yet succinct review. There is an extensive body of empirical research that supports the use of harm reduction tenets in preventing, modifying, and treating alcohol-related problems. For a historical review of this literature, consult Heather and Robertson (1983), Rosenberg (1993), and Marlatt (1998; 1983).

For a more recent review of the relevant literature, consult Marlatt and Witkiewitz (2002), Witkiewitz and Marlatt (2006), and Marlatt, Larimer, and Witkiewitz (2011).

Research addressing high-risk drinking from a harm reduction perspective became prominent in the 1970s when harm reduction approaches were introduced as *controlled drinking* or *drinking in moderation* (Sobell & Sobell, 1995). Until then, most alcohol treatment programs in the US utilized the familiar 12-step approach introduced by Alcoholics Anonymous (Peele, 1989). To date, HRT approaches to alcohol abuse include availability of alcohol, taxation, educational campaigns, laws on drinking and driving, and a range of other formal and informal alcohol interventions (Herring, Thom, Beccaria, Kolind, & Moskalweicz, 2010).

Researchers often maintain that harm-related alcohol consumption can be "reduced by teaching skills, modifying the environment, and promoting public policies to reduce the risks of drinking" (Larimer et al., 1998, p. 69). Prevention interventions that aim to reduce the harm experienced by risky consumers of alcohol continue to show effectiveness in educating people about the consequences associated with alcohol consumption (Larimer et al., 1998). According to Mosher (1999), by acknowledging that most people drink alcohol, this audience is more likely to listen and adhere to less harmful drinking behaviors. The purpose of acknowledging the behavior is to provide education and prevention without irritating and provoking negative attitudes and behaviors among target audience members.

Even though a variety of work has been done to move beyond abstinence-only programming, Sobell and Sobell (2006) commented that moderation goals (i.e., harm reduction strategies) are still more controversial in the US than in other countries. For example, Peele (1998) found in a survey of 450 private-sector alcohol/chemical dependency programs in the US that approximately 93% utilized a 12-step treatment approach. Historically, researchers that were initially focused on alcohol treatment programs were former alcoholics and held personal beliefs that they needed to remain abstinent to defeat previous alcohol consumption behaviors (Nowinski, Baker, & Carroll, 1999; Pattison, Sobell, & Sobell, 1977).

However, a plethora of literature supports harm reduction approaches to alcohol-related problems from issues of reducing harm associated with binge drinking on college campuses to tertiary prevention strategies for those who already have an alcohol dependency. Research continues to expand around the area of drinking in moderation and other harm-reducing behaviors, as examples in this chapter illustrate. According to researchers (e.g., Saladin & Santa Ana, 2004; Sobell & Sobell, 2006; Rosenberg, 1993) the problem is not the lack of research on this issue, but rather the lack of dissemination of the research findings to promote the use of alcohol harm reduction interventions.

Engaging in harm-reducing conversations with those who participate in high-risk drinking behaviors and/or abuse alcohol is an important aspect of harm reduction interventions. Particularly, research indicates that using a harm reduction approach by emphasizing that a moderate consumption of alcohol is acceptable can be more effective among those who do not have a medical or legal record related to their drinking behaviors (Sobell & Sobell, 2000). For example, *Moderation Management* is a national self-help group that supports but does not require abstinence from alcohol (Witkiewitz & Marlatt, 2006). Individuals who join this group tend to drink less, have fewer problems related to their alcohol consumption behaviors, and more often abstain from alcohol over a period of time, even if that was not their original goal (Hodgins, Leigh, Milne, & Gerrish, 1997; Humphreys & Klaw, 2001). Moderation Management is just one example that supports reducing alcohol consumption over time. To date, several harm reduction interventions exist and continue to evolve to reduce the negative consequences associated with high-risk drinking. In the following section we provide a historical overview of such interventions.

Abridged History of Harm Reduction Interventions Addressing High-Risk Drinking

Since a one-size-fits-all intervention does not yet exist for harm reduction strategies, these original interventions have been adapted over time and some have taken on different names at varying locations. You will notice that the interventions listed below focus more on interaction at the intrapersonal and/or interpersonal levels. The tenets of humanistic value, pragmatism, empowerment, and goal setting in communication with the target audiences are already evident in these interventions but community collaboration could be encouraged in future modifications of such programs.

- *Life Skills Training Program.* A program designed to target risky behaviors (i.e., cigarette smoking, alcohol use, and marijuana use) among elementary and junior high school students. The program teaches students about the effects of drugs, how to respond to peer pressure, promotes self-esteem, and involves communication with parents about these risky behaviors (Botvin, 1985).
- *Alcohol Misuse Prevention Study (AMPS).* An alcohol misuse prevention program for elementary through high school students. AMPS is administered in elementary school and then again in high school. This program recognizes and discusses the effects of alcohol use, consequences of high-risk drinking, and social pressures that lead to high-risk drinking. The program aims to increase knowledge about high-risk drinking, improve self-efficacy

to say no to alcohol, and reduce increased rates of alcohol use (Office of Juvenile Justice and Delinquency Prevention, 2014). This program has been evaluated, enhanced, and revised several times (e.g., Shope, Elliot, Raghunathan, & Waller, 2001; Shope, Copeland, & Dielman, 1994; Shope, Dielman, Butchart, Campanelli, & Koska,1992).

- *School Health and Alcohol Harm Reduction Project (SHAHRP) in Australia.* A classroom-based harm reduction intervention that provides students with skill-based training, alcohol education, and activities to encourage positive health behavior change (Marlatt & Witkiewitz, 2002). Pre-tests and post-tests are administered to assess knowledge about and attitude toward alcohol, risky consumptions behaviors, and risks of alcohol consumption (National Drug Research Institute, 2013). This program has been adapted and used for a variety of student populations (e.g., McBride, Farringdone, & Kennedy, 2007; McKay, McBride, Sumnall, & Cole, 2012).
- *Brief Alcohol Screening and Intervention for College Students (BASICS).* A commonly used harm reduction prevention program designed to reduce alcohol consumption and/or address high-risk drinking behaviors among college students. The course is typically administered in two, one hour waves. The manual provides information about how to talk with students about their high-risk drinking, health risks of alcohol use, and protective strategies to reduce these health risks (Dimeff, Baer, Kivlahan, & Marlatt, 1999). BASICS was first implemented in 1992 but since then has been used at over 1,100 locations, reaching over 20,000 individuals (National Registry of Evidence-based Programs and Practices, 2013). Colleges continue to adapt and utilize this program since evaluations continue to support its effectiveness in reducing high-risk drinking behaviors and reducing alcohol-related harm including fewer blackouts and physical fights (e.g., Baer, Kivlahan, Blume, McKnight, & Marlatt, 2001; Mastroleo et al., 2009; McBride, Midford, Farringdone, & Phillips, 2000).

Initial evaluations of these interventions showed an increased awareness of harmful consequences in response to risky and dangerous drinking behaviors. The evaluation of these harm reduction programs provides encouragement about the effectiveness of such education efforts that strive to reduce harm experienced by adolescent and young adult alcohol drinkers (Larimer et al., 1998). Several researchers concluded that showing humanistic value and pragmatism by acknowledging that most adolescents and young adults drink alcohol, students are more likely to listen and adhere to less harmful drinking behaviors. However, additional research showed that most brief interventions were not as effective as long-term interventions (Babor et al., 2003; Herring et al., 2010; Kaner et al., 2007) indicating the importance of longevity in programming.

Also, because abstinence-based interventions may be too extreme, particularly for at-risk populations, HRT techniques often are defined and used with these groups (Eshrati et al., 2008). One example considered alcohol consumption among adolescents and college students (Whiteside, Cronce, Pedersen, & Larimer, 2010). The researchers combined motivational interviewing strategies, cognitive-behavioral skills training, and personalized feedback to prevent heavy drinking among young adults. In order to effectively communicate with students, the researchers developed rapport with the target group of students, discovered individual motives for drinking, established how they compared their drinking to their peers' drinking, and assessed current readiness to change drinking behaviors. Recommendations were different for everyone, based on individual risks and behaviors. Thus, the HRT tenets can help communicate with these at-risk populations and can help identify and dismantle social norms within individuals' surrounding environments (Logan & Marlatt, 2010). More about the use of HRT during alcohol abuse interventions, with a focus on the college population, is discussed further during the second short case study.

Evaluation of Harm Reduction Theory Research and Application

As the examples in this section indicate, HRT research can focus on several health issues including NEPs to prevent the transmission of HIV/AIDS, smoking and other addictions, and alcohol abuse. Although HRT interventions are systematically designed based on a harm reduction philosophy, HRT remains difficult to empirically evaluate and advance in consistent application. To address this, we change our focus and discuss how to most appropriately advance HRT beyond the traditional and stagnant techniques commonly used in health promotion research and practice.

Although HRT interventions often lack rigorous empirical evaluation, they seem to reduce negative consequences associated with risky health behaviors (Shepard, 2007). For example, Ritter and Cameron (2006) reviewed approximately 650 harm reduction studies that included pre-test and post-test data or had control group comparisons. The results illustrated efficacy for harm reduction interventions to reduce alcohol-related road trauma but not solely alcohol reduction interventions. For tobacco, as our review of harm reduction products showed, this area is still controversial but shows promise for future interventions. Regarding NEPs, economic and outreach data shows effectiveness in reducing risky behaviors. In the few studies we discussed previously, HRT interventions appeared to offer substantial benefits during follow-up dialogue with the target audience. Although research encourages the creation of HRT interventions, "almost no research and funding has tried to establish appropriate measures of HRT and evaluate its worth" (Rogers & Ruefli, 2004, p. 2).

In response, most interventions that incorporate harm reduction strategies do not have a means to empirically or consistently evaluate effectiveness.

The positive outcomes of initial harm reduction interventions encouraged expansion. However, the absence of a reliable evaluation tool poses a barrier to tracking and improving the utility of HRT interventions. HRT is in need of rigorous evaluation tools to analyze past, current, and future interventions (Marlatt, 1998). Evaluating the effectiveness of harm reduction interventions is especially challenging because it "requires the selection of a set of criteria for evaluating outcomes, and the recognition of the hierarchical nature of harm reduction goals" (O'Hare, 1992, p. xvii).

For example, Ksobiech's (2004a) analysis of NEPs focused on methodological problems common in NEP evaluation studies. The greatest concern stemming from NEP evaluation literature is that many studies were primarily descriptive (e.g., hours worked, number/type of locations, demographics of individuals, and number of needles distributed) (Ksobiech, 2004b). This type of evaluation, or process tracking, lacks the data to show whether NEPs are effective in reducing risky drug and sexual behaviors, or increasing HIV/AIDS knowledge (Ksobiech, 2004a). Also, there is not agreement about the appropriate length of time between baseline and follow-up measurements across different harm reduction intervention studies. It is necessary for researchers to compare some concrete measurements of NEP and other harm reduction interventions to help modify and improve future harm reduction efforts.

Another barrier to evaluating HRT interventions is that, in comparison, abstinence interventions are fairly easy to evaluate (i.e., has the individual refrained from the risky health behavior and if so for how long?). HRT interventions are more complex because they involve the selection of goals and behaviors from a plethora of harm-reducing options (Newcombe, 1992). Therefore, a gap remains in the empirical development and evaluation of HRT interventions. It is important to involve clients in generating valid outcome measures that are culturally relevant, incremental, and hierarchical (Ruefli & Rogers, 2004).

Our review of interventions guided by HRT shows that harm reduction efforts can focus on individuals, small groups, organizations, communities, and/or policymakers. According to Bigler (2005), this broad use makes HRT appropriate to practice in almost every social service or health care setting. However, we also discussed the barriers encountered during HRT research due to its controversial, inconsistent, and perhaps impractical use as a theory. In this book we argue that the conceptual tenets of HRT make it better suited as a metatheory. Specifically, other health behavior theories can provide developmental and evaluative assistance to the application and operationalization of the broad tenets of HRT, filling a gap in HRT research, while HRT also provides guidance in the implementation of humanistic, pragmatic interventions.

To instigate how HRT can be applied as a metatheory in tandem with health behavior theories, we present two short case studies in which HRT was used concurrently with other health promotion theories. The success of these case studies helps build support for considering harm reduction as a metatheory in health promotion research and practice.

EXAMPLE OF HARM REDUCTION RESEARCH IN PRACTICE: HIV TEST COUNSELING[1]

Besides focusing on safer injection practices to reduce the risk of HIV transmission, as we discussed earlier with the case of NEPs, harm reduction approaches also are utilized to reduce the sexual transmission of HIV. Examples of such initiatives promote consistent condom use and communication about sexual intentions before engaging in sexual activity. These interventions can take the form of health campaigns that persuade individuals to use condoms and/or through individual test counseling that discusses methods to help prevent infecting other people with HIV. The first example in this chapter highlights a study that integrated HRT with HIV-test-counseling practices. Although not explicitly applied as a metatheory, the tenets of HRT were used to reframe an HIV-test-counseling protocol to aid prevention communication with the target audience of individuals at risk for HIV, which illustrates the metatheoretical utility of HRT.

HIV-test counseling is defined as combining personalized counseling with knowledge of HIV status to motivate an individual to change behaviors in order to prevent the transmission of HIV (Denison, O'Reilly, Schmid, Kennedy, & Sweat, 2007). HIV-test counseling is a commonly used method to promote safer sex and other harm-reducing behaviors to prevent exposure to and/or transmission of HIV. Longitudinal studies revealed that a personalized approach to HIV-test counseling showed much promise in reducing risky sexual behaviors (Hollander, 2001). However, after reviewing common HIV-test-counseling protocols with support from client reactions during counseling sessions, Mattson and Basnyat (2008) argued that these HIV-test-counseling sessions lacked genuine, empathetic, individualized interaction with clients.

Despite the implementation of revised CDC guidelines in 2001 that focused on risk reduction, assessing personal risk, and focusing on skill-building activities (CDC, 2001), Mattson (1999, 2000; Mattson & Basnyat, 2008) contended that HIV-test-counseling protocols were vague and were compromising an opportunity to more effectively communicate with clients. Although the revised guidelines encouraged a more tailored approach, it was difficult for counselors to incorporate because counseling sessions continued to be assessment-laden both before and after testing. In addition, as transcripts analyzed by Mattson and Basnyat (2008) indicated, because clients provided predominantly close-ended "no" responses to a majority of counselor questions, it is possible clients did not trust and/or feel safe discussing their risky sexual behaviors with counselors.

In an effort to employ a more client-centered approach to HIV-test counseling, Mattson (2000) reasoned that HRT has the "theoretical and practical vitality to reduce the relevant harms of HIV/AIDS through HIV-test-counseling discourse that empowers and promotes clients' agency" (p. 339). HRT is a suitable fit for HIV-test counseling because it promotes that individuals have choices about their health behaviors (Rosenberg, 2003). In Figure 2.1, the ways that Mattson and Basnyat (2008) utilized central tenets of HRT to inform future applications of HIV-test counseling are highlighted.

Research in Practice Illustration
Using Harm Reduction to Inform HIV-Test-Counseling Practices

Humanistic Value → Recognize individuals' health decisions and respects their rights to make their own choices.

- **Example in Practice:** "The counselor would accept the client's situation and behaviors without attaching judgment, regardless of whether the counselor approves of the situation or behavior" (p. 150).

Pragmatism → Accept that individuals engage in risky health and safety behaviors and focus on ways to minimize their risk of negative consequences as a result of those behaviors.

- **Example in Practice:** "Counselor accepting unconditionally that individuals engage in risky behaviors and rather than eliminating the cause (i.e., unsafe sex), they would focus on reducing the negative effects of the risk such as negotiating relevant skills to employ in the future, increase general knowledge, and provide access to condoms" (p. 151).

Focus on Immediate Harm → Do not exclude nor assume the goal of abstinence.

- **Example in Practice:** "For HIV testing counseling, the focus of the discussion would not be on how individuals placed themselves at risk for HIV but rather on how to cope with the outcome of that behavior because of the understanding that behavior is a multifaceted phenomenon and impacts the community within which it is embedded" (p. 151).

Prioritizing Goal Setting (i.e., empowerment) → Focus attention on immediate health consequences and provide many choices to alleviate the possibility of those consequences.

- **Example in Practice:** "During an HIV-test-counseling session this translates into the client, rather than the counselor, being the primary agent for reducing the harm of risky behaviors to the self and other. The counselor mostly listens and offers healthier options for consideration by the client" (p. 151).

Balancing Costs and Benefits (i.e., community collaboration) → Encourage a cost-benefit analysis that extends to the individual, community, and society so everyone benefits.

- **Example in Practice:** "For HIV test counseling, this means providing immediate, personalized care to the individual that would help curb the long-term use of community resources such as mental health and other health care services" (p. 151).

Figure 2.1 Research in Practice Illustration: Using Harm Reduction to Inform HIV-Test-Counseling Practices. *Source*: Adapted from Mattson and Basnyat, 2008.

After considering the ways that the tenets of HRT could inform current protocols used during HIV-test-counseling sessions, the authors proposed an integrated framework to further enhance the standardized protocols.

Developing an HIV-Test Counseling and Harm Reduction Integrated Framework

Mattson and Basnyat (2008) drew upon other integrative models and strategies to conceptualize their integration of HRT with HIV-test counseling. Specifically, to inform their model they referred to integrative harm reduction models by Roche et al. (2001) and MacCoun (1998), which focused on a collaborative, overarching approach to decreasing drug abuse. Depicted in Figure 2.2, the resulting model integrated the tenets of HRT with the CDC's current HIV-test-counseling protocol. Mattson and Basnyat argued that using HRT with CDC's current risk reduction objectives further centralizes the concerns of clients by focusing on aspects of respect, empowerment, and developing and addressing immediate goals based on current barriers an individual may be facing.

Further, the researchers claimed that by "infusing" HRT tenets within the HIV-test-counseling protocol, counselors became more mindful of harm reduction and as a result, the tenets permeated the discussion with clients (p. 157) while still communicating accurate information with this at-risk audience. Figure 2.3 juxtaposes a traditional HIV-test-counseling session with a reframed excerpt from an HIV-test-counseling session to illustrate the differences in communication between the client and counselor when the session is infused with HRT.

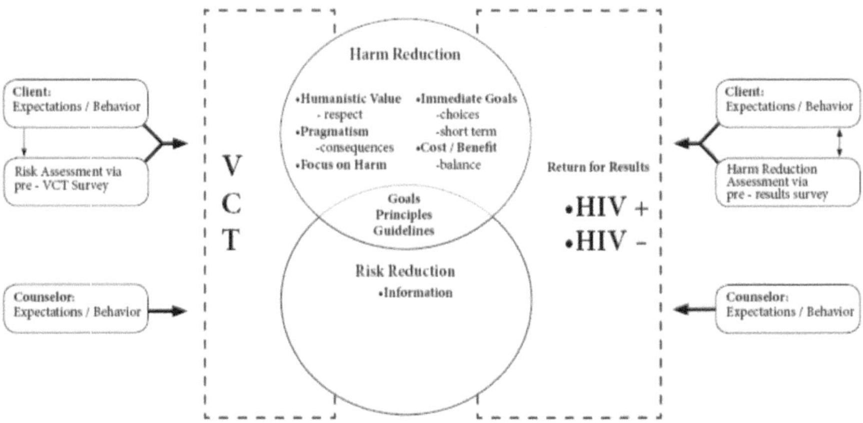

Figure 2.2 Integrated Harm Reduction Model of HIV-Test Counseling. *Source*: Used with permission from Mattson & Basnyat, 2008.

Research in Practice Illustration
Infusing Harm Reduction Into HIV-Test Counseling

Traditional Excerpt 1 (p. 138)	HRT Reframed Excerpt 1 (p. 157)
Healthcare Provider (HP): Okay, looking back now are you comfortable with the choices you made Client (C): Pregnancy is big deal, it changes your life but AIDS pretty much kills you, so no, I guess I was focusing on the wrong thing. HP: So, what will happen if this comes up again, you meet someone you are attractive to him and he is attracted to you C: No, I wouldn't sleep with him unless I was in a relationship HP: He offers a relationship and things are going well, so do you have unprotected sex with him C: Yeah, well, I don't know. I wouldn't have unprotected sex unless I knew. First of all I would still be on birth-control but that doesn't affect AIDS, hmm. I would want to know if he has been tested HP: Okay, so he shows you a piece of paper and oh he's everything, totally groovy, he's shows you the lab result and has been tested negative, he tells you he has only been with few other women in his life and that you are so beautiful. That's all going great and you know you have been tested negative. Do you have unprotected sex with him? C: I mean I guess I would, I would feel guilty if I didn't HP: Are you telling me what you think I want to hear or what you believe C: Obviously, unless I didn't trust him HP: You trust him from the short amount of time he seems very trustworthy and very honest C: Yes I would do the same HP: Ok, let's talk about the holes in that particular process. It would seem from the outside that it wasn't necessarily a bad thing. You are entering into a relationship, you are monogamous, he's tested you are tested, you talk about the past and he admits about the people he has been with in the past and the people you have been with and you do all that stuff so what's the problem?	Healthcare Provider (HP): Okay, looking back now are you comfortable with the choices you made [actual discussion] Client (C): Pregnancy is big deal, it changes your life but AIDS pretty much kills you, so no, I guess I was focusing on the wrong thing. HP: I understand why you would be focused on just pregnancy but you are also right, if you are or intend to have unprotected sex, you should also be concerned about AIDS. But what will you do if this situation happens again, where you meet someone you are attracted to? C: It's not like I would sleep with him unless I was in a relationship. HP: That's great but what if he offers you a relationship? C: I would make sure that I either had protected sex or make sure I know his sexual history and want to make sure he has been tested. I am on birth control but it's not like that's protecting me from AIDS. HP: That's true; you should make sure he has been tested. But, you should also keep in mind that doesn't mean he is 100% safe either. Because the tests are only valid from 6 months after the last intercourse, so you also want to make sure he has been tested after his last relationship and/or intercourse. C: That's good to know otherwise I would have felt guilty not to have unprotected sex, after seeing his papers. HP: You know, you always have a choice and perhaps, if you feel uncomfortable or guilty you should consider asking him to wait until both of you are tested. C: Well, I wouldn't have unprotected sex if I didn't trust him. HP: Yes, that might be the case. But, what if it is just someone you have recently met? In this case, for you to trust him you might need for him to be tested first and using protection until then. Of course, if you have been with the same partner for a longer time then you might be able to trust him since you already know his history. C: Yes I would do the same

Figure 2.3 Research in Practice Illustration: Infusing Harm Reduction Into HIV-Test Counseling. *Source*: Adapted from Mattson and Basynat, 2008.

This example from HIV-test-counseling practice showcases a different health topic and situation in which HRT can be used to guide and improve an already existing protocol that had not achieved optimal behavior change success in the past. By reframing the current CDC HIV-test-counseling protocol, health communication with clients may be perceived as less judgmental and standardized, and hopefully result in healthier behaviors.

Next, we discuss another health issue to which HRT has been regularly applied. That is, to reduce negative consequences of high-risk alcohol consumption.

EXAMPLE OF HIGH-RISK ALCOHOL CONSUMPTION AND HARM REDUCTION PROGRAMMING IN HIGHER EDUCATION USING THE SOCIAL ECOLOGICAL MODEL[2]

Previously in this chapter we discussed ways that HRT has been utilized as a strategy for addressing alcohol consumption in the form of high-risk drinking, alcoholism, and other alcohol-related problems and associated consequences. Although harm reduction research pertaining to alcohol-related problems has focused on a variety of audiences from underage youth who consume alcohol to individuals who are alcohol-dependent, we focus on harm reduction strategies for traditional college-aged students. Because the case study we present focuses on alcohol consumption among the college population during our *Research in Practice Illustrations*, we use the term "high-risk drinking" throughout this particular review; this terminology is common on college campuses. *High-risk drinking* typically refers to excessive and/or underage alcohol consumption behaviors (National Institute on Alcohol Abuse and Alcoholism [NIAAA], 2002). In the following section we provide a general discussion of alcohol programming in the college setting including how this programming has advanced over time in part due to guidance by the Social Ecological Model (SEM) (McLeroy, Bibeau, Steckler, & Glance, 1988). Then, we discuss how alcohol programming that is framed by the SEM can be further enhanced and targeted for college students when infused with the tenets of harm reduction.

High-risk drinking continues to be a problem on college campuses nationwide. Specific to college students, heavy drinkers more often miss class, fall behind in school, black out, engage in unprotected sex, get into arguments and/or physical fights, damage property, and get in trouble with local authorities (Wechsler, Molnar, Davenport, & Baer, 2000). When applying tenets of harm reduction independently, researchers have focused on environmental strategies such as interventions and access, and target the individual to engage in personal harm reduction strategies either by using a designated driver, consuming less alcohol in one place, and watching your drink(s) throughout the night so no one tampers with your beverage (Martens, Ferrier, & Cimini, 2007).

Another example of a harm reduction approach to reduce consequences of high-risk drinking is reported by Rosenberg and colleagues (2011). These researchers proposed 17 protective strategies for college students to engage in while consuming alcohol (i.e. the Alcohol Safety and Health Strategies). Strategies include staying with a trusted friend, letting your friends know where you are going if you decide to leave, using a condom if you engage in sexual activity, avoiding (or) not carrying a weapon or using drugs while drinking, and walking away from arguments with other people. These researchers found that a majority of students who participated in the study were moderately confident that they could employ several of the harm reduction strategies on the list. Rosenberg et al. (2011) argued that colleges and universities could use the generated list to determine which protective strategies students are not efficacious in and develop targeted interventions to increase skills and confidence in those specific protective strategies.

College students themselves recognize the need for such educational/interventional programming aimed at reducing negative alcohol-related consequences. For instance, after conducting a qualitative investigation into the strategies college students employ to safeguard themselves and others when drinking, Howard and colleagues (2007) asserted, "In terms of informational and behavioral needs, students expressed both frustration at being taught only to abstain from drinking and genuine interest in acquiring specific kinds of knowledge and skills. Salient among their concerns was knowing how to drink responsibly . . ." (p. 252). Previous investigations (Barry & Goodson, 2011a) suggested that college students believe there are seven distinct themes associated with responsible drinking: refraining from drinking and driving; drinking in moderation; monitoring and limiting consumption; pacing one's drinking rate; knowing one's personal limit; taking precautions to avoid intoxication; and planning ahead. Unfortunately, at-risk drinkers report less confidence, and lower intentions, to enact many of these protective behavioral strategies the next time they consume alcohol (Barry, Howell, & Dennis, 2011). Moreover, those who drink more believe these behaviors should occur with less frequency and report greater perceived barriers (Barry & Goodson, 2011b). Previous research identified numerous contextual factors (e.g., next day responsibilities, participation in drinking games, financial considerations) that influence one's decision to implement responsible drinking behaviors (Barry & Goodson, 2012). As this review illustrates, a large base of empirical evidence exists that incorporates harm reduction to address college drinking behaviors.

Besides using HRT to uncover several barriers to managing one's drinking behaviors, the *Social Ecological Model* (SEM) often is used to help understand and recognize that students' drinking behaviors are influenced by multiple spheres of influence from the individual level to the surrounding environment level. Each level is used to help develop and guide more systematic and comprehensive strategies to address students' risky drinking behaviors. A description of each SEM level is outlined in Figure 2.4.

Further, examples of ways that college and university campuses have used the SEM to inform alcohol prevention initiatives in the past are highlighted in Table 2.1.

When DeJong and Langford (2002) discussed the SEM as a framework to address high-risk drinking at Institutions of Higher Education (IHE), they observed that most campuses had focused their prevention efforts on intrapersonal and interpersonal factors. They argued, "less attention has been paid to factors in the local community that affect student alcohol use; calls by campus officials for changes in state or federal policy remain rare" (p. 141). However, a lack of community and policy involvement is not as common in higher education initiatives to prevent high-risk drinking.

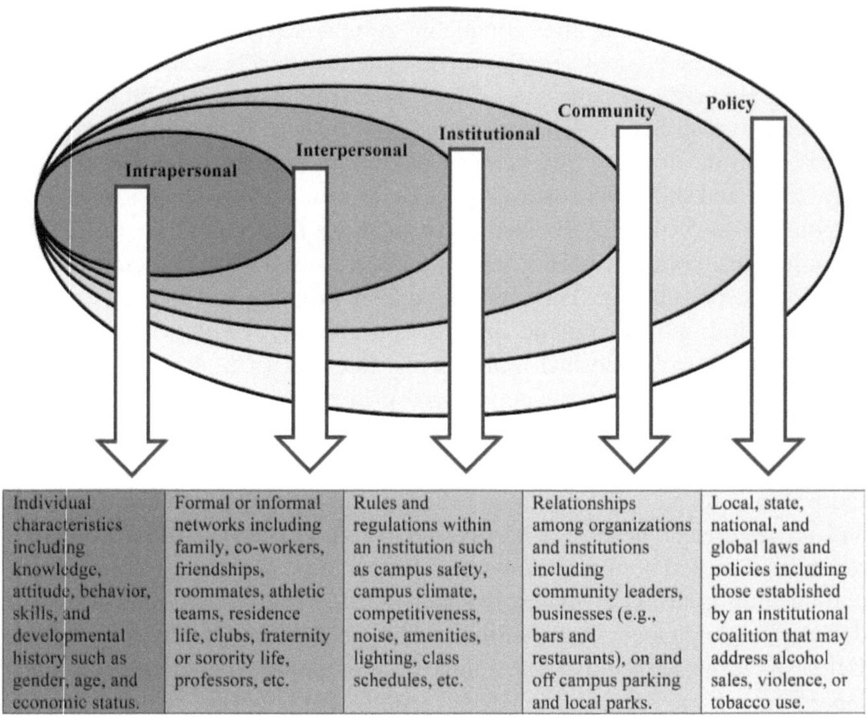

Figure 2.4 Social Ecological Model. *Source*: Adapted from McLeroy, Steckler, Bibeau, & Glanz, 1988.

Table 2.1 A Social Ecological Framework to Address Alcohol Consumption on College and University Campuses

1. *Intrapersonal*. Motivational feedback interviews, individual counseling, knowledge of the effects of alcohol consumption on academics and potentially participation in clubs and athletics, and first-year orientation activities addressing alcohol consumption.
2. *Interpersonal*. Peer-to-peer or parent-student communication.
3. *Institutional*. Not allowing on-campus advertising for alcohol-promoting activities, medical amnesty policies, sponsoring alcohol-free activities.
4. *Community*. Encouraging bars, liquor stores, and off-campus party locations to check students' IDs, campus/community coalitions.
5. *Policy*. Establishing and following through on-campus policies, state, and federal laws that are in place.

Source: Adapted from DeJong and Langford, 2002.

In 1976, the first report about risky drinking among college students was released by the *National Institute on Alcohol Abuse and Alcoholism* [NIAAA] (2002). Since then, the researchers and practitioners have learned more about the variety of external and internal factors that affect students' drinking behaviors. Specifically, three years of discussions and intensive research culminated in the NIAAA report, *A Call to Action: Changing the Culture of Drinking at U.S. College* (2002). In this report, recommendations, presented as the four tiers of effectiveness, were identified that further supported the importance of addressing all areas in the SEM when addressing high-risk drinking on college campuses. The four tiers, now used to guide alcohol-related initiatives on campuses, are outlined in Table 2.2 as a preface to the alcohol-related harm reduction strategies discussed later in this chapter.

As the strategies within these four tiers indicate, these strategies need to be observed from the intrapersonal through policy levels of the SEM to accurately identify and respond to students' perceived barriers to reducing risky alcohol consumption. In addition, within these tiers harm reduction terminology plays a key role in reducing high-risk drinking on college campuses through the strategies listed (e.g., using safe-ride programs acknowledges that students will engage in heavy drinking).

Many of these strategies were implemented on campuses with the thought of harm reduction or the SEM, but not always with a conscious effort to integrate the two frameworks. We argue that integrating these two frameworks can result in accurate and nonjudgmental communication with students through a variety of outlets. Specifically, the tenets of HRT can be utilized as a metatheory to inform the areas of the SEM when devising communication methods to target college students' risky drinking behaviors. In this section, we illustrate examples of how the tenets of HRT, integrated with the SEM, may help reduce the negative consequences of college drinking from

Table 2.2 The Four "Tiers" of Effectiveness

1. *Evidence of Effectiveness Among College Students*
   Strategies
   - Combine cognitive-behavioral skills training with norms clarification and motivational enhancement interventions.
   - Offer brief motivational interventions.
   - Challenge alcohol expectancies.
2. *Evidence of Success with General Populations that Could be Applied to College Environments*
   Strategies
   - Better enforce minimum drinking age laws.
   - Implement, increase publicity, and enforce other laws to reduce driving under the influence.
   - Restrict alcohol retail outlet density.
   - Increase prices and taxes on alcohol.
   - Promote responsible policies in social and commercial settings.
   - Form a campus and community coalition that involves major stakeholders.
3. *Evidence of Logical and Theoretical Promise, But Require more Comprehensive Evaluation*
   Strategies
   - Adopt campus policies that may reduce high-risk alcohol use (e.g., Friday exams).
   - Increase enforcement at campus-based events that promote excessive drinking.
   - Increase publicity about and enforcement of underage drinking laws on campus.
   - Enforce disciplinary action.
   - Develop and disseminate marketing campaigns.
   - Use safe-ride programs.
   - Regulate happy hours and alcohol sales.
   - Inform new students and parents about alcohol policies before arriving on campus.
4. *Evidence of Ineffectiveness*
   Strategies
   - Use of informational, knowledge-based interventions only.
   - Provide Blood Alcohol Content (BAC) content feedback to students.

Source: Adapted from NIAAA, 2002, pp. 16–23.

institutional and community perspectives, since these advancements in community collaboration are more recent on many campuses. In some examples below, we showcase a community and university collaborative effort at Purdue University, led by the Student Wellness Office located within the Student Health Center on campus.

Using the SEM and Harm Reduction Tenets to Reduce High-Risk Drinking

In 2001, Purdue University's Student Wellness Office (SWO) formed the *Campus Community Bar Retail Coalition* (CCBRC). The mission of this group, provided below, demonstrates a strong emphasis on community collaboration, humanistic value, and pragmatism to help facilitate a safer drinking environment for students.

> As participants in the Campus Community Bar Retailer Coalition, we recognize that high-risk alcohol behaviors occur in and around our campus community and must be addressed. We believe that these behaviors are best addressed by collaboration between alcohol retailers, law enforcement, campus and community. (CCBRC, 2014)

CCBRC Meetings are held on a quarterly basis. The city's Police Chief co-facilitates these meetings with the Health Advocacy Coordinator of SWO. Key stakeholders from several organizations that can impact students' drinking behaviors attend the meetings. On average, 35–55 stakeholders attend each quarter. Meetings often are held in the city library or a local bar frequented by students. Refer to the list of participating organizations below.

General List of CCBRC Attendees

- Prosecutor's Office
- City of West Lafayette (including city council members and city officials, such as the mayor)
- Several campus offices
- Student groups
- Community agencies
- Three police agencies
- Legislators
- Campus-area bars and package stores
- Area business owners

Notice on the list of participants that depending on their role in the community or on campus, they can address different levels of the SEM to facilitate a safer drinking environment. For example, student groups may work to address factors at the institutional level such as promoting safe-ride programs while police agencies work with bar owners at the community and policy levels to ensure checking of identification, over-service, and occupancy issues.

Based on the CCBRC's mission, this group operates from a harm reduction standpoint to address college drinking at the individual, institutional, community, and policy levels. In being realistic about students' drinking behaviors and realizing the variety of internal and external influences that affect those behaviors, the CCBRC has positioned itself to target students using a variety of nonjudgmental and immediate strategies. In the following case study illustrations, we highlight how the campus/community works together in other ways to focus on how a harm reduction approach guided activities carried out within particular levels of the SEM. Notice in the illustrations that the HRT tenet of community collaboration has an overarching presence which guides the harm reduction strategies implemented. In other words, a variety of individuals work together to create "enabling environments" to facilitate safer and healthier behaviors (Rhodes, 2002).

Hosting Safer Parties for Off-Campus Students

Toward the beginning of the school year, several groups collaborate in the West Lafayette/Purdue University community to distribute safe party magnets to students (Figure 2.5). This partnership reaches residents of apartment complexes and houses near campus. City officials, residents, police, campus officials, and students deliver magnets to apartment complexes and travel door-to-door to distribute safer party tips (example follows) and discuss ways

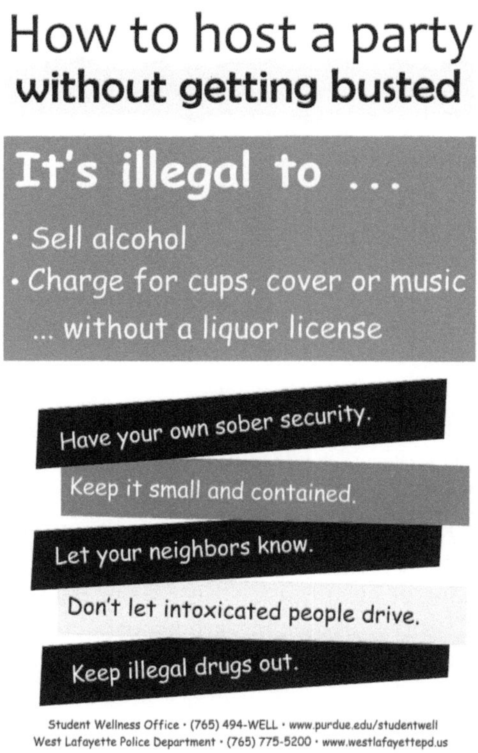
How to host a party
without getting busted
It's illegal to ...
• Sell alcohol
• Charge for cups, cover or music
... without a liquor license
Have your own sober security.
Keep it small and contained.
Let your neighbors know.
Don't let intoxicated people drive.
Keep illegal drugs out.
Student Wellness Office • (765) 494-WELL • www.purdue.edu/studentwell
West Lafayette Police Department • (765) 775-5200 • www.westlafayettepd.us

Figure 2.5 Purdue University Safer Party Magnet Example. *Source*: Used with permission from Purdue University Student Wellness Office.

to host a more responsible party, while acknowledging that alcohol will be available at the parties. In one year this group may distribute up to 8,500 magnets.

Figure 2.6 further outlines how the tenets of HRT were integrated into practice during this safer drinking initiative.

This initiative required collaboration among student groups, campus representatives and the city. Police reported that arrests were down, and during student interviews on safe parties, several students cited specific implementation strategies from the magnets as ways they host safer parties.

21st Birthday Cards

Another initiative that was practiced on this campus is the dissemination of birthday cards to students on their 21st birthday. Several universities have distributed some form of 21st birthday cards that list protective strategies to

Research in Practice Illustration
HRT Informing Communication via the SEM at the Community Level: Party Magnets

Following are examples of how the tenets of harm reduction are acknowledged and/or practiced in this collaborative effort to promote safer parties.

Humanistic Value → Recognize and accept that students may choose to engage in risky drinking behaviors and respect their rights to make their own choices.

- **Example in Practice:** By distributing information to students about safer parties, this group acknowledges that parties are being hosted, students are making the decision to drink, and may engage in heavy drinking.

Pragmatism → Accept that students engage in risky situations that involve alcohol consumption and focus on ways to minimize their risk of negative consequences as a result of those choices.

- **Example in Practice:** The magnets provide realistic strategies to reduce potentially negative consequences of hosting a party during which alcohol will be available. For example, asking an individual to keep parties small and contained is a realistic recommendation for hosting a safer, more contained party.

Immediacy and Goal Setting → Provide strategies to reduce risky behaviors and consequences of those behaviors.

- **Example in Practice:** These magnets provide several protective strategies that students can use that night to reduce their chances of being reprimanded by local authorities as a result of hosting/attending a party. All of the strategies on the magnet can be enacted immediately and with relative ease, making it more likely students will act upon the advice.

Empowerment → Provides choices to individuals, allowing them to choose and implement short-term strategies.

- **Example in Practice:** The magnets provide several ideas that students can choose to initiate to protect themselves if they decide to host a party. Allowing students to choose one or more strategies may empower them to be more in control of their situation.

Figure 2.6 Research in Practice Illustration: HRT Informing Communication via the SEM at the Community Level—Party Magnets. *Source*: Adapted with permission from Loew, Orstad, and Maylath, 2013.

prevent high-risk drinking on students' 21st birthdays. For example, Neighbors, Lee, Lewis, Fossos, and Walter (2009) conducted a randomized prevention intervention in which some students received a web-based 21st birthday card that listed protective strategies such as limiting drinking games, knowing where your drink is, and avoiding drinks that contain multiple shots. Strategies contained within the cards were adapted from the BASICS program previously discussed and the cards also displayed normative information about drinking on campus.

Another example of a harm reduction initiative led by members of Purdue University's Student Wellness Office, Student Government, and the President's Office, included the distribution of 21st birthday cards to students. The 21st birthday card encouraged that, if students chose to drink, to drink responsibly. During the 2011 school year, 4,587 cards were sent to students to

Research in Practice Illustration
HRT Informing Communication via the SEM at the Institutional Level: 21st Birthday Cards

Humanistic Value → Recognize that students may choose to engage in risky drinking behaviors and respect their rights to make their own choices.

- **Example in Practice:** This birthday card states, "If you choose to drink, please drink responsibly." This line does not judge all students as drinkers, or assumes that everyone will consume alcohol just because they legally can. However, it also acknowledges that some students may choose to drink and instead of telling students to abstain from alcohol, this birthday card simply encourages them to do so responsibly.

Pragmatism → Accept that students engage in risky drinking behaviors and focus on ways to minimize their risk of negative consequences as a result of alcohol consumption.

- **Example in Practice:** The inside of the card also provides realistic strategies to engage in to reduce potentially negative consequences of partying and drinking. For example, asking an individual to eat food before going out is a much more realistic alternative than asking that person not to drink.

Immediacy and Goal Setting → Provide coping strategies to begin reducing risky behaviors and consequences of those behaviors.

- **Example in Practice:** The birthday card lists 10 protective strategies that students can use that night to provide a safer birthday celebration. The strategies on the card, ranging from driving sober to drinking water, can be employed immediately and with relative ease, making it more likely students will adhere to the advice. (See results of evaluation that follows)

Empowerment → Provides choices to students, allowing them to choose and implement short-term, pragmatic goals.

- **Example in Practice:** The birthday card offers several options that students can choose to initiate to protect themselves throughout their birthday. Encouraging students to choose one or more strategies may empower them to be more in control of their situation. In addition, not all of the strategies may be applicable to everyone. For example, a student may not have a car on campus and as a result, not be driving. So, listing strategies that encompass a variety of situations is a method utilized in the birthday card as well.

Figure 2.7 Research in Practice Illustration: HRT Informing Communication via the SEM at the Institutional Level—21st Birthday Cards. *Source*: Adapted with permission from Loew, Orstad, and Maylath, 2013.

encourage them to celebrate their 21st birthday in a safe and responsible way. Refer to the tenets below to see how an HRT perspective can inform targeted, persuasive feedback for students. In Figure 2.7, we highlight the 21st birthday card program that was implemented at Purdue University, which was a collaboration between SWO and several student groups.

This intervention occurred within and across the intrapersonal, interpersonal, and the institutional levels of the SEM. Integrated with a harm reduction approach, this program was effective in decreasing students' risky drinking behaviors on their 21st birthday. Figure 2.8 lists the ten harm reduction, or proactive strategies that were listed on the back of the birthday card.

This harm reduction initiative was first evaluated in spring 2011. Students who received the 21st birthday card that year participated in a survey in which they responded about the drinking behaviors and protective strategies they used the night they celebrated their 21st birthday. General results indicated that receiving the intervention significantly reduced students' BAC levels on their 21st birthday. In particular, the researchers found the most success for those students who intended to reach higher BAC levels during their birthday, indicating the importance of personalized feedback, including protective strategies, to reduce intentions and actions to engage in ultimately risky behaviors. Key findings are listed below.

Results from Initial Evaluation of 21st Birthday Card Program

- 71% remembered receiving the card
- 6% said they drank *less* alcohol because of the card
- 59% said the program should continue
- 55% consumed 0–8 drinks when they celebrated their 21st birthday
- 61% had a sober driver when they celebrated their 21st birthday
- 91% celebrated with friends they could trust
- 24% alternated between alcoholic and nonalcoholic drinks throughout the evening
- 40% limited the amount of alcohol they consumed
- 82% ate food throughout the evening

These results indicate that students utilized some or all of the strategies listed on the birthday card. This nonjudgmental, realistic approach to modifying behaviors throughout the night may have resulted in fewer students receiving DUIs (driving under the influence), getting alcohol poisoning, or getting into trouble with law enforcement. For more information about this initiative, visit www.purdue.edu/21birthday.

These are just a few examples of harm reduction initiatives that took place at one university. These examples illustrate that a university coalition can

Top Ten 21st Birthday Tips

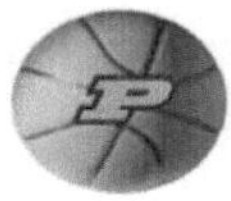

10. Don't be stupid. How about...doing 21 push-ups...eating 21 jalapeno poppers or hitting 21 shots...with a basketball. ***But 21 shots of alcohol? Bad idea.***

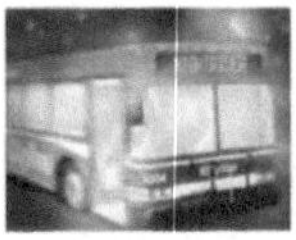

9. Sober driver, Sober driver, Sober driver. How many times do we have to say this?

8. Celebrate with friends you trust—the ones who have enough sense to keep you from losing control, out of jail, or will call for an ambulance if you need it. They might even buy you a gift.

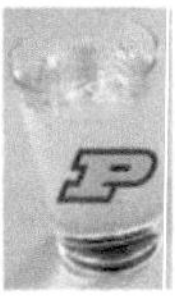

7. Can you say "alternate"? If you alternate between alcoholic and non-alcoholic drinks throughout the night (we're partial to thirst-quenching water), your body will thank you. Alcohol dehydrates the body. Water helps.

6. Do we have to send you back to kindergarten for this message, again? Don't take a drink from a stranger or leave your drink unattended. There just might be a special dose of a date-rape drug inside (but remember that alcohol is THE #1 date rape drug).

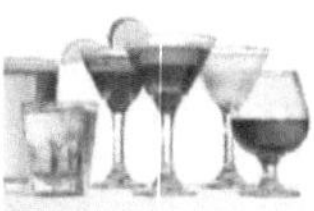

5. All drinks are not created equally . . . Usually, a drink is one 12 oz. beer, one shot of 80-proof liquor, or one 4 oz. glass of wine. But, even within each category, there are varying alcohol contents, e.g. regular beer has more alcohol than lite beer, and tequila has more alcohol than schnapps. If you don't know how much alcohol you're drinking, ask your server!

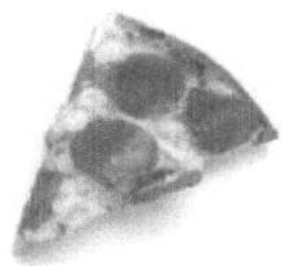

4. Eat birthday cake, nachos, or pizza before you go out. Food fills you up and slows alcohol absorption, too.

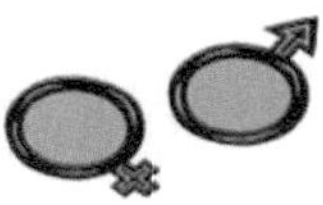

3. Alcohol is sexist! It treats men and women differently due to body size, composition and hormones.

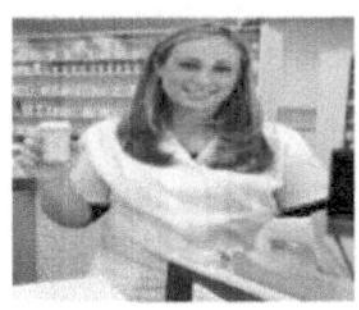

2. Ask your friendly pharmacist to wish you a happy birthday. Some medications should not be combined with alcohol. Your pharmacist will tell you if you can drink safely.

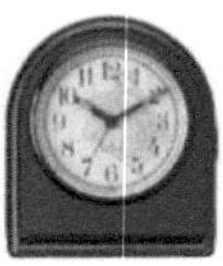

1. Whoa. Slow down! Enjoy all 1,440 minutes of your birthday. Take your time. You don't want to just remember the first fifteen minutes, do you?

Card content and design by Student Wellness Office

Figure 2.8 Purdue University 21st Birthday Card Proactive Strategies. *Source*: Used with permission from Purdue University Student Wellness Office.

promote efforts at the institutional, community, and policy levels to encourage change at levels of the SEM. Initiatives led by the CCBRC influenced the institutional and community levels by making the physical environment safer, limiting accessibility of alcohol through restricted drink promotions and more organized identification carding practices. At the same time these efforts built community capacity. Notice that collaboration, an overarching tenet of HRT, is crucial to guiding and influencing strategies to reduce high-risk drinking at the broader levels of the SEM, showcasing the integration between the theory (i.e., SEM) and proposed metatheory (i.e., HRT).

For example, pragmatism and immediacy were highly emphasized in efforts to reduce high-risk drinking among the student population by determining realistic changes that students may be willing to make immediately in their drinking behaviors. In addition, although the CCBRC is not made up of members of the target population, student voices were incorporated in harm reduction efforts by including students in the development of products and events that promote less risky alcohol consumption. However, further integrating students who engage in high-risk drinking behaviors may enhance student empowerment in the future.

Now that we provided two examples in which harm reduction served as an overarching framework in combination with other health behavior theories and programs, we further discuss the feasibility and utility of harm reduction as a metatheory. We begin building harm reduction as metatheory to inform motorcycle safety.

HARM REDUCTION RESEARCH TO PRACTICE: STARTING WITH MOTORCYCLE SAFETY

As a part of the first chapter we discussed some of the barriers that prevent the consistent and accepted use of HRT in research and practice. One of the barriers we mentioned was the misunderstanding of HRT being applied as a strategy to legalize and promote drug use. Predominantly, HRT has been used as a method to prevent negative consequences of drug abuse. This application has been controversial over the years. Some researchers argue that, in order to gain empirical support, HRT must be used to address less politically-charged public health issues (Reid, 2002; Stevenson, 1994). The case study throughout this book focuses on the public health issue of motorcycle safety, which is a less politically-charged issue than illegal drug and alcohol abuse. Traffic policies already incorporate HRT tenets to reduce the risks of injury while driving. Examples of harm reduction strategies for traffic safety include setting speed limits, passing laws requiring the use of seatbelts and helmets, establishing a minimum age for alcohol consumption, and reducing the allowable blood alcohol concentration for legal driving (Transportation Research Board, 1998).

In the next section we begin conceptualizing and framing HRT as an overarching, guiding framework in qualitative health and safety research with a focus on motorcycle safety as the case example. This discussion provides a foundation for the rest of the book. While crafting this qualitative research design, we also offer a summary of the content covered in this chapter to further support and organize how we came to our conclusion to propose HRT as a metatheory in health and safety research.

Designing a Harm Reduction Metatheory Empirical Research Project

A research project cannot begin without a research idea, which provides the foundation for conceptualizing the project. In the preface, you read how and why we decided to focus both on motorcycle safety and HRT as areas of inquiry for our research area and specific project. We were interested in the utility of HRT in health communication campaigns. Particularly, we wanted to study ways to expand the use of HRT and improve the effectiveness of health communication for a variety of health and safety issues, starting with motorcycle safety. The first step to designing a research project is to become familiar with the literature. According to Corbin and Strauss (2008), "the more familiar one is with the literature, the more readily one can identify the inconsistencies, contradictions, or gaps in current theory" or other areas of inquiry (p. 69). After consulting the literature, we discovered that previous studies successfully utilized HRT during interventions, but sustaining harm reduction initiatives posed challenges in subsequent research. In the first two chapters, we identified two primary challenges to sustaining harm reduction initiatives in previous projects.

First, as we discussed in this chapter, literature indicated that typically HRT interventions were not fully evaluated for strengths and weaknesses, making it difficult to know if these strategies reduced harm for the target audience (Rogers & Ruefli, 2004). Research showed that HRT lacked rigorous evaluation tools to analyze past, current, and future interventions (Marlatt, 1998). Evaluating the effectiveness of interventions remained a challenge because no set of criteria for evaluating outcomes and the recognition of the hierarchical nature of harm reduction goals existed or was even close to being operationalized (O'Hare, 1992). Prior research encouraged the creation and implementation of HRT interventions, but research and funding did not emphasize measurement of the tenets of HRT to evaluate interventions (Rogers & Ruefli, 2004), which was restricting the reliability of harm reduction programming.

In addition to the lack of consistent evaluations, another barrier we discussed in the first chapter was the controversial history of harm reduction initiatives. The Trojan horse metaphor was commonly used to pejoratively describe HRT. Hall (2007) argued that in the United States, HRT is considered a Trojan Horse for drug legalization (p. 338). HRT is considered a Trojan horse because HRT acknowledges that people use illegal drugs and HRT interventions may approve of and even encourage people continuing to use drugs. Consequently, although HRT initiatives may initially seem positive they actually are detrimental to society (DuPont & Ford, 2000; Marlatt, 1998). Therefore, when health practitioners use the term HRT to discuss the reduction of negative health outcomes due to risky health behaviors such as drug use, the public may perceive this language as tantamount to legalizing drugs. Relatedly, one of the primary problems with the Trojan horse metaphor is its implication that harm reduction initiatives exclusively focus on drug use (Marlatt, 1998).

From this literature review, we drew two conclusions. First, an assessment of the tenets of HRT (i.e., humanistic value, pragmatism, immediacy/goal setting, empowerment, and community collaboration), with a specific focus on their potential to be evaluated, was necessary. And, second, another health-oriented behavior, besides illicit drug use, needed to be incorporated into a study of the tenets, to initiate more positive, less controversial discourse surrounding HRT. Upon further research into the tenets and numerous iterations into ways to advance the application of HRT, we determined that HRT may be impractical as a theory. However, the conceptual tenets of HRT seemed better suited as a metatheory. Coupled with applied health behavior theories, we wondered if HRT at a metatheoretical level would advance research and practice. This metatheoretical approach and specific terms will be discussed in the next chapter.

SUMMARY

The foundational research into HRT we discussed in Chapter 1 and Chapter 2 was necessary to discover a niche within health promotion research and practice. This phase of designing a qualitative research project is known as planning (Lindlof & Taylor, 2002) and serves to focus goals on a research area and potential problem(s) to address. Based on what we determined to be the problem of HRT in current research and practice, we decided that our path of inquiry should be the use of qualitative research to advance metatheoretical understanding of communication and intervention among at-risk populations. Besides our literature review and theoretical approach to qualitative inquiry, personal experiences and current opportunities also influenced the health issue we address in this project. The motorcycle-related death and accident we described in the Preface cued our interests in motorcycle safety. In addition, the Motorcycle Safety Campaign at Purdue University provided an opportunity to build knowledge and make personal connections in this area of health and human safety. Therefore, metatheory, personal experiences, and viable opportunities all served to influence our research ideas, which culminated into a research project that we designed, implemented, and now are presenting results about in this book to further the future application of harm reduction.

How we developed our research project was highlighted to illustrate the thought process that occurred to conceptualize the development of a metatheory before progressing to the design of our harm reduction empirical research project. In the next chapter, we continue to set the foundation for our goal of integrating harm reduction metatheory by offering a primer on metatheory building. Harm reduction metatheory is discussed in tandem with another health behavior theory and the public health issue of motorcycle safety.

NOTES

1. Adapted with permission from Mattson and Basnyat, 2008.
2. Adapted with permission and in collaboration with Loew, Orstad, and Mayalth, 2013.

REFERENCES

Audrey, S., Holliday, J., & Capbell, R. (2006). It's good to talk: Adolescent perspectives of an informal, peer-led intervention to reduce smoking. *Social Science & Medicine, 63,*(12), 320–334.

Babor, T. F., Caetano, R., Casswell, S., Edwards, G., Giesbrecht, N., Graham, K., et al. (2003). *Alcohol: No ordinary commodity*. Oxford: Oxford University Press.

Baer, J. S., Kivlahan, D. R., Blume, A. W., McKnight, P., & Marlatt, G. A. (2001). Brief intervention for heavy-drinking college students: 4-year follow-up and natural history. *American Journal of Public Health, 91*(8),1310–1316.

Barry, A. E., & Goodson, P. (2012). Contextual factors influencing college students' decision to drink responsibly. *Substance Use & Misuse, 47*(10), 1172–1184.

Barry, A. E., & Goodson, P. (2011a). How college students conceptualize and practice responsible drinking. *Journal of American College Health, 59*(4), 304–312.

Barry, A. E., & Goodson, P. (2011b). Development and testing of the CHORDS: Characteristics of responsible drinking survey. *American Journal of Health Promotion, 25*(6), e11–e21.

Barry, A. E., Howell, S. M., & Dennis, M. (2011). Evaluating impaired drivers' confidence and intention to "(Please) drink responsibly." *Journal of Safety Research, 42*(2), 137–142.

Bigler, M. O. (2005). Harm reduction as a practice and prevention model for social work. *The Journal of Baccalaureate Social Work, 10*(2), 69–86.

Botvin, G. J. (1985). The Life Skills Training program as a health promotion strategy: Theoretical issues and empirical findings. *Special Services in the Schools, 1,* 9–23.

Bullen, C., McRobbie, H., Thornley, S., Glover, M., Lin, R., & Laugesen, M. (2010). Effect of an electronic nicotine delivery device (e-cigarette) on desire to smoke and withdrawal user preferences and nicotine delivery: Randomized cross-over trial. *Tobacco Control. 19,* 98–103.

Campus Community Bar Retail Coalition (2014). Working together to address high-risk alcohol behaviors. Retrieved from http://www.purdue.edu/ccbrc/ on April 6, 2014.

Centers for Disease Control and Prevention (2013, September 6). Notes from the Field: Electronic Cigarette Use Among Middle and High School Students—United States, 2011–2012. Morbidity and Mortality Weekly Report (MMWR). Retrieved March 23, 2014 from http://www.cdc.gov/mmwr/preview/mmwrhtml/mm6235a6.htm.

Centers for Disease Control and Prevention (CDC). (2005). Update: syringe exchange interventions-United States, 2002. *Morbidity and Mortality Weekly Report*; *54*(27), 673–676.

Centers for Disease Control and Prevention (CDC) (2001). *Revised guidelines for HIV counseling, testing, and referral.* Atlanta, GA: Author.

Central Eastern European Harm Reduction Network (CEEHRN) (2004). *Scaling up provision of anti-retrovirals to drug users in Central and Eastern Europe and Central Asia.* Vilnius: CEEHRN.

Cooper, H., Moore, L., Gruskin, S., Krieger, N. (2005). The impact of a police drug crackdown on drug injectors' ability to practice harm reduction: A qualitative study. *Social Science & Medicine, 61*, 673–684.

Corbin, J., & Strauss, A. (2008). *Basics of qualitative research* (3rd Ed.). Thousand Oaks, CA: Sage.

DeJong, W., & Langford, L. M. (2002). A typology for campus-based alcohol prevention: Moving toward environmental management strategies. *Journal of Studies on Alcohol, 14,* 140–147.

Denison, J. A., O'Reilly, K. R., Schmid, G. P., Kennedy, C. E., & Sweat, M. D. (2007). HIV voluntary counseling and testing and behavioral risk reduction in developing countries: A meta-analysis, 1990–2005. *AIDS Behavior, 23,* 363–373.

Dhand, A. (2006). The roles performed by peer educators during outreach among heroin addicts in India: Ethnographic insights. *Social Science & Medicine, 63,* 2674–2685.

Dielman, T., Shope, J. T., Butchart, A. T., & Campanelli, P. C. (1986). Prevention of adolescent alcohol misuse: An elementary school program. *Journal of Pediatric Psychology, 11,* 259–282.

Dimeff, L. A., Baer, J. S., Kivlahan, D. R., & Marlatt, G. A. (1999). *Brief Alcohol Screening and Intervention for College Students (BASICS): A harm reduction approach.* New York, NY: Guilford Press.

Drucker, E., Lurie, P., Wodak, A., & Alcabes, P. (1998). Measuring harm reduction: The effects of needle and syringe exchange programs and methadone maintenance on the ecology of HIV. *AIDS, 12*(Suppl A), S217–5230.

DuPont, R. L., & Ford, B. (2000). *The selfish brain: Learning from addiction.* Hazeldon Publishing.

Eshrati, B., Asl, R. T., Dell, C. A., Afshar, P., Millson, P. M., Kamali, M., Weekes, J. (2008). Preventing HIV transmission among Iranian prisoners: Initial support for providing education on the benefits of harm reduction practices. *Harm Reduction Journal, 5*(21). Published online 2008 June 9. Available from http://www.harmreductionjournal.com/content/pdf/1477-7517-5-21.pdf.

Etter, J. F. (2010). Electronic cigarettes: A survey of users. *BMC Public Health, 10,* 231.

Fairchild, A. L., Bayer, R., & Colgrove, J. (2013). The renormalization of smoking? E-cigarettes and the tobacco "endgame". *The New England Journal of Medicine.* Doi:10.1056/NEJMp1313940.

Gartner, C. E., Hall, W. D., Vos, T., Bertram, M. Y., Wallace, A. L., & Lim, S. S. (2007). Assessment of Swedish snus for tobacco harm reduction: an epidemiological modelling study. *The Lancet, 369*(9578), 2010–2014.

Hall, W. (2007). What's in a name: *Addiction, 102,* 691–692.

Harrison, E. (2011). Harm reduction gives snus key role in reducing cigarette smoking. Retrieved March 23, 2014, from http://www.swedishmatch.com/en/Media/Articles/Harm-reduction-gives-snus-key-role-in-reducing-cigarette-smoking/.

Heather, N., & Robertson, I. (1983). *Controlled drinking* (2nd Ed). New York: Methuen.

Herring, R., Thom, B., Beccaria, F., Kolind, T., & Moskalewicz, J. (2010). Alcohol harm reduction in Europe. In T. Rhodes & D. Hedrich (Eds.), *European Monitoring Centre for Drugs and Drug Addiction (EMCDDA), Harm reduction: evidence, impacts, and challenges* (pp. 275–301). Scientific Monographs Series No. 10, Luxembourg: Publications Office of the European Union.

Hodgins, D. C., Leigh, G., Milne, R., & Gerrish, R. (1997). Drinking goal selection in behavioral self-management treatment of chronic alcoholics. *Addictive Behaviors, 22*(2), 247–255.

Hollander, D. (2001). Personalized HIV test counseling and testing show promise in reducing risk behaviors. *International Family Planning Perspectives, 27*(1), 49–50.

Howard, D. E., Griffin, M., Boekeloo, B., Lake, K., & Bellows, D. (2007). Staying safe while consuming alcohol: A qualitative study of the protective strategies and informational needs of college freshmen. *Journal of American College Health, 56*(3), 247–254.

Humphreys, K., & Klaw, E. (2001). Can targeting non-dependent problem drinkers and providing internet-based services expand access to assistance for alcohol problems? A study of the Moderation Management self-help/mutual aid organization. *Journal of Studies on Alcohol, 62*, 528–532.

Inciardi, J.A., & Harrison, L.D. (2000). *Harm reduction: National and international perspectives*. California: Thousand Oaks Press.

Kaner, E. F., Beyer, F., Dickinson, H. O., Pienaar, E., Campbell, F., Schlesinger, C., Heather, N., Saunders, J., & Burnand, B. (2007). Effectiveness of brief alcohol interventions in primary care populations. *Cochrane Database of Systematic Reviews, 18*(2), CD004148.

Ksobiech, K. (2004a). Assessing and improving needle exchange programs: Gaps and problems in the literature. *Harm Reduction Journal, 1*(4). Available at http://www.harmreductionjournal.com/content/pdf/1477–7517-1–4.pdf.

Ksobiech, K. (2004b). Return rates for needle exchange programs: A common criticism answered. *Harm Reduction Journal, 1*(2). Available at http://www.harmreductionjournal.com/content/pdf/1477–7517-1–2.pdf.

Larimer, M. E., Marlatt, G. A., Baer, J. S., Quigley, L. A., Blume, A. W., & Hawkins, E. H. (1998). Harm reduction for alcohol problems: Expanding access to and acceptability of prevention treatment services. In G. A. Marlatt (Ed.), *Harm Reduction: Pragmatic approaches to managing high-risk behaviors* (pp. 69–121). New York: Guilford Press.

Lindlof, T. R., & Taylor, B. C. (2002). *Qualitative communication research methods* (2nd Ed.). Thousand Oaks, CA: Sage Publications.

Littlejohn, S. W., & Foss, K. A. (2005). *Theories of human communication.* Belmont, CA: Thomson Wadsworth.

Loew, T., & Maylath, N. (2014). Purdue University student wellness office alcohol harm reduction initiatives. Personal communication. April 2013.

Logan, D. E., & Marlatt, G. A. (2010). Harm reduction therapy: A practice-friendly review of research. *Journal of Clinical Psychology, 66*(2), 201–214.

MacCoun, R. J. (1998). Toward a psychology of harm reduction. *American Psychologist, 53,* 1199–1208.

Marlatt, G. A. (1998). *Harm reduction: Pragmatic strategies for managing high-risk behaviors.* New York: The Guilford Press.

Marlatt, G. A. (1983). The controlled drinking controversy: A commentary. *American Psychologist, 38,* 1097–1110.

Marlatt, G. A., Larimer, M. E., & Witkiewitz, K. A. (2011). *Harm Reduction: Pragmatism strategies for managing high-risk behaviors* (2nd Eds.). New York: The Guilford Press.

Marlatt, G. A., & Witkiewitz, K. (2002). Harm reduction approaches to alcohol use: Health promotion, prevention, and treatment. *Addictive Behaviors, 27*, 867–886.

Martens, M. P., Ferrier, A. G., & Cimini, M. D. (2007). Do protective behavioral strategies mediate the relationship between drinking motives and alcohol use in college students? *Journal of Studies on Alcohol and Drugs, 68,* 106–114.

Mastroleo, I., Geisner, M., Grossbard, J. R., Tollison, S. J., Lostutter, T. W., Montoya, H. (2009). A randomized clinical trial evaluating a combined alcohol intervention for high-risk college students. *Journal of Studies on Alcohol and Drugs*, *70,* 555–567.

Mattson, M. (2000). Empowerment through agency-promoting dialogue: An explicit application of harm reduction theory to reframe HIV test counseling. *Journal of Health Communication, 5,* 333–347.

Mattson, M. (1999). Toward a reconcepualization of communication cues to action in the Health Belief Model: HIV testing counseling. *Communication Monographs, 66*, 240–263.

Mattson, M., & Basnyat, I. (2008). Infusing HIV test counseling practice with harm reduction theory: An integrated model for voluntary counseling and testing.

In T. Edgar, S. Noar, & V. Freimuth (Eds.). *Communication perspectives for HIV/AIDS in the 21st century* (pp. 137–167). New York: Lawrence Erlbaum Associates.

McBride, N., Farringdon, F., & Kennedy, C. (2007). Research to practice - formal dissemination of the School Health Harm Reduction Project (SHAHRP) in Australia. *Drug and Alcohol Review, 26*(6), 665–672.

McBride, N. T., Midford, R., Farringdon, F., & Phillips, M. (2000). Early results from a school alcohol harm minimization study: The School Health and Alcohol Harm Reduction Project. *Addiction, 95*(7), 1021–1042.

McKay, M. T., McBride, N. T., Sumnall, H. R., & Cole, J. C. (2012). Reducing the harm from adolescent alcohol consumption: Results from an adapted version of SHAHRP in Northern Ireland. *Journal of Substance Use, 17*(2), 98–121.

McLeroy, K. R., Bibeau, D., Steckler, A., & Glance, K. (1988). An ecological perspective on health promotion programs. *Health Education Quarterly, 15*(4), 351–377.

National Drug Research Institute (2013). *School Health and Alcohol Harm Reduction Project: An evidence-based program to reduce alcohol related harm in young people.* Retrieved from http://ndri.curtin.edu.au/research/shahrp/about/index.cfm on April 5, 2014.

National Institute on Alcohol Abuse and Alcoholism (NIAAA, 2002). *A call to action: Changing the culture of drinking at US colleges.* National Institutes of Health. US Department of Health and Human Services. Available at http://www.collegedrinkingprevention.gov/media/taskforcereport.pdf.

National Registry of Evidence-based Programs and Practices (2013). *Intervention summary for Brief Alcohol Screening and Intervention for College Students (BASICS).* Retrieved from http://www.nrepp.samhsa.gov/ViewIntervention.aspx?id=124 on April 5, 2014.

Neighbors, C., Lee, C. M., Lewis, M. A., Fossos, N., & Walter, T. (2009). Internet-based personalized feedback to reduce 21st birthday drinking: A randomized controlled trial of an event-specific prevention intervention. *Journal of Consulting and Clinical Psychology, 77*(1), 51–63.

Newcombe, R. (1992). The reduction of drug-related harm: A conceptual framework for theory, practice, and research. In P. O'Hare, R. Newcombe, A. Matthews, E.C. Buning, & E. Drucker (Eds.), *The reduction of drug-related harm* (pp. 1–15). New York, NY: Routledge.

Newcombe, R. (1987). High time for harm reduction. *Druglink, 2*(1), 10–11.

Nichter, M., Nichter, M., Adrian, S., Goldade, K., Tesler, L., Muramoto, M. (2008). Smoking and harm-reduction efforts among postpartum women. *Qualitative Health Research, 18*(9), 1184–1194.

Nowinski, J., Baker, S., & Carroll, K. (1999). Twelve step facilitation therapy manual: A clinical research guide for therapists treating individuals with alcohol abuse and dependence. Project MATCH monograph vol. 1. Rockville, Maryland: National Institute on Alcohol Abuse and Alcoholism. Available at http://pubs.niaaa.nih.gov/publications/ProjectMatch/match01.pdf.

Office of Juvenile Justice and Delinquency Prevention (2014). OJJDP Model Programs Guide. Alcohol Misuse Prevention Study (AMPS). Retrieved from https://www.crimesolutions.gov/ProgramDetails.aspx?ID=304 on April 5, 2014.

O'Hare, P.A., (1992). A note on the concept of drug-related harm. In P. O'Hare, R. Newcombe, A. Matthews, E.C. Brunig, & E. Drucker (Eds.), *The reduction of drug-related harm.* New Fetter Lane, London: Routledge.

Pattison, E. M., Sobell, M. B., & Sobell, L. C. (1977). *Emerging concepts of alcohol dependence.* New York: Springer.

Peele, S. (1989). *Diseasing of America: Addiction treatment out of control.* Lexington, MA: Lexington Books.

Peele, S. (1998). Ten radical things NIAAA research shows about alcoholism. *The Addictions Newsletter,* 5–6, 17–19.

Reid, R. J. (2002). Harm reduction and injection drug use: Pragmatic lessons from a public health model. *Health and Social Work, 27*(3), 223–226.

Rhodes, T. (2002). The "risk environment": A framework for understanding and reducing drug-related harm. *International Journal of Drug Policy, 13,* 85–94.

Rhodes, T., & Hedrich, D. (2010). Harm reduction and the mainstream. In T. Rhodes & D. Hedrich (10th Ed.), *European Monitoring Centre for Drugs and Drug Addiction Monographs: Harm reduction evidence, impacts, and challenges* (pp. 19–33). Luxembourg: Publications Office of the European Union.

Ritter, A., & Cameron, J. (2006). A review of the efficacy and effectiveness of harm reduction strategies for alcohol, tobacco and illicit drugs. *Drug and Alcohol Review, 25,* 611–624.

Robson, G., & Marlatt, G. A. (2006). Harm reduction and alcohol policy. *International Journal of Drug Policy, 17,* 255–257.

Roche, A., Evans, K., & Staton, W. (2001). Harm reduction: Road less traveled to the Holy Grail. *Addiction, 92,* 1207–1212.

Rogers, S. J., & Ruefli, T. (2004). Does harm reduction programming make a difference in the lives of highly marginalized, at-risk drug users? *Harm Reduction Journal, 1*: 7. Available at http://www.harmreductionjournal.com/content/pdf/1477-7517-1-7.pdf.

Rosenberg, H. (1993). Prediction of controlled drinking by alcoholics and problem drinkers. *Psychological Bulletin, 113,* 129–139.

Rosenberg, H., Bonar, E. E., Hoffmann, E., Kryszak, E., Young, K. M., Kraus, S. W., Ashrafioun, L., Bannon, E. E., & Pavlick, M. (2011). Assessing University students' self-efficacy to employ alcohol-related harm reduction strategies. *Journal of American College Health, 59*(8), 736–742.

Rosenburg, J. (2003). Not all Ohio physicians offer HIV testing during standard prenatal care. *Perspectives on Sexual and Reproductive Health, 35*(4), 194–195.

Ruefli, T., & Rogers, S. J. (2004). How do drug users define their progress in harm reduction interventions? Qualitative research to develop user-generated outcomes. *Harm Reduction Journal, 1*: 8. Available at http://www.harmreductionjournal.com/content/pdf/1477–7517-1–8.pdf.

Saladin, M. E., & Santa Ana, E. J. (2004). Controlled drinking: More than just a controversy. *Current Opinion Psychiatry, 17,* 175–187.

Sarang, A., Stuikyte, R., & Bykov, R. (2007). Implementation of harm reduction in Central and Eastern Europe and Central Asia. *International Journal of Drug Policy, 18,* 129–135.

Shepard, B. (2007). Harm reduction outreach services and engagement of chemically dependent homeless people living with HIV/AIDS: An analysis of service utilization data to evaluation program theory. *Einstein Journal of Biology and Medicine, 23,* 26–32.

Shope, J. T., Dielman, T. E., Butchart, A. T., Campanelli, P. C., & Kloska, D. D. (1992). An elementary school-based alcohol misuse prevention program: A follow-up evaluation. *Journal of Studies on Alcohol, 53*(2),106–21.

Shope, J. T., Copeland, L. A., & Dielman, T. E. (1994). Measurement of alcohol use and misuse in a cohort of students followed from grade 6 through grade 12. *Alcoholism: Clinical And Experimental Research, 18*(3), 726–33.

Shope, J. T., Elliott, M. R., Raghunathan, T. E., & Waller, P. F. (2001). Long-term follow-up of a high school misuse prevention program's effect on students' subsequent driving. *Alcoholism: Clinical and Experimental Research, 25,* 403–410.

Siegel, M. B., Tanwar, K. L., & Wood, K. S. (2011). Electronic cigarettes as a smoking cessation tool: Results from an online survey. *American Journal of Preventative Medicine, 40,* 472–475.

Sobell, M. B., & Sobell, L. C. (1995). Controlled drinking after 25 years: How important was the great debate? *Addiction, 90,* 1149–1153.

Sobell, M. B., & Sobell, L. C. (2000). Stepped care as a heuristic approach to the treatment of alcohol problems. *Journal of Consulting and Clinical Psychology, 68,* 573–579.

Sobell, M. B., & Sobell, L. C. (2005). Obstacles to adoption of low risk drinking goals in the treatment of alcohol problems in the United States: A commentary. *Addiction Research and Theory, 14*(1), 19–24.

Springer, E. (1991). Effective AIDS prevention with active drug users: The harm reduction model. *Journal of Chemical Dependency Treatment, 4*(2), 141–157.

Stafford, N. (2007). Using words: The harm reduction conception of drug use and drug users. *International Journal of Drug Policy, 18,* 88–91.

Stevenson, R. (1994). Harm reduction, rational addiction, and the optimal prescribing of illegal drugs. *Contemporary Economic Policy, 12,* 101–108.

Stimson, G. V. (2007). Harm reduction-coming of age: A local movement with global impact. *International Journal of Drug Policy, 18,* 67–69.

Stimson, G. V., & O'Hare, P. (2010). Harm reduction: Moving through the third decade. *International Journal of Drug Policy, 21,* 91–93.

Stratton, K., Shetty, P., Wallace, R., & Bondurant, S. (2001). Clearing the smoke: Assessing the science base for tobacco harm reduction – an executive summary. *Tobacco Control, 10,* 189–195.

Subata, E., & Stuikyte, R. (2006). Substitution drug treatment in Central and Eastern Europe and Central Asia: Regulation and practices.

Swedish Match (2013, October 14). New look for General snus is unveiled in US. Retrieved March 23, 2014 from http://www.swedishmatch.com/en/Media/Pressreleases/Press-releases/Other/New-look-for-General-snus-is-unveiled-in-the-US/.

Transportation Research Board, National Research Council, Committee for Guidance on Setting and Enforcing Speed Limits (1998). Managing Speed: Review of Current Practice for Setting and Enforcing Speed Limits. Special Report #254.

Washington, D.C.: National Academies Press. Available at http://onlinepubs.trb.org/onlinepubs/sr/sr254.pdf.

Tucker, J. A., Donovan, D. M., & Marlatt, G. A. (1999). *Changing addictive behavior: Bridging clinical and public health strategies*. New York: The Guilford Press.

U.S. Food and Drug Administration (2009). *Electronic cigarettes*. Retrieved from http://www.fda.gov/newsevents/publichealthfocus/ucm172906.htm on April 5, 2014.

Van Den Berg, C., Smit, C., Brussel, G. V., Coutinho, R., & Prins, M. (2007). Full participation in harm reduction programmes is associated with decreased risk for human immunodeficiency virus and hepatitis C virus: Evidence from the Amsterdam Cohort Studies among drug users. *Addiction, 102*(9), 1454–1462.

Wallis, S. E. (2010). Toward a science of metatheory. *Integral Review, 6*(6), 73–120.

Wechsler, H., Molnar, B. E., Davenport, A. E., & Baer, J. S. (2000). College alcohol use: A full or empty glass? *American Journal of College Health, 47,* 247–252.

Whiteside, U., Cronce, J. M., Pedersen, E. R., & Larimer, M. E. (2010). Brief motivational feedback for college students and adolescents: A harm reduction approach. *Journal of Clinical Psychology, 66,* 150–163.

Witkiewitz, K., & Marlatt, G. A. (2006). Overview of harm reduction treatment for alcohol problems. *International Journal of Drug Policy, 17,* 185–294.

Wodak, A., & McLeod, L., (2008). The role of harm reduction in controlling HIV among injecting drug users. *AIDS, 22*(Suppl 2), S81–92.

Chapter 3

Improving the Theoretical Utility of Harm Reduction

A Motorcycle Safety Exemplar

In the previous chapter, we introduced various health and safety issues for which HRT has been applied in practice. In addition, we illustrated how HRT has been applied concurrently with other health behavior theories, which sparked our interest in further integrating HRT as a metatheory in our own research and practice. We proposed HRT as a metatheory in health and safety research as a viable solution to the controversial, applicable, and evaluative dilemmas that have been encountered to date. Then, we introduced our rationale for choosing motorcycle safety as an illustrative example throughout the book. The purpose of this chapter is to provide you with more detail of the process we undertook to conceptualize HRT as an integrative metatheory and how each tenet of HRT can guide a component of the Reconceptualized Health Belief Model (RHBM; Mattson, 1999). Hopefully detailing this research approach will persuade you that metatheorizing is feasible and applicable for other health and safety research projects. The following objectives guide this chapter:

- Provide an overview of theory and metatheory
- Review and compare individual-level health behavior theories and justify why one of these theories has more potential to benefit from harm reduction metatheoretical guidance
- Discuss the integration of harm reduction tenets and components from the Reconceptualized Health Belief Model
- Use examples from motorcycle safety to further support and clarify how one tenet of harm reduction can strengthen the application of a theoretical component

We begin by defining theory and metatheory, respective to health and safety research.

PROPOSING HARM REDUCTION THEORY AS A METATHEORY

Currently, harm reduction is discussed as a theory in public health promotion and behavioral literature. According to Littlejohn and Foss (2005) a *theory* is, "in its broadest sense any organized set of concepts, explanations, and principles of some aspect of human experience" (p. 17). A theory assists in examining, organizing, and representing facts (Littlejohn & Foss, 2005) whereas a metatheory is an examination and analysis of theories (Weinstein & Weinstein, 1992). Wallis (2010) determined in his review that a *metatheory* is the study of theory including, "the development of an overarching combination of theory, as well as the development and application of themes for analysis that reveal underlying assumptions about theory and theorizing" (p. 78). Further, Hjorland (1998) offered the following: "Metatheoretical assumptions are thus broader and less specific than theories. They are more or less conscious or unconscious assumptions behind theoretical, empirical, and practical work" (p. 607).

Wallis (2010) argued that the complex local and global issues society faces cannot be met with existing social science theories. Rather than continually trying to think of new theories, Wallis probed researchers to consider other ways to advance research and address important societal problems. We argue that enhancing our social scientific metatheoretical base may help to increase the theoretical complexity and rigor available to current health and safety research.

In our current project we used harm reduction metatheory to examine the underlying assumptions and components of another theory in order to strengthen "theoretical consciousness" (Poonamallee, 2010, p. 190; Ritzer, 1988) while providing an alternate framework for qualitative research methodology (Abrams & Hogg, 2004). There are several approaches to metatheorizing. Whatever approach you decide on, the metatheorizing process is likely to be rigorous and time consuming. Detailing our entire metatheorizing process is beyond the scope of this book since we are focused on how to enhance the utility of harm reduction, specifically in qualitative research and practice. This book details how you can apply harm reduction as a metatheory in your own research. However, for a complete discussion of the eight phases used to conceptualize and develop HRT as a metatheory, refer to Haas (2012). The next section introduces individual-level health behavior theories that we initially considered as possibilities to empirically validate HRT as a metatheory in health and safety research and practice.

A REVIEW OF APPLICABLE HEALTH BEHAVIOR THEORIES

Although HRT has been practiced at individual, community, and societal levels, this book emphasizes the application of harm reduction metatheory on an individual level. In other words, we are focusing on behavior changes that are within the control of the individual, instead of behavior change within a community or society. Rimer (2008) suggested that, to effectively and accurately measure the impact of interventions, it is necessary to first understand the role of the individual in changing health behavior. In addition, it is more practical for metatheorizing to begin at the individual level of analysis because addressing micro problems at the individual level may allow health campaign practitioners to glean more effective strategies for how to address macro problems at the societal level (MacCoun, 2009; Hall, 2007). Finally, focusing on the individual at a micro level may be more amenable to initially advancing HRT in health and safety research and practice.

However, the results of the motorcycle safety research project discussed throughout this book demonstrate that, after empirically studying HRT as a metatheoretical framework for individual-level analysis, metatheorizing can be designed and expanded to the community and societal levels, to address health and safety problems. Therefore, we recognize and discuss some ways that the external environment can influence and facilitate healthier behaviors of the individual, relative to motorcycle safety.

Health behavior theories that consider behavior at the individual level include the Health Belief Model (HBM), the Theory of Reasoned Action/Planned Behavior (TRA/TPB), and the Transtheoretical Model and Stages of Change (TTM/SCM) (Glanz, Rimer, & Viswanath, 2008). Although metatheories can guide an integration of several theories, simultaneously addressing different concepts of each theory (Wallis, 2010), the motorcycle safety research project illustrated throughout this book focuses on one theory to analyze and evaluate the metatheoretical possibilities of HRT. Therefore, our initial analysis to determine and use an applicable theory utilizes a deconstructive approach (Dervin, 1999) in which one theory is examined for its components. To provide justification for our choice of one particular theory, we discuss four theories and conclude with an explanation of why the RHBM is better suited to initially complement harm reduction metatheory in the current research project. Although the outcome of our analysis identified the RHBM for this study, a subsequent analysis with a different health issue may reveal a different result.

The Health Belief Model and the Reconceptualized HBM

The *Health Belief Model* (HBM) was developed in the 1950s to explain the adoption of or failure to practice health-related behaviors, such as screening tests or vaccinations (Becker, 1974; Rosenstock, 1974). Since then, the HBM has been used to understand why individuals engage in a variety of health-related behaviors, including why they accept preventive health services or why they do or do not adhere to health recommendations and treatment (Champion & Skinner, 2008; Janz & Becker, 1984). The HBM assumes that individuals are rational decision makers and can make their own choices (Wundersitz, Hutchinson, & Woolley, 2010).

This assumption is consistent with HRT, which also assumes that individuals can and should make their own decisions (Reid, 2002). Initially the HBM consisted of the following components: perceived susceptibility to the health problem, perceived severity of the health problem, perceived benefits, and perceived barriers to practicing the recommended health behavior (Becker, 1974; Rosenstock, 1974).

In addition to the perceived benefits and perceived barriers in the HBM, perceived self-efficacy (Bandura, 1982) is a crucial component of the HBM (Mattson, 1999). According to Mattson (1999), "If individuals are confident in their capability to perform healthy behaviors, they are more likely than those who are not to fulfill that self-perception" (p. 243). Previous harm reduction studies support this point, showing that individual compliance when reducing negative behaviors is likely to be higher among those with greater self-efficacy (Carey et al., 2007; Larimer & Cronce, 2007). Because of its association with increased compliance, self-efficacy often is incorporated into concepts of MI and goal setting, both discussed in the first chapter as aspects of HRT. The components of the RHBM are expanded on in a later section in order to more clearly explain potential connections to the tenets of HRT.

Even though the HBM is the most commonly used theory in health campaign research (Rimer, 2008), it is necessary to consider a common criticism of the HBM. During its first two decades, some research criticized the HBM because in order to initiate behavior change people often need some sort of stimulus or trigger to begin thinking about changing their behaviors (Janz & Becker, 1984). This stimulus is termed a cue to action. An individual who is primed for action may not engage in the targeted behavior(s) without an adequate and persuasive cue to stimulate that behavior (Rosenstock, 1974). The cue to action may be internal (e.g., knowing someone who was in an accident while driving a motorcycle) or external (e.g., a health campaign message or media coverage of a motorcycle accident). Unfortunately, Janz and Becker (1984) noted, "few HBM studies have attempted to assess the contribution of cues to predicting health actions" (p. 3). Currently, cues to action are considered vital to the predictive power of the HBM and to behavior change.

The *Reconceptualized Health Belief Model* (RHBM; Figure 3.1; Mattson, 1999) originated from the HBM. Based on research indicating the critical role cues to action play in the HBM, Mattson (1999) proposed the Reconceptualized HBM (RHBM), which centralized cues to action within the model. The RHBM differs from the HBM in that the RHBM "recognizes that individual beliefs, perceptions, and behaviors about health and illness are socially constructed and contingent upon interaction with others" (Mattson, 1999, p. 258). Communication, whether it is through media outlets, health campaigns, counseling, or interpersonal dialogue, is the cue that prompts individuals to assess their risk(s) and decide whether or not to act. By recognizing that individuals who are engaging in risky health behaviors often need a cue to action to stimulate decision-making behaviors (Witte, Stokols, Ituarte, & Schneider, 1993), the RHBM is more ideally suited to be guided by the proposed metatheory of HRT. The other components of the HBM are the same in the RHBM (Figure 3.1).

Although previously the RHBM has not been used in tandem with HRT, one study combined the HBM with harm reduction concepts. According to the researchers (Eshrati et al., 2008), within a harm reduction context, the HBM "provides a systematic framework for examining the reasoning behind an individual's choice to decrease, maintain, or increase their high-risk

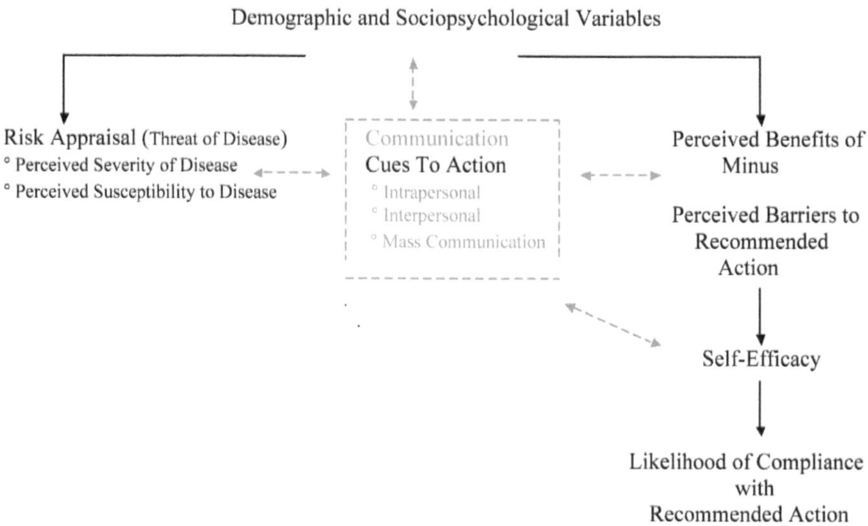

Figure 3.1 Reconceptualized Health Belief Model. *Source*: Adapted from Mattson, 1999.

behavior(s)" (p. 2). Their intervention was designed to increase harm reduction programming in order to reduce prisoners' risks of contracting and spreading HIV/AIDS. The study found that educational harm reduction initiatives that promote strategies designed to reduce the risk of HIV transmission may decrease prisoners' high-risk behaviors.

Eshrati et al. (2008) discovered that perceived benefits was the only component of the HBM that was significantly associated with the reduction of high-risk behaviors. This finding makes sense because according to the HBM benefits must exceed barriers for preventive behavior to occur (Brown, DiClemente, & Reynolds, 1991). In particular, prisoners noticed a decrease in their high-risk behaviors when they believed the strategies presented to them would effectively reduce their risk or seriousness of the negative impact. This study showed that even if projects aim to reduce key barriers, health messages (i.e., cues to action) that relay the benefits of changing a behavior are crucial to the effectiveness of HRT interventions.

In addition, a plethora of research exists that utilizes the HBM to predict traffic safety behaviors related to bicycle helmet use and risky driving practices (Elliot, 2010; Germeni et al., 2010; Jacques, 1994; Lajunen & Rasanen, 2004; Ross, Ross, Rahman, & Cataldo, 2010; Von, Ebert, Ngamvitroj, Park, & Kang, 2004; Yagil, 2000). For example, Jacques (1994) demonstrated that bicyclists' helmet use depended mostly on bicyclists' motivation to use helmets rather than environmental, exposure, or cost-related factors. Further, Arnold and Quine (1994) found that the components of the HBM explain 53% of variance in bicycle helmet use. In addition, a study by Lajunen and Rasanen (2004) found that perceived barriers and cues to action were the strongest predictors of helmet use, whereas the other components of the HBM predicted less of the variance in behaviors. Because cues to action was the strongest predictor of helmet use among bicyclists, we felt this was another reason why the RHBM may be a more useful framework for predicting and promoting motorcyclists' safety behaviors on the road, including why motorcyclists are unwilling to use a helmet, even if they own a helmet.

However, some studies also indicated a gap in the health messages disseminated through the HBM, suggesting that improvements are needed in future research. For example, a study that targeted farm worker safety found that farmers considered farm equipment injuries to be severe and thought they were capable of participating in safer health behaviors (Peterson et al., 1994). However, the farmers did not find resonance in the tailored safety messages, and as a result, their perceived susceptibility to accidents remained the same or decreased (Peterson et al., 1994). The motorcycle safety exemplar that we present in this book demonstrates how integrating HRT tenets into health and safety research can aid the development of accurate, targeted messages so the relevant components of the RHBM can be heightened within the target audience.

Theory of Reasoned Action/Theory of Planned Behavior

The *Theory of Reasoned Action/Planned Behavior* (TRA/TPB) is used in a variety of contexts when predicting volitional (i.e., at-will) behaviors, with subjective norms or attitude playing the greater role, depending on the context and targeted behavior (Ajzen, 2001). *Normative influence*, also known as *subjective norms*, is an individual's beliefs about whether influential others think they should perform the target behavior (Fishbein & Ajzen, 1975). Normative influence is composed of *normative beliefs*, or what others expect you to do, and *motivation to comply*, or how important it is to follow through on what is expected (Ajzen & Fishbein, 1980).

The concept of normative influence does not neatly fit with the tenets of HRT because the central tenets of HRT do not focus on what other people want or think individuals should do. Instead, HRT aims to induce healthy behavior change through empowering individuals to change on their own, despite what others may think. Even when harm reduction counseling occurs, clients are encouraged to make their own decisions based on what they think is possible, not what the counselor or others think is possible (Logan & Marlatt, 2010).

Another important component of TRA/TPB is attitude. *Attitude* toward a specific health behavior is the degree to which adopting the behavior is positively or negatively valued by the individual (Fishbein & Ajzen, 1975). Attitudes are affected by the strength of beliefs, the expected outcome, and belief evaluation, the values, judgments, and worth of the anticipated outcome if the behavior is performed (Fishbein & Ajzen, 1975). The concept of attitude is more relevant to HRT than normative beliefs. However, TRA/TPB does not tease out the varying aspects of attitude. Instead, the RHBM separates cognitive components related to attitude (e.g., perceived susceptibility and perceived barriers). Therefore, simply including the concept of attitude toward a behavior, as in TRA/TPB, may not fully tap into predicting and facilitating steps toward behavior change. Wundersitz et al. (2010) emphasized the same point when they stated, "The model (HBM) is broader than the TPB because it also includes different emotional responses: perceived susceptibility and perceived seriousness of the consequence" (p. 13).

Later, Ajzen and colleagues added perceived behavioral control to the TRA in order to account for factors that were outside individuals' control and may affect behaviors (Ajzen, 1991; Ajzen & Driver, 1991; Ajzen & Madden, 1986). *Perceived behavioral control* is determined by control beliefs concerning the availability of facilitators or barriers to behavioral performance, balanced with an individual's perceived power (i.e., self-efficacy) to control their own behavior (Ajzen, 1991). With the addition of perceived behavioral control, the TPB was conceived. Although TPB may account for more variability in behavior by addressing self-efficacy, which also is included in the tenets of HRT, it does not justify using this theory rather than the RHBM because of the complexity of the attitude component that the TPB does not as thoroughly address.

In addition, when considering a theory for our metatheoretical integration, we had to consider the health and safety issue of focus—motorcycle safety. Previous research on traffic safety utilized the TPB to predict motorcyclists' intentions to speed (Elliot, 2010) and skaters' and bicyclists' intention to wear safety gear (Deroche, Stephan, Castanier, Brewer, & LeScanff, 2009; Lajunen & Rasanen, 2004). Results indicate that the aspects of the TPB can predict variance in adhering to safety guidelines. Specifically, the most significant results were achieved when researchers added and accounted for additional factors, not originally included in the TPB, such as self-identity, social identity, and locus of control (Elliot, 2010).

In other motorcycle safety studies, researchers divided attitude into multiple components, in order to more accurately measure this research variable (Elliot, 2010). In addition, research that empirically tested both the TRA/TPB and the HBM discovered that the TRA predicted two behavioral factors of motorcyclists while the HBM predicted five behavioral factors of motorcyclists (Rutter & Quine, 1994; Rutter, Quine, & Chesham, 1995). Therefore, the TRA/TPB was not fully supported by data with regard to predicting motorcycle and other traffic safety behaviors (Deroche et al., 2009) in part because researchers have not sufficiently pinpointed the concept of attitude (Avery & MacKinnon, 1996; Lajunen & Rasanen, 2004).

Further, some research using the TPB found that significant results were dependent on age of the participants (Ajzen, 1991). This finding was consistent in several studies focusing on traffic safety behaviors (Holland & Hill, 2007; Lajunen & Rasanen, 2004; O'Callaghan & Nausbaum, 2006) in which subjective norm and attitude continually varied when studies focused on teenagers and/or adults.

For the reasons presented in this section, we determined that using the TRA/TPB is not the most applicable fit for initially considering HRT as a metatheory to guide health behavior theory. In the next section, the Transtheoretical Model/Stages of Change is considered as another possible theory for inclusion in an integrative metatheory with HRT.

Transtheoretical Model/Stages of Change Model

The *Transtheoretical Model/Stages of Change Model* (TTM/SCM) emerged from theories of psychotherapy and behavior change. The TTM/SCM incorporates individuals' stages of change, which are both behavioral and cognitive, with processes of change across health issues (Prochaska, Redding, & Evers, 2008). This five-stage process provides a framework to help determine someone's readiness to change behavior. By identifying where an individual is at in this behavior change cycle, health and safety interventions can be tailored to the individual's "readiness" to progress toward a healthier lifestyle. These stages are as follows (Prochaska & DiClemente, 1992, 1986, 1984):

1. *Precontemplation.* Individuals do not perceive a problem in their behavior and not considering a change in behavior.
2. *Contemplation.* Individuals begin to consider that there is a problem with their behavior and they begin thinking about the pros, cons, benefits, and barriers to behavior change. They may struggle with ambivalence.
3. *Preparation.* Individuals decide to make a change in behavior and begin preparing for this change in the near future.
4. *Action.* Individuals begin to modify their behaviors and continue to make changes over time. Examples include avoiding certain people or situations or substituting activities.
5. *Maintenance.* Individuals work to prevent relapse. Individuals who maintain a change for more than 6 months are considered to be in this stage. Seeking communicative support is important.

Previous research attempted to integrate HRT and the TTM/SCM with a focus on substance abuse or alcohol abuse (Connors et al., 2001; DiClemente & Prochaska, 1998; DiClemente, 1996; Procheska & DiClemente, 1983; Marlatt, 1998). A basic assumption when utilizing aspects of HRT and the TTM/SCM together is that, when trying to reduce a risky behavior, HRT approaches recognize that individuals' risky health behaviors vary along a continuum from abstinence to problematic use (Connors, Donovan, & DiClemente, 2001) much like the TTM/SCM recognizes that individuals' health behavior varies along a continuum from precontemplation to contemplation to preparation for change (Prochaska & DiClemente, 1992, 1986, 1984). However, previous research did not determine how HRT influenced the process of behavior change, despite recommendations to do so, indicating an integrative gap between these two theories (Connors et al., 2001).

Our review of research identified two barriers to the ongoing association between HRT and the TTM/SCM. First, research that integrates these two theories tends to focus on substance abuse or alcohol abuse. Other risky health behaviors also can and should be addressed from a harm reduction standpoint and to move beyond some of the initial barriers we identified to applying HRT more regularly into health and safety research. Perhaps shifting from the TTM/SCM to a different theory will facilitate an emphasis on addressing additional health behaviors. Second, although many studies integrated HRT and the TTM/SCM to reduce risky health behaviors, these studies did not extend HRT into health and safety research and practice. Consequently, we concluded that integrating a different theory with HRT was needed to create a wider space for HRT to influence health and safety research and practice and perhaps inform how HRT could more appropriately guide the TTM/SCM in future studies. Therefore, we felt that integrating HRT with the RHBM can more specifically illustrate how HRT facilitates behavior change within the context of motorcycle safety.

Based on our justification for the inclusion of the RHBM in this project, rather than other individual-level theories, and discussing how the components of the RHBM were used in previous traffic safety research, the next section supports the conceptualization process of harm reduction metatheory in reference to guiding the RHBM.

DESIGNING HARM REDUCTION AS A METATHEORY TO THE RECONCEPTUALIZED HEALTH BELIEF MODEL

So far we discussed reasons to integrate HRT and the RHBM in an effort to propose harm reduction as a metatheoretical perspective to the RHBM. Through this metatheoretical framework, HRT and the RHBM can be used in tandem to help inform, educate, and persuade individuals about the health risks of their behavior through a variety of communication cues including campaigns, counseling, and training. This framework, which we empirically studied with motorcyclists who engaged in risky driving behaviors, illustrated and proposed that individuals may make safer driving decisions by initiating the HRT tenets to respond to the components of the RHBM (i.e., cues to action, perceived susceptibility, perceived severity, perceived benefits, perceived barriers) (Mattson, 1999). The subsequent sections detail this metatheoretical framework. Each subsection highlights a tenet of HRT and integrates it with a component of the RHBM while using motorcycle safety as a case example. You will notice that we utilize a tenet of HRT to enhance how a specific component of the RHBM may reveal at-risk motorcyclists' attitudes and behaviors toward motorcycle safety. Figure 3.2 visually depicts the integration between harm reduction metatheory and the RHBM follows this explanation of the integrated metatheoretical tenets with the theoretical components.

Humanistic Value Guiding Cues to Action

Emphasis on cues to action in the RHBM offers an apt starting point to integrate the tenets of HRT into the process of health behavior change.

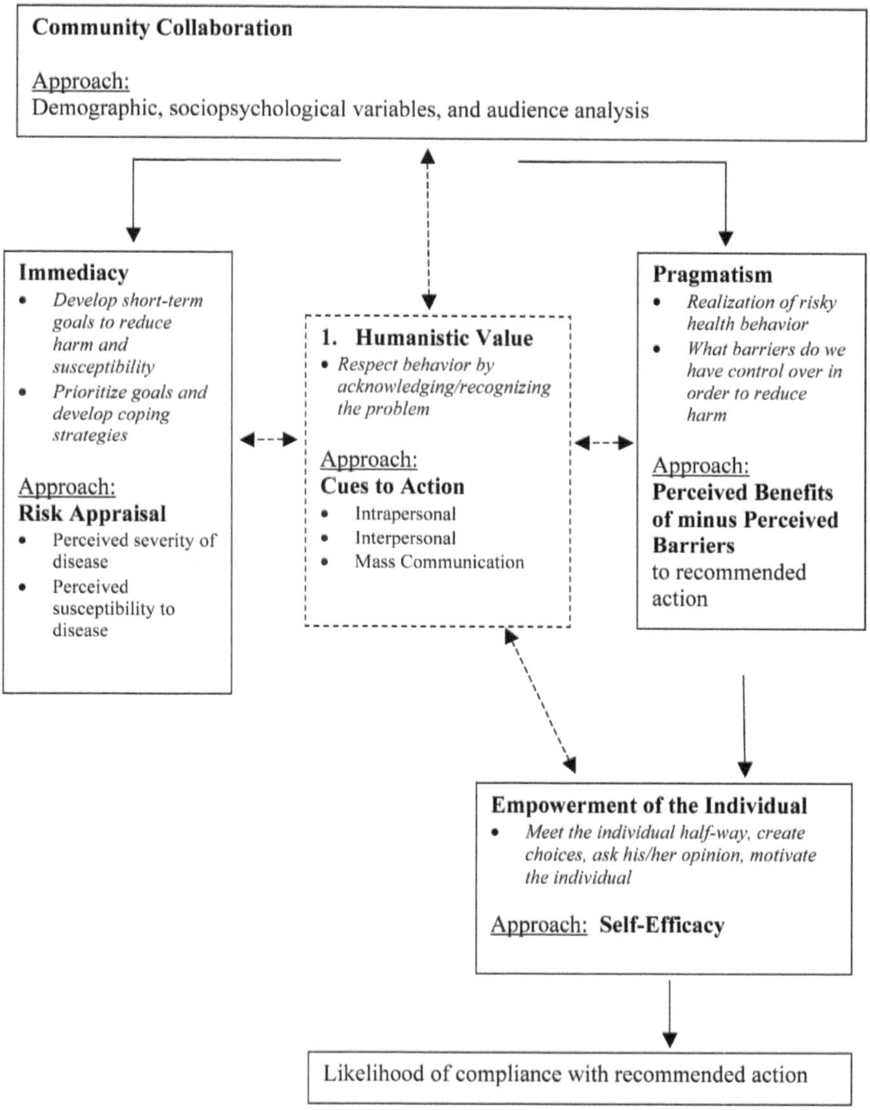

Figure 3.2 Proposed Integrative Model of Harm Reduction as Metatheory to the Reconceptualized Health Belief Model. *Source*: Haas, 2012.

Specifically, the humanistic concept of HRT ties in with the concept of cues to action in the RHBM. As humanistic value indicates, it must be recognized that a problem exists and the individual engaging in a risky health behavior should be treated with respect (Bigler, 2005; Brocato & Wagner, 2003; Riley & O'Hare, 2000). Communication, such as health messages on a billboard or a conversation with a friend or family member, can serve as a cue to action for an individual (Mattson, 1999). A cue to action, whether within a written message or within interpersonal dialogue, can initiate recognition of the problem and acknowledge that something needs to be done to address the problem. In the RHBM, cues to action play a dual role in problem recognition and behavior change initiation for an individual. Mattson (1999) framed cues to action as an important first step in the RHBM, which complements HRT since humanistic value is the first step to successful HRT programming (Marlatt, 1998). The cues to action emphasis in the RHBM also emphasizes meeting individuals where they are at while working toward making some progress rather than no progress, which is another tenet of HRT (Logan & Marlatt, 2010; Reid, 2002). Cues to action also are important because these cues trigger the other four components of the model (Aldoory & Bonzo, 2005).

Regarding motorcycle safety, humanistic value serves as recognition of the risky driving behaviors that motorcyclists may participate in on the road. Practicing humanistic value, HRT encourages individuals to respect the choices motorcyclists make and, instead of criticizing their behavior, strive to raise awareness about their safety behaviors and meet motorcyclists where they may be at in regards to safety behavior change.

Cues to action refer to any trigger motorcyclists receive to practice safety behaviors while riding a motorcycle. For example, cues to action such as owning a helmet and keeping a helmet with the keys to the motorcycle, viewing a persuasive message about safety on the road, or having a conversation with someone about motorcycle safety behaviors can be primed by a variety of communication mediums. At times, individuals may just need to be reminded that first, they have a helmet and second, they should wear it when riding a motorcycle (Lajunen & Rasanen, 2004). However, a news story about a local motorcycle accident also may serve as a cue to action for a motorcyclist. A newspaper story can be utilized by a campaign, family member, or friend to cue other motorcyclists. A motorcycle safety campaign can be considered a cue to action as well (Aldoory & Bonzo, 2005) because a communication campaign has an indirect effect on attitude change and behavior outcomes (Peterson et al., 1994; Witte et al., 1993).

To be consistent with the tenets of HRT, when initiating cues to action toward motorcyclists, it is important to do so with nonjudgmental strategies. After individuals receive a cue to action, they may contemplate the perceived benefits and barriers of modifying current behaviors. Continuing to be realistic about behaviors that are most applicable in terms of personal modification is important. However, a pragmatic approach is more likely to be effective after humanistic value (i.e., acceptance of the behavior) is recognized, supporting the need for humanistic value to be the preliminary guiding tenet for initiating health behavior change toward reducing harm. This aspect of realistic behavior change is discussed in the next section.

Pragmatism Guiding Perceived Benefits and Perceived Barriers

Within HRT, pragmatism is the notion of being realistic about individuals' behaviors and focusing on initial harm-reducing behaviors that are associated with their risks (Heather, 2006; Reid, 2002). In the RHBM, perceived benefits and barriers also predict whether or not behavior change occurs. *Perceived benefits* are "an individual's beliefs regarding the effectiveness of strategies designed to decrease vulnerability or reduce the threat of illness" (Brown et al., 1991, p. 51). *Perceived barriers* are "the assessment of potential negative consequences that may result from taking particular health actions" (Brown et al., 1991, p. 51). In order for an individual to adopt the preventive or less risky behavior, the benefits must exceed the barriers.

When individuals are encouraged to evaluate the pros and cons of changing current behaviors and replacing those behaviors with healthier or safer behaviors the concept of pragmatism is critical. Being practical about setting goals to address the barriers that individuals can overcome is necessary for individuals to overcome the obstacles in their own way. The comprehensive definition of HRT previously offered utilizes concepts from MI that may be useful when assessing the perceived barriers and benefits within a target audience. Acknowledging barriers to healthy behavior change and responding to those barriers by working with individuals to develop a hierarchy of realistic goals may help consistently maintain healthier behavior changes.

So, when assessing benefits and barriers, emphasizing pragmatism while trying to initiate behavior change should be helpful. With reference to our motorcycle safety exemplar, initiating a realistic attitude with motorcyclists about what they more easily can and cannot do at the present time may be beneficial and not as overwhelming for this target audience. Specifically, addressing what barriers motorcyclists have control over may be a useful starting point. For example, perceived barriers can be as simple as difficulty finding a comfortable helmet or finding a helmet that looks good when worn while riding. It may be that helping a particular motorcyclist find a comfortable, attractive helmet are the only barriers to overcome for this individual to start wearing a helmet while riding. Utilizing a realistic, noncritical approach to unveil barriers that motorcyclists perceive to practicing safer riding behaviors is a crucial step in knowing what types of communication are needed about motorcycle safety to address those barriers. Importantly, Lajunen and Rasanen's (2004) study showed that peers and parents play crucial roles in individuals' intentions to wear a bicycle helmet. In response, these researchers provided specific recommendations to create a campaign that aims at changing peers' and parents' attitudes toward safety behaviors. This same logic may be applicable to motorcycle helmets.

Behavioral evaluation also consists of perceived benefits, such as increasing safety behaviors on the road and preventing injuries if motorcyclists are in an accident (Lajunen & Rasanen, 2004). A difficulty with perceived benefits is that individuals often perceive more benefits from engaging in riskier driving behaviors than safer driving behaviors. For example, motorcyclists may speed or tailgate in order to get to their destination faster. In addition, high sensation seekers often engage in risky driving behaviors, such as speeding, to feel a thrill (Zuckerman, 1994). Communicating in a way that combats thrill-seeking behaviors among those who already think they are good drivers can be difficult. However, our proposed model uses pragmatism as a tool to inform conversations with at-risk motorcyclists to help this particular audience identify more benefits to driving within the speed limit. In addition, these pragmatic conversations may help necessitate discussions about perceived risk and severity of negative outcomes while riding a motorcycle. This acknowledgment also can probe the development of other short-term goals.

Immediacy and Goal Setting Guiding Perceived Susceptibility and Perceived Severity

As previously discussed, HRT focuses on the consequences of immediate goals by understanding current, risky health or safety behaviors and how those behaviors impact the individual or their community (Mattson & Basnyat, 2008). Once a cue to action is received, individuals usually assess the severity of a particular health threat and how susceptible they are to that health threat. Brown and colleagues (1991) defined *perceived severity* as the perception of the seriousness of the health threat and *perceived susceptibility* as an individual's perception of risk relative to that health threat. The RHBM predicts that as an individual's perception of risk regarding negative health outcome increases, the chances that the individual will comply with a prevention behavior also increases (Mattson, 1999).

Essentially then, the RHBM predicts that if cues to action are strong enough and individuals assess their perceived risk as being high, they are more likely to act and comply with the recommended health behavior. To be realistic for the individual and increase compliance, it is important to focus on short-term goals for target audience members. Through the concepts of immediacy and balancing goals, HRT suggests that individuals assess what they can do at any particular point in time to reduce short-term harm (Reid, 2002). By prioritizing goals individuals start on a path toward reducing risky health behaviors and decreasing their susceptibility to the health threat (Reid, 2002). HRT can positively influence the perceived risk aspect of the RHBM because it supports practitioners as they encourage individuals to develop steady, realistic, achievable goals toward healthier lifestyles.

When applied to the case of motorcycle safety, the RHBM emphasizes risk appraisal and behavioral evaluation (Rosenstock, 1974, 1966). *Risk appraisal* includes perceived susceptibility, such as the probability of getting in a motorcycle accident or being cited for unsafe driving (Fernandes, Hatfield, & Job, 2006). Perceived susceptibility is considered a determinant of risky driving behavior, however, it is difficult to engage motorcyclists' thinking about susceptibility because they often consider themselves invulnerable to injury and/or death. This is consistent with traffic safety research which found that most people possess illusory invulnerability, meaning they consider themselves less likely than the average person to be injured or killed in a crash (Chua & Job, 1999; Job, 1990). In addition, perceived severity was affected by individuals' tendency to think that they were better drivers than other people (Job, 1990). The results of this research were significant particularly among young male drivers and motorcyclists (Chua & Job, 1999; Job, 1990). However, strong cues to action may help motorcyclists begin reassessing their perceived susceptibility to crashes and techniques that they can use to realistically reduce the likelihood of a negative consequence.

If cues to action are targeted and persuasive enough, motorcyclists may perceive higher susceptibility to harm and undergo a change regarding personal risk assessment. To progress from a mindset that perceives higher susceptibility toward behavior change, incorporating the immediacy and goal setting tenets of HRT may be beneficial. Dialogue with motorcyclists about what is in their immediate control to lower their susceptibility to an accident can occur through one-on-one conversations, health campaign messages, news stories, or press releases following major motorcycle crashes. For example, if a motorcyclist owns a helmet but only wears it occasionally, it may be possible to influence that motorcyclist to wear the helmet at all times after a major motorcycle crash occurs that is covered in the news or is talked about among friends. At these times motorcyclists may be more susceptible to motorcycle safety and more likely to engage in health behaviors to reduce their immediate risk for serious injury, such as wearing a helmet and taking more time to assess their situational awareness at intersections. Encouraging motorcyclists to practice realistic, practical driving behaviors can serve as immediate coping responses. However, in order to change and maintain safer behaviors, the target audience must feel confident in both the effectiveness of the target behavior and their ability to perform the behavioral task.

Empowerment Guiding Self-efficacy

Empowerment is essential to initiating and maintaining behavior change. Creating choices for individuals is one of the ways to encourage individuals to follow through with suggested recommendations (Shepard, 2007). In addition, talking with individuals, helping to assess strengths and weaknesses, and in essence, making sense of the behaviors helps individuals believe in the possibility of change (Miller & Rollnick, 1991). This concept of believing in the possibility of change is referred to as self-efficacy (Bandura, 1977), another component of the RHBM. More specifically, *self-efficacy* is individuals' perceptions that they can successfully complete the safer behavior that is necessary to reduce harm associated with a targeted riskier behavior (Bandura, 1977; Brown et al., 1991). Forming communication relationships with individuals is imperative to increasing their self-efficacy. When self-efficacy is perceived to be low, and when risk perceptions increase, personal intentions may unconsciously decrease because individuals perceive they have no other alternatives and instead react defensively (Rogers, 1975, 1983; Rogers & Mewborn, 1976).

Because self-efficacy is an important component of the RHBM and health behavior change, it is essential that this aspect of the model also receive more guidance. The HRT tenet empowerment is a good check for how well health practitioners and other communicators help individuals build confidence and facilitate behavior change. Empowerment, which involves providing choices during communication with individuals to offer multiple options, developing response scripts for when temptation occurs, and pinpointing what interferes with practicing healthier or safer behaviors all can serve as tools to increase self-efficacy.

When applied to the case of motorcycle safety, the HRT tenet of empowerment can increase motorcyclists' perceptions that they can successfully practice the safety behaviors necessary to reduce potential harms associated with driving a motorcycle. Utilizing the notion of empowerment during conversations with motorcyclists may include providing them with choices toward safer driving behaviors. For example, if motorcyclists cannot afford to buy a full set of safe riding gear (i.e., boots, pants, jacket, gloves, eye protection, helmet), it may be appropriate to ask them if there are items they can afford immediately. Also, providing motorcyclists with talking points for situations when they sense peer pressure from other motorcyclists to not wear their safety gear may also be empowering for motorcyclists. Creating a plethora of choices and useful tools for motorcyclists may increase their self-efficacy to practice safer behaviors.

Now that most of the tenets of HRT were discussed relative to the components of the RHBM, the next section discusses community collaboration as a tenet of HRT that can facilitate aspects of and progression during multiple aspects of the RHBM such as communicating with individuals or disseminating a health campaign or intervention.

Community Collaboration Guiding Formative Research and Audience Analysis

The community aspect is necessary to consider and involve in all aspects of a health campaign or intervention. Cooperation with the community is essential in creating enabling environments for individuals whether through public policy or removing structural barriers that impede behavior change (Rhodes & Hendrich, 2010; WHO, 1986). As Blankenship and colleagues (2006) emphasized, health campaigns and interventions should seek to remove contextual or environmental barriers to facilitate harm reduction efforts. Rather, interventions should be designed to enable influential social and environmental conditions to help protect the individual from increased susceptibility to harm.

Community collaboration can facilitate all aspects of the RHBM in regards to motorcycle safety. For example, collaborating with media organizations such as local newspapers and community partners can help initiate more targeted cues to action among motorcyclists. If a journalist or editor agrees to run a story about motorcycle safety alongside accident coverage, this may serve as a targeted cue to action for an individual. Likewise, perceived susceptibility can be addressed in news articles or campaign messages by stating what motorcyclists can do immediately to reduce potential harm while driving a motorcycle. For instance, perceived barriers to safety by motorcyclists may be reduced by making the environment more user-friendly, such as fixing potholes in local roads and providing ample parking for motorcycles. These efforts likely require collaboration with community organizations and policymakers.

In addition to considering potential partnerships in the community, it also is important for health researchers and practitioners to continually assess the demographic and sociopsychological aspects of target audience members. With regard to motorcycle safety, previous research that collected demographic and psychological data showed that these variables accounted for 44% of the variance for law and rule-breaking behavior among motorcyclists (Elliot et al., 2003). Specifically, gender and age influenced motorcyclists' behavior on the road. More specifically, the influence of gender was mediated by the perceived benefits of feeling safe, which was found among male motorcyclists. Age was mediated both by perceived barriers to and perceived susceptibility to having an accident in addition to the perceived benefit of having more fun on the road (Elliot et al., 2003). This research shows that audience analysis within the community is crucial. Awareness of the audience is an ongoing task during any health or safety intervention. We argue that community collaboration can be incorporated into aspects of each component of the RHBM to acknowledge the external stimuli that facilitate safe and risky behaviors. Thus, the community collaboration aspect is an overarching concept that ties the other components of the integrative metatheory together.

The conceptual model in Figure 3.2 visually depicts the integrated model of HRT as a metatheory to the Reconceptualized Health Belief Model (Figure 3.2).

SUMMARY OF CONCEPTUALIZING HARM REDUCTION METATHEORY

This chapter detailed one way to conceptualize a metatheory for application in health and safety research. In this chapter, we focused on possible health-oriented theories and models for inclusion in the metatheory (Edwards, 2010). Multiple theories including the Theory of Reasoned Action/Theory of Planned Behavior, Transtheoretical Model/Stages of Change, the Health Belief Model, and the Reconceptualized Health Belief Model were involved in this review as possibilities for inclusion in HRT as a metatheory. This process was equivalent to Ritzer's (1992) *metatheorizing for understanding*, which emphasizes possessing a representative lens on the metatheory by analyzing relevant theories.

We succinctly collated the results of our review of theories and chose the components that best fit the proposed metatheoretical lens (Edwards, 2010). Engaging in this process initially revealed and then justified why the RHBM was well suited to be guided by HRT. Then we highlighted the integration of HRT and the RHBM as a model that could be used to empirically study harm reduction as a metatheory. We offered a visual model to illustrate how HRT can guide the RHBM during research projects. In the chapters to follow we continue to detail and support harm reduction as a metatheory by offering motorcycle safety Research Project in Practice Illustrations.

The next chapter begins detailing the methodology used to empirically examine harm reduction as a metatheory. Since there are few resources that explain how to pragmatically apply a metatheory in research, we spend time highlighting basics principles of qualitative research, noting the differences that are present when incorporating a metatheory.

REFERENCES

Abrams, D., & Hogg, M. A., (2004). Metatheory: Lessons from social identity research. *Personality and Social Psychology Review, 8*(2), 98–106.

Ajzen, I. (2001). Nature and operation of attitudes. *Annual Review of Psychology, 52*, 27–58.

Ajzen, I. (1991). The theory of planned behavior. *Organizational Behavior and Human Decision Processes, 50*, 179–211.

Ajzen, I., & Driver, B. L., (1991). Prediction of leisure participation from behavioral, normative, and control beliefs: An application of the theory of planned behavior. *Leisure Sciences, 13*, 185–204.

Ajzen, I., & Fishbein, M. (1980). *Understanding attitudes and predicting social behavior.* Englewood Cliffs, NJ: Prentice-Hall.

Ajzen, I., & Madden, T. J. (1986). Prediction of goal-directed behavior: Attitudes, intentions, and perceived behavioral control. *Journal of Experimental Social Psychology, 22*, 453–474.

Aldoory, L., & Bonzo, S. (2005). Using communication theory in injury prevention campaigns. *Injury Prevention, 11*, 260–263.

Arnold, L. N., & Quine, L. (1994). Predicting helmet use among schoolboy cyclists: An application of the Health Belief Model. In D. R. Rutter & L. Quine (Eds.), *Social psychology and health: European perspectives* (pp. 101–130). Aldershot: Avebury.

Avery, R., & MacKinnon, D. P. (1996). Injuries and use of protective equipment among college in-line skaters. *Accident Analysis and Prevention, 28*, 779–784.

Bandura, A. (1977). Self-efficacy: Toward a unifying theory of behavioral change. *Psychological Review, 84*, 191–215.

Bandura, A. (1982). Self-efficacy mechanism in human agency. *American Psychologist, 37*, 122–147.

Becker, M. H. (1974). The health belief model and personal health behavior. *Health Education Monographs, 2*, 324–473.

Bigler, M. O. (2005). Harm reduction as a practice and prevention model for social work. *The Journal of Baccalaureate Social Work, 10*(2), 69–86.

Blankenship, K. M., Friedman, S. R., Dworkin, S., & Mantell, J. E. (2006). Structural interventions: Concepts, challenges, and opportunities for research. *Journal of Urban Health, 83*, 59–72.

Brocato, J., & Wagner, E. F. (2003). Harm reduction: A social work practice model and social justice agenda. *Health & Social Work, 28*(2), 117–125.

Brown, L., DiClemente, R., & Reynolds, L. (1991). HIV prevention for adolescents: The utility of the Health Belief Model. *AIDS Education and Prevention, 3*, 50–59.

Carey, K. B., Scott-Sheldon, L. A. J., Carey, M. P., DeMartini, K. S. (2007). Individual-level interventions to reduce college student drinking: A meta-analytic review. *Addictive Behaviors, 32*, 2469–2494.

Champion, V. L., & Skinner, C. S. (2008). The health belief model. In K. Glanz, B. K. Rimer, & K. Viswanath. *Health behavior and health education: Theory, research, and practice* (4th Ed., pp. 45–65). San Francisco, CA: Jossey-Bass.

Chua, F. J., & Job, R. F. S. (1999). Event-specific versus unitary causal accounts of optimism bias. *Journal of Behavioural Medicine, 22*, 457–490.

Connors, G. J., Donovan, D. M., & DiClemente, C. C. (2001). *Selecting and planning interventions: Substance abuse treatment and the stages of change.* New York: The Guilford Press.

Deroche, T., Stephan, Y., Castanier, C., Brewer, B. W., & LeScanff, C. (2009). Social cognitive determinants of the intention to wear safety gear among adult in-line skaters. *Accident Analysis and Prevention, 41,* 1064–1069.

Dervin, B. (1999). On studying information seeking methodologically: The implications of connecting metatheory to method. *Information Processing & Management, 35*(6), 727–750.

DiClemente, R. J. (1996). Prevention and harm reduction for chemical dependency: A process perspective. *Clinical Psychology Review, 19,* 473–486.

DiClemente, R. J., & Prochaska, J. O. (1998). Toward a comprehensive, transtheoretical model of change: Stages of change and addictive behaviors. In W. R. Miller & N. Heather, *Treating addictive behaviors* (2nd Ed., pp. 3–24). New York: Plenum Press.

Edwards, M. G. (2010). *Organisational transformation for sustainability: An integral metatheory.* New York: Taylor & Francis Group.

Elliot, M. A. (2010). Predicting motorcyclists' intentions to speed: Effects of selected cognitions from the theory of planned behavior, self-identity, and social identity. *Accident Analysis and Prevention, 42,* 718–725.

Elliot, M. A., Baughan, C. J., Broughton, J., Chinn, B., Grayson, G. B., Khoules, J., Smith, C. R., & Simpson, H. (2003). *Motorcycle safety: A scoping study.* [Report No. TRL581]. Transport Research Laboratory.

Eshrati, B., Asl, R. T., Dell, C. A., Afshar, P., Millson, P. M., Kamali, M., Weekes, J. (2008). Preventing HIV transmission among Iranian prisoners: Initial support for providing education on the benefits of harm reduction practices. *Harm Reduction Journal, 5*(21). Published online 2008 June 9. doi: 10.1186/1477-7517-5-21. Available from http://www.harmreductionjournal.com/content/pdf/1477-7517-5-21.pdf.

Fernandes, R. F., Hatfield, J., & Job, R. F. S. (2006). *Examination of different predictors of different risky driving behaviors in young NSW drivers.* Final Report for the Motor Accidents Authority of NSW. Retrieved November 27, 2010, from http://www.irmrc.unsw.edu.au/documents/predictors%20of%20risky%20drving%20report.pdf.

Fishbein, M., & Ajzen, I. (1975). *Belief, attitude, intention, and behavior: An introduction to theory and research.* Reading, MA: Addison-Wesley.

Germeni, E., Lionis, C., Kalampoki, V., Davou, B., Belechri, M., & Petridou, E. (2010). Evaluating the impact of a school-based helmet promotion program on eligible adolescent drivers: Different audiences, different needs? *Health Education Research, 25,* 865–876.

Glanz, K., Rimer, B. K., & Viswanath, K. (2008). *Health behavior and health education: Theory, research, and practice* (4th Ed.). San Francisco, CA: Jossey-Bass.

Haas, E. J. (2012). *Toward harm reduction as a metatheory for health communication campaigns: An empirical study of harm reduction metatheory and the reconceptualized health belief model addressing motorcycle safety.* Unpublished doctoral dissertation. West Lafayette, IN: Purdue University.

Heather, N. (2006). Controlled drinking, harm reduction and their roles in the response to alcohol-related problems. *Addiction Research and Theory, 14,* 7–18.

Hjorland, B. (1998). Theory and metatheory of information science: A new interpretation. *Journal of Documentation, 54*(5), 606–621.

Holland, C., & Hill, R. (2007). The effect of age, gender, and driver status on pedestrians' intentions to cross the road in risky situations. *Accident Analysis and Prevention, 39,* 224–237.

Jacques, L. B. (1994). Rates of bicycle helmet use in an affluent Michigan County. *Public Health Reports, 109,* 296–301.

Janz, N. K., & Becker, M. H. (1984). The health belief model: A decade later. *Health Education Quarterly, 11*(1), 1–47.

Job, R. F. S. (1990). The application of learning theory to driving confidence: The effect of age and the impact of random breath testing. *Accident Analysis and Prevention, 22*, 97–107.

Lajunen, T., & Rasanen, M. (2004). Can social psychological models be used to promote bicycle helmet use among teenagers? A comparison of the Health Belief Model, Theory of Planned Behavior and Locus of Control. *Journal of Safety Research, 35,* 115–123.

Larimer, M. E., & Cronce, J. M. (2007). Identification, prevention, and treatment revisited: Individual-focused college drinking prevention strategies: 1999–2006. *Addictive Behaviors, 32*, 2439–2468.

Littlejohn, S. W., & Foss, K. A. (2005). *Theories of human communication.* Belmont, CA: Thomson Wadsworth.

Logan, D. E., & Marlatt, G. A. (2010). Harm reduction therapy: A practice-friendly review of research. *Journal of Clinical Psychology, 66*(2), 201–214.

MacCoun, R. J. (2009). Toward a psychology of harm reduction. In G.A. Marlatt & K. Witkiewitz. *Addictive behaviors: New readings on etiology, prevention, and treatment* (pp. 137–158). Washington, DC: American Psychological Association.

Marlatt, G. A. (1998). *Harm reduction: Pragmatic strategies for managing high-risk behaviors.* New York: The Guilford Press.

Mattson, M. (1999). Toward a reconcepualization of communication cues to action in the Health Belief Model: HIV testing counseling. *Communication Monographs, 66*, 240–263.

Mattson, M., & Basnyat, I. (2008). Infusing HIV test counseling practice with harm reduction theory: An integrated model for voluntary counseling and testing. In T. Edgar, S. Noar, & V. Freimuth (Eds.). *Communication perspectives for HIV/AIDS in the 21st century* (pp. 137–167). New York: Lawrence Erlbaum Associates.

Miller, W. R., & Rollnick, S. (1991). *Motivational interviewing: Preparing people to change addictive behavior.* New York, NY: The Guilford Press.

O'Callaghan, F., & Nausbaum, S. (2006). Predicting bicycle helmet wearing intentions and behavior among adolescents. *Journal of Safety Research, 37,* 425–431.

Peterson, T. R., Witte, K., Enkerlin-Hoeflich, E., Espericueta, L., Flora, J. T., Florey, N., Loughran, T., & Stuart, R. (1994). Using informant directed interviews to discover risk orientation: How formative evaluations based on interpretive analysis can improve persuasive safety campaigns. *Journal of Applied Communication Research, 22,* 199–215.

Prochaska, J. O., & DiClemente, C. C. (1983). Stages and processes of self-change of smoking: Toward an integrative model of change. *Journal of Counseling and Clinical Psychology, 51,* 390–395.

Prochaska, J. O., & DiClemente, C. C. (1984). *The transtheoretical approach: Crossing the traditional boundaries of therapy.* Malabar, FL: Krieger.

Prochaska, J. O., & DiClemente, C. C. (1986). Toward a comprehensive model of change. In W.R. Miller & N. Heather (Eds.), *Treating addictive behaviors: Processes of change* (pp. 3–27). New York: Plenum Press.

Prochaska, J. O., & DiClemente, C. C. (1992). Stages of change in the modification of problem behaviors. In M. Hersen, R.M. Eisler, & P.M. Miller (Eds.), *Progress in behavior modification* (Vol. 28, pp. 183–218). Sycamore, IL: Sycamore Publishing Co.

Prochaska, J. O., Reddings, C. A., & Evers, K. E. (2008). The transtheoretical model and stages of change. In K. Glanz, B.K. Rimer, & K. Viswanath (4th Ed.), *Health behavior and health education: Theory, research, and practice* (pp 97–122). San Francisco, CA: Jossey-Bass.

Poonamallee, L. (2010). *Advaita* (Non-dualism) as metatheory: A constellation of ontology, epistemology, and praxis. *Integral Review, 6*(3), 190–200.

Reid, R. J. (2002). Harm reduction and injection drug use: Pragmatic lessons from a public health model. *Health and Social Work, 27*(3), 223–226.

Rhodes, T., & Hedrich, D. (2010). Harm reduction and the mainstream. In T. Rhodes & D. Hedrich (10th Ed.), *European Monitoring Centre for Drugs and Drug Addiction Monographs: Harm reduction evidence, impacts, and challenges* (pp. 19–33). Luxembourg: Publications Office of the European Union.

Riley, D., & O'Hare, P. (2000). Harm reduction: History, definition, and practice. In J.A. Inciardi & L.D. Harrison (Eds.), *Harm reduction: National and international perspectives* (pp. 1–26). Thousand Oaks, CA: Sage.

Rimer, B. K. (2008). Models of individual health behavior. In K. Glanz, B.K. Rimer, & K. Viswanath (4th Ed.), *Health behavior and health education: Theory, research, and practice* (pp. 41–43). San Francisco, CA: Jossey-Bass.

Ritzer, G. (1988). Sociological metatheory: A defense of a subfield by a delineation of its parameters. *Sociological Theory, 6*(2), 187–200.

Ritzer, G. (1992). *Metatheorizing: Key issues in sociological theory.* London: Sage.

Rogers, R. W. (1975). A protection motivation theory of fear appeals and attitude change. *Journal of Psychology, 91,* 93–114.

Rogers, R. W. (1983). Cognitive and physiological processes in fear appeals and attitude change: A revised theory of protection motivation. In J. Cacioppo & R. Petty (Ed.), *Social Psychophysiology* (pp. 153–176). New York: Guilford Press.

Rogers, R. W., & Mewborn, C. R. (1976). Fear appeals and attitude change: Effects of a threat's noxiousness, probability of occurrence, and the efficacy of coping responses. *Journal of Personality & Social Psychology, 34,* 54–61.

Rosenstock, I. M. (1966). Why people use health services? *Milbank Memorial Fund Quarterly, 44,* 94–124.

Rosenstock, I. M. (1974). Historical origins of the health belief model. *Health Education Monographs, 2,* 328–335.

Ross, T. P., Ross, L. T., Rahman, A., & Cataldo, S. (2010). The bicycle helmet attitudes scale: Using the health belief model to predict helmet use among undergraduates. *Journal of American College Health, 59,* 29–36.

Rutter, D. R., & Quine, L. (1994). Age and experience in motorcycling safety. *Accident Analysis and Prevention, 28,* 15–21.

Rutter, D. R., Quine, L., & Chesham, D. J. (1995). Predicting safe riding behavior and accidents: Demography, beliefs, and behaviour in motorcycling safety. *Psychology and Health. 10,* 369–386.

Von, D., Ebert, S., Ngamvitroj, A., Park, N., & Kang, D. (2004). Predictors of health behaviors in college students. *Journal of Advanced Nursing, 48(*5), 463–474. doi: 10.1111/j.1365-2648.2004.03229.x.

Wallis, S. E. (2010). Toward a science of metatheory. *Integral Review, 6*(6), 73–120.

Weinstein, D., & Weinstein, M. A. (1992). The postmodern discourse of metatheory. In G. Ritzer (Ed.), *Metatheorizing* (pp. 135–150). Newbury Park, CA: Sage.

Witte, K., Stokols, D., Ituarte, P., & Schneider, M. (1993). Testing the health belief model in a field study to promote bicycle safety helmets. *Communication Research, 20,* 564–586.

Wundersitz, L. N., Hutchinson, T. P., & Woolley, J. E. (2010). Best practice in road safety mass media campaigns: A literature review. Centre for automotive safety research: Case report series CASR074. Retrieved December 5, 2010, from http://casr.adelaide.edu.au/casrpubfile/972/CASR074.pdf.

Yagil, D. (2000). Beliefs, motives and situational factors related to pedestrians' self-reported behavior at signal-controlled crossings. *Transportation Research Part F, 3,* 1–13.

Zuckerman, M. (1994). *Behavioral expressions and biosocial bases of sensation seeking.* Cambridge: Cambridge University Press.

Chapter 4

A Qualitative Approach to Applying Harm Reduction Metatheory

The previous chapter discussed aspects of the metatheorizing process we engaged in to conceptualize and justify *HRT* as an integrative metatheory. We explained how each tenet of HRT could be used to guide a component of the Reconceptualized Health Belief Model (*RHBM*). Now that the metatheory is proposed, it is necessary to empirically test the utility of the framework. In order to demonstrate how you can evaluate the feasibility of a proposed metatheory, this chapter provides guidance for utilizing and assessing the usefulness of metatheory during a research project, particularly during data analysis. Since there are few resources that explain how to pragmatically apply a metatheory in research, we highlight basic aspects of qualitative interviewing methodology to elucidate this research approach. We use harm reduction metatheory and motorcycle safety as a research project in practice illustration to guide the following chapter objectives:

- Define in-depth interviewing
- Conceptualize in-depth interviews as contextualized conversations
- Design a qualitative research project and frame theory-driven research questions
- Discuss how to structure an interview protocol using metatheory
- Explain the dual role of metatheory during the qualitative interview
- Explain how to analyze qualitative data using a metatheoretical framework

We begin by defining in-depth interviews and conceptualizing in-depth interviews as contextualized conversations.

IN-DEPTH INTERVIEWING FOR QUALITATIVE RESEARCH

In our harm reduction project we take a qualitative approach to research meaning that our goal is primarily to understand rather than explain a phenomenon. In particular, we focus on in-depth interviews to empirically study harm reduction as a metatheory. *In-depth interviews* are an inductive mode of research and are most appropriate for questions of an exploratory nature or questions that require rich, thick description. In other words, qualitative research questions that ask about what and how social processes are enacted rather than why social processes are enacted in everyday life necessitate the use of in-depth interviews.

In their discussion of in-depth interviewing as a social form unique from other types of interpersonal interaction (e.g., job interviews and counseling sessions), Johnson and Rowlands (2012) argued that although this form of interpersonal interaction may resemble talking among friends, it is different than friendship because the interviewer intends to use the information gathered from the interaction for some other purpose. That purpose usually involves gathering deep information about lived experience, values, perspectives, decisions, and cultural knowledge. The term "deep" has several meanings pertaining to in-depth interview methodology. We discuss four particular meanings below.

First, one meaning is that deep understandings are held by the real-life members of or participants in an activity, event, or place. If the interviewer is not a member or participant but wants to achieve the same deep level of knowledge and understanding as the members or participants, in-depth interviewing can assist the researcher in learning the meanings of participants' actions. If the interviewer is a current or former member, in-depth interviewing can be used to explore or check the interviewers' own understandings and determine if these understandings are shared by others. This exploration involves reflexivity by the researcher. Lived experience and member status are no longer stigmatized by social scientists and many consider experience a relative advantage (Lofland, Snow, Anderson, & Lofland, 2006).

Second, deep understandings penetrate further into commonsense understandings by exploring the context and boundaries of a perception or experience to uncover what may be hidden from ordinary view. For example, in the research project presented throughout this book, we conducted in-depth interviews with motorcyclists to explore their experiences of and meanings for riding a motorcycle. The third meaning is that deep understandings can reveal how the interviewers' own commonsense assumptions, practices, and ways of communicating influence how they interview and understand the data. The fourth meaning is that deep understandings allow the researcher to ". . . grasp and articulate the multiple views, perspectives on, and meanings of some activity, event, place, or cultural object" (Johnson & Rowlands, 2012, p. 102). Now that we discussed the similarities and differences of interviews and everyday conversations, we argue for thinking about and practicing in-depth interviews as contextualized conversations, particularly when utilizing the tenets of HRT while conversing with participants.

Comparing and Contrasting Interviews with Conversations

Following Spradley (1979), Stage and Mattson (2003) contrasted traditional ethnographic, in-depth interviews with conversations and challenged qualitative researchers to reconceptualize interviews as less researcher dominated and more like *contextualized conversations*. We chose to take this approach during our in-depth interviews with motorcyclists. These interviews typically consist of three phases. During the first phase, the researcher explains the explicit purpose of the interview, including why the interview is occurring, the goal of the interview, and the direction of the interview. The expressed purpose of the interview is from the interviewer's perspective.

In the second phase, the interviewer uses a series of ethnographic explanations to explicate how the goal of the interview will be achieved. These interviewer-directed explanations take the form of project explanations, recording explanations, native language explanations, interview explanations and question explanations. During *project explanations*, the interviewer tells the interviewee what aspects of the interviewee's experience are germane to the research project. Through *recording explanations* the interviewer discusses how the interviewee's responses will be recorded. *Native language explanations* encourage the interviewee to express their responses in their own words. The interviewer lays out the trajectory of the interview through *interview explanations* including an outline of questions, which is presented during *question explanations*.

During the third phase, the interviewer asks a variety of questions to guide and accomplish the purpose of the interview. Descriptive questions are most common during interviews. According to Spradley (1979), there are two types of descriptive questions; grand-tour questions and mini-tour questions. *Grand-tour questions* ask interviewees to provide verbal descriptions of aspects or features that are relevant to the focus of the study. *Mini-tour questions* are utilized as a tool to obtain more specific details. However, it is common to encounter various other names for and types of interview questions. For instance, Rubin and Rubin (2012) emphasized three types of questions including main questions, probes, and follow-up questions. *Main questions* address the research questions and structure of the interview. *Probes* help manage the interview and elicit detail. *Follow-up questions* explore and test ideas that come up during the interview.

Rubin and Rubin (2012) also discussed the similarities and differences between what they term responsive interviewing and ordinary conversations. During *responsive interviewing*, a relationship is created to address research questions and during the interview, the researcher responds to and asks follow-up questions based on what they hear from the interviewee. In this sense, the interviewee is considered a conversational partner. However, *ordinary conversations* occur within the context of an ongoing relationship, are usually informal and social in nature, and occur to maintain the relationship. Conversations usually lack explicit purpose, are based on common understanding, avoid repetition, balance turn taking, use abbreviations, and exhibit curious ignorance by both parties (Stage & Mattson, 2003). When complemented by the assets of conversations, interviews become more participant-respectful and insightful to the project. Stage and Mattson (2003) suggested three conversational techniques to incorporate into interviews to enhance participant respect, including problematizing the research context, redefining interviewer and interview participant roles, and contextualizing interviews. These three techniques, which are consistent with harm reduction objectives, are discussed in turn.

Problematizing the research context refers to the need for researchers to understand rather than ignore any particular event or phenomena within the larger social milieu. Burawoy (1991) discussed the need to understand how external forces shape present social situations. In other words, an interview need not focus exclusively on the direct experience of an interviewee. If an interviewee refers to historical texts or local lore on the topic explored during the interview, the researcher has a responsibility to consider and seek to understand the interviewee's experience in relation to the referenced texts, customs, and events.

In addition to a responsibility to understand events as they are framed by a larger social context, there is need to address issues surrounding the notion of knowledge creation including who is afforded the opportunity to create knowledge in the process of research. Tanno and Jandt (1994) argued for *redefining interviewer* and *interview participant roles* such that the interviewee is a coproducer with the interviewer in the creation of knowledge. They also stressed the need to extend the research process to include participant groups as research peers. Blurring the roles between researcher and participant provides those who will be defined an opportunity to participate in their portrayal. Researchers must recognize the power of their position as researcher, accept the responsibility that comes with portraying others, and learn to share the power of representation.

Why, you might be wondering, should qualitative researchers have an obligation to address these concerns? Lincoln and Guba (1985, adapted from pg. 39) outlined two distinct characteristics of naturalistic research and two of these characteristics speak directly to this question:

- *Characteristic 1: Natural Settings*—Realities are wholes that cannot be understood in isolation from their contexts, nor can they be fragmented for separate study of the parts.
- *Characteristic 2: Human Instrument*—The researcher elects to use himself or herself as well as other humans as the primary data-gathering instruments. There is an understanding that all instruments interact with respondents and objects but that only the human instrument is capable of grasping and evaluating the meaning of that differential interaction.

Therefore, researchers cannot assume that merely doing research with humans in a natural setting as a human instrument to gather information results in good interview data. To believe that merely going through the motions of interviewing in a particular way yields the rich promise of the interview method is to be ensnared in a research trap (Watzlawick, 1984). To avoid such traps, researchers need to heed these cautions and not separate the goals and methods of the research project from the context in which the study is embedded. Also, interviewers must carefully and respectfully build relationships with participants.

We provided some focused information about in-depth interviews in order to illustrate the approaches we took during our interviews with motorcyclists. This content, such as involving the interviewee in the conversation, are important aspects of communicating from a harm reduction perspective. Thus, we wanted to illustrate the similarities in communicating from a harm reduction perspective and performing one's job as a qualitative researcher. The next section discusses crafting research questions using harm reduction tenets and with metatheory in mind.

Crafting Research Questions

There are several approaches to developing research questions. According to Rubin and Rubin (2011), if the research topic is inspired by the literature, moving from a research topic to research questions should flow rather naturally. Several researchers have provided guidance for developing research questions. However, because we are exploring a new research approach integrating harm reduction as metatheory, we briefly review the development of research questions. A succinct checklist adapted from other qualitative research books follows and you can easily refer to these resources as needed in the future.

Checklist for developing research questions:

- Match to the research problem (Rubin & Rubin, 2011)
- Frame in an open-ended, probing format (Lindlof & Taylor, 2002)
- Provide enough flexibility to in-depthly explore the research problem (Corbin & Strauss, 2008)

- Do not imply causality (King & Horrocks, 2010)
- Use vocabulary that embeds the conceptual framework being studied (Wengraf, 2001)
- Provide an opening to insert yourself in the research setting and recruit participants (Lindlof & Taylor, 2002)

In this book we encourage metatheoretical integration to determine a research problem and potential solution. Therefore, we focus on developing metatheory/theory-driven research questions. To explain this process, we turn to the motorcycle safety exemplar and how we developed research questions to assess the feasibility of harm reduction as a metatheory, while still adhering to guidelines for developing effective research questions to guide our project.

After we conceptualized HRT as a metatheory, we knew this framework needed to be empirically studied. According to Edwards (2010), "A key reason that overarching theory in particular has struggled to gain scientific credibility is its lack of a solid methodological basis" (p. 46). In other words, formal evaluation of the research and design was absent in the development of metatheory within the field of scientific inquiry. The proposed qualitative methodology for this empirical study aimed to evaluate the fit and usefulness of HRT as a metatheory. Literature reviews conducted during this metatheory-conceptualization phase helped focus our area of inquiry. Ultimately, the literature surrounding HRT and the RHBM helped frame the theory-driven research questions presented in Figure 4.1.

Now that we presented our research questions, we return to the checklist provided for developing research questions and discuss how these guidelines were adapted to account for the harm reduction, metatheoretical aspect of this research project. Although this discussion pertaining to research questions may be a review, the content should be useful if you decide to apply harm reduction in your future research, incorporate a metatheory, or both.

First, we needed to phrase the research questions in a way that addressed the research problems we identified from our literature review in Chapter 1 and Chapter 2 and subsequently in a way that would help resolve these problems (Rubin & Rubin, 2011). To accurately address the problems that we identified, we proposed that HRT may serve as a metatheory in health and safety research. In Chapter 3 we conceptualized that one tenet of HRT may guide one component of the RHBM. Therefore, RQ1 and the five subsets of RQ1 were phrased to assess the metatheoretical feasibility of HRT. Then, RQ2 and RQ3 further probed the problems associated with accurate health and safety communication and interventions, and whether or not HRT as a metatheory could result in more realistic methods to target at-risk populations. Therefore, these research questions were informed by the literature review of HRT.

Research in Practice Illustration
Metatheory-driven Research Questions (RQ)

RQ1: In what ways can Harm Reduction Theory (HRT), in tandem with the Reconceptualized Health Belief Model (RHBM), guide interviews with motorcyclists about their safety behaviors while driving a motorcycle?
RQ1a: In what ways can the HRT tenet *humanistic value* inform the RHBM component cues to action to encourage motorcyclists to discuss their current safety behaviors while driving a motorcycle?
RQ1b: In what ways can the HRT tenet *pragmatism* inform the RHBM components perceived benefits and perceived barriers to encourage motorcyclists to discuss their current safety behaviors while driving a motorcycle?
RQ1c: In what ways can the HRT tenet *immediacy/goal setting* inform the RHBM components risk susceptibility and severity to encourage motorcyclists to discuss their current safety behaviors while driving a motorcycle?
RQ1d: In what ways can the HRT tenet *empowerment* inform the RHBM component self-efficacy to encourage motorcyclists to discuss their current safety behaviors while driving a motorcycle?
RQ1e: In what ways can the HRT tenet *community collaboration* inform the formative research practiced by motorcycle safety campaign practitioners to encourage motorcyclists to discuss their current safety behaviors while driving a motorcycle?
RQ2: In what ways can interviews with motorcyclists that were guided by HRT, in tandem with the RHBM, assist in developing realistic motorcycle safety messages?
RQ3: What implications do the results from RQ1 and RQ2 provide for considering HRT as a metatheory for health and safety campaigns/interventions?

Figure 4.1 Research in Practice Illustration: Metatheory-driven Research Questions (RQ).

Second, Lindlof and Taylor (2002) indicated that research questions should be "open-ended probes that, with the benefit of theoretical reasoning and some scene casing, orient the investigator's interests to the scene" (p. 88). Thus, besides maintaining project flexibility, the open-ended nature of questions also transitions researchers into the scene they are studying to collect data. The research questions in this research project were constructed in an open-ended format via the phrases "In what ways . . ." and "What implications . . . ." This format provided us the opportunity to freely probe each interview participant about the ways a tenet of HRT may guide a component of the RHBM while discussing safety behaviors. The open-ended nature of this wording also added flexibility to the interviews which is another guideline for developing theory-driven research questions (Corbin & Strauss, 2008). However, even though the questions were open-ended and allowed for rich dialogue, the focus on one HRT tenet guiding one component of the RHBM, with an emphasis on participants' safety behaviors, provided direction during the project. If we did not narrow the potential relationships between the metatheory and theory or narrow the health issue in advance of the interviews, the study may have been too broad resulting in the gathering of unmanageable data.

In addition, King and Horrocks (2010) argued that qualitative research questions should not focus on causation between components of a theory but instead, focus on participants' experiences with reference to a particular behavior. These authors stated, "while qualitative research questions should not seek to establish causality, they may focus on perceptions of causality from the perspective of research participants" (p. 26). In our case, asking participants how specific harm reduction initiatives may guide their motorcycle safety decisions probed at-risk motorcyclists' perceptions of their behavior choices.

Finally, Wengraf (2001) indicated that theory-driven research questions need to include vocabulary that embeds the conceptual framework being studied. In our project, the research questions needed to include language that embedded the metatheoretical framework being studied, by incorporating concepts from the proposed metatheory and theory. We inquired about two theories (i.e., Harm Reduction Theory and the Reconceptualized Health Belief Model) and integrated vocabularies from these previously conceptualized theories to inquire about a potential metatheoretical framework. In addition, the research questions were written in a way that described the potential connection between the metatheory and theory. Therefore, the research questions were worded in a way that, according to Wengraf (2001), may develop new explanations (i.e., theories), which may in turn create partially new vocabularies (i.e., conceptual frameworks). According to Wengraf (2001), theory-driven research questions are "couched in terms of conceptual frameworks used by previous researchers" and contain "concepts that are researcher-friendly and that advance conceptual frameworks and the theory or theories within the field" (p. 84). Accordingly, our research questions were based on previous conceptual frameworks but were worded in a way that could advance both HRT and the RHBM by considering the possibility of a metatheory.

Now that we stressed the importance of crafting research questions, with an emphasis on (meta)theory-driven research questions that also seek to advance harm reduction, the next section discusses developing an interview protocol using the tenets of harm reduction as a guiding framework.

DEVELOPING A HARM REDUCTION INTERVIEW PROTOCOL

We adhered to best practices when constructing our interview protocol including the development of an introduction, main questions, probing questions, and a closing. Since several other books (for examples see: King & Horrocks, 2010; Kvale, 2009; Lindlof & Taylor, 2002; Rubin & Rubin, 2011) detail the types of questions to ask (and not ask) during an interview, we instead feature how a metatheory informed the development of a harm reduction interview protocol. Following we provide examples of how our proposed metatheoretical framework structured and guided this process.

A semi-structured interview guide was used for our study that assessed the feasibility of harm reduction as a metatheory. A semi-structured interview guide was employed rather than a structured interview guide to bring us closer to the intimate understandings of participants' social worlds, including allowing us to carryout out the interviews as contextualized conversations, as discussed earlier (Hermanowicz, 2002; Mattson & Stage, 2003). Table 4.1 provides an abridged view of how we employed the harm reduction tenets as a metatheoretical framework throughout the development of questions and facilitation of our interviews with motorcyclists.

According to Rubin and Rubin (2011) an interview guide that is informed by a theory inquires about behaviors implied by the theory (highlighted in Table 4.1: Column 3). Our interview guide was structured differently in that the metatheoretical tenets of harm reduction were utilized to engage the components of the RHBM throughout the interview (highlighted in Table 4.1: Column 2). Specifically, we adapted questions to include a harm reduction perspective while eliciting participants' attitudes and opinions relative to the components of the RHBM. The interview guide had seven sections including an introduction, one section to assess each of the five harm reduction tenets with a component of the RHBM, and a conclusion. Next we discuss each section of the harm reduction interview protocol.

Introducing the Interview Topic

A qualitative interview typically begins with an introduction of the researcher to the participant and an explanation of the interview topic. The concept of harm reduction metatheory did not affect how the introduction to participants was structured because the focus of the introduction was to signal participants toward our desire to learn about their motorcycle safety attitudes and behaviors. We justified why our research project and the motorcyclists' insights were important. Two excerpts from our introductory discussion with motorcyclists follow:

> As you may know, motorcycles are becoming a more popular mode of transportation, making motorcyclists an important audience to understand. I would like to determine if particular communication materials, such as health messages, may influence safety behaviors so we can find more effective ways to interact with motorcyclists and others in their personal networks.

> Today, we will talk about your account of what it is like to ride a motorcycle including barriers that you encounter to practicing safer riding behaviors. We also will focus on safety behaviors in which you participate before and during your motorcycle rides, including any benefits or drawbacks to engaging in these behaviors. Your responses will be included with other motorcyclists' responses.

Table 4.1 Implementing a Harm Reduction Metatheoretical Framework for Qualitative Interviews

Metatheory Framework	*Using Metatheory Tenet to Inform Researcher Perspective*	*Using Metatheory Tenet to Inform Theory*	*Theoretical Component*
Humanistic Value	Acknowledge risky behaviors and respectfully communicate toward the participants.	Probe how other outlets respond to risky behaviors and the participants' reaction to these responses.	Probe cues to action that target risky behaviors.
Pragmatism	Continue not to judge behaviors and instead have a realistic conversation about the behaviors within the participant's control.	Be realistic toward participants about their ability to change risky behaviors by discussing barriers both within/not within their control.	Probe perceived barriers to and perceived benefits of practicing behaviors.
Immediacy/Goal Setting	Encourage the discussion of short-term behavior choices participants make upon receiving cues to action.	Explore what situations have caused or may cause short-term or long-term changes due to increased susceptibility to accidents or injuries.	Probe perceived susceptibility toward harm and perceived severity of the incident.
Empowerment	Maintain a positive attitude toward participants by encouraging them to share all of the safer choices they make, and probe whether these changes motivate additional behaviors.	Discuss choices participants feel exist to being safer and their ability to adapt behaviors, if desired, and allow participants to choose a desirable option.	Assess participants' confidence to initiate and sustain behavior(s); provide with skills needed to succeed.
Community Collaboration	Treat participants as experts when soliciting feedback about the target audience and stakeholders who can help the environment to facilitate behavior change.	What people or groups may be influential in both minimizing barriers for this audience and persuading the audience to change behaviors.	Consider the demographic and socio-psychological characteristics of the audience, and how organizations and stakeholders can target these characteristics.

The purpose of these introductory statements was to inform participants' that their feedback is essential to making the roads safer for motorcyclists. After introducing participants to the research topic, we emphasized that the conversation was confidential and that they could discontinue the interview at any time. Although the introduction to the interview did not contain information about the metatheory that was guiding the research project, a tenet of the metatheory was incorporated into the introduction for each of the five corresponding interview segments, as explained in the next section.

Engaging Harm Reduction Metatheory during the Interview

In addition to the general introduction, there was a brief opening to each of the five sections of the interview that corresponded with the tenets of the proposed harm reduction metatheory. These openings included harm reduction terminology in an effort to build participants' trust, increase their comfort in responding to questions, and encourage reflexivity during the interview (highlighted in Table 4.1: Column 1). Throughout this section of the book, we provide examples of these introductions in combination with the construction of sample interview questions.

The main questions within each of the five sections that corresponded with HRT tenets were open-ended and included additional probing questions to more fully understand participants' responses (Berg, 2004). Besides being guided by the tenets of HRT to inform and structure interview questions, we consulted literature including Mattson's (1999) RHBM scales to survey HIV-test clients and Ross et al.'s (2010) Health Belief Model (*HBM*) scales to predict safety behaviors among bicyclists. We adapted survey items into open-ended interview questions to assess motorcyclists' current safety behaviors and their ability to adjust their at-risk behaviors. Following, we provide examples of how we used metatheory to adapt interview questions within the five tenet sections of the interview guide.

Humanistic Value Informing Cues to Action Interview Questions

After the introduction to the interview, we began with the humanistic value/cues to action section of the interview. The introduction to this section is provided in Figure 4.2, which also includes a mental note for the researcher.

Including this mental note for the researcher reminded us to be nonjudgmental toward participants and their behaviors and helped ensure participants' comfort in sharing their at-risk, and sometimes illegal

Research in Practice Illustration

Humanistic value interview section
Mental note for the researcher: Ensure that the participant knows that, even though he/she may engage in risky behaviors while riding a motorcycle, I still respect the individual.

Application of tenet in practice: Probing cues to action
"I know that motorcyclists, including you, may regularly engage in risky behaviors while riding. I recognize that these behaviors exist and do not judge you for these behaviors. Rather I'd like to learn from you. I would like to ask you some questions about how other people respond to your safety behaviors and how you react to their responses."

Figure 4.2 Research in Practice Illustration.

behaviors while driving a motorcycle. If you apply humanistic value as a metatheoretical tenet in your own research, this mental note can serve as a reminder for any health issue. For example, if you were interviewing underage college students about their alcohol consumption behaviors, it would be important to maintain a nonjudgmental attitude toward their alcohol consumption behaviors, despite potential participants being under 21 years of age. A judgmental or critical attitude may result in participants not trusting you and sharing only a few of their personal experiences. In our research project, emphasizing humanistic value was crucial in setting the stage for the entire interview discussion. In adhering to the tenet of humanistic value, it was important for us to immediately communicate that we expect participants to practice risky behaviors and that we do not judge those behaviors, rather we want to understand how and why participants make these specific health and safety choices (Marlatt, 1998; Mattson & Basnyat, 2008).

After the introduction to this section of the interview, we proceeded with other questions guided by academic literature. For example, Ross et al. (2010) identified family and friends as a strong cue to action for bicyclists to practice safer behaviors when they bicycle. Therefore, one question in the interview protocol was, "How do your family and friends respond to your motorcycle safety behaviors?" This was followed by the probing question, "How do their responses make you feel?" Asking participants to discuss if and how their family and friends communicate their viewpoints (e.g., positive, emotional, judgmental) allowed us to gauge family and friends as a cue to action to persuade motorcyclists to change behavior. We took a similar approach to develop questions to assess media as a possible cue to action for participants. Participants discussed if the way the media portrays motorcycle safety is positive or negative, and if the format of media messages influences their safety behaviors.

Pragmatism Informing Perceived Benefits and Perceived Barriers Interview Questions

The next section utilized the HRT tenet pragmatism to inform questions about participants' perceived benefits of driving their motorcycle safer in addition to perceived barriers to driving their motorcycle safer. The introduction for this section of the interview is illustrated in Research Project in Practice Illustration Figure 4.3.

During this section of the interview, it was important for us to maintain a realistic attitude toward participants about their current safety behaviors while driving a motorcycle. By maintaining a pragmatic attitude, it was easier to probe participants to discuss what behavior choices they thought were impossible to achieve or that may result in more harm than good (Stronach, 2003). In addition to us being realistic about participants' current safety behaviors, the introduction to this section communicated the importance of participants being honest during the interview about the safety decisions they make while driving a motorcycle.

After the introduction to this section, we proceeded with other interview questions. First, we asked questions to assess if participants were cognizant of their safety behaviors while driving a motorcycle. The answers to these questions helped us understand whether participants were pragmatic about their safety choices in reference to how they define what it means to be safe on their motorcycle. These questions are displayed in Research Project in Practice Illustration Figure 4.4.

After gauging participants' perceptions of how they define motorcycle safety, we continued with interview questions designed from academic literature that utilized components of the RHBM to assess health and safety behaviors of other audiences. For example, Mattson (1999) studied the types of persuasive message strategies HIV-test counselors use to gain client

Research in Practice Illustration

Pragmatism

Mental note for the researcher: Accept that participants engage in risky motorcycling behaviors but rather than focusing on changing all of their behaviors, gauge their perceptions of current barriers to being safer and focus on challenging realistic barriers to reduce potential harm.

Use of tenet in practice: Probing perceived barriers and perceived benefits

"Now I am interested in hearing about your general view of motorcycle safety, any benefits you think exist to practicing safer behaviors on the road, and barriers that may prevent you from being safer. In this section I will continue not to judge your safety behaviors and instead, want to have a conversation about the behaviors that are realistic and within your control."

Figure 4.3 Research in Practice Illustration.

Research in Practice Illustration

Pragmatism Excerpt from Interview Guide

1. What is your definition of motorcycle safety?
2. Explain some intentional safety choices that you make **before** you ride your motorcycle.
3. Explain some intentional safety behaviors that you practice **during** your motorcycle rides.
4. Explain some intentional risky choices that you make **before** you ride your motorcycle
5. Explain some intentional risky behaviors you practice **during** your motorcycle rides.

Note for research: Loop back in data analysis to see if the participant consciously/unconsciously practice behaviors listed in their own definition of motorcycle safety.

Figure 4.4 Research in Practice Illustration.

compliance to practice safer sex. Her survey instrument was comprised of questions to understand clients' perceived benefits and barriers to practicing safer sex. Examples of questions used to assess clients' perceived barriers to practicing safer sex included: "The disadvantages of using safer-sex practices are a real problem," and "The use of a condom jeopardizes a relationship" (Mattson, 1999, p. 247). In another example from the literature about bicycle helmet safety, Ross et al. (2010) included questions about perceived barriers to wearing a bicycle helmet such as: "I would feel embarrassed wearing a bicycle helmet," "Wearing a helmet makes me look foolish if no one else is wearing one," "Wearing a helmet is too hot," and "A bicycle helmet is not worth the cost" (p. 32).

We began this section of the interview with some broad questions about barriers to safety and then we honed in on some common barriers to practicing safer behaviors identified in the literature. Examples of questions we asked include: "What barriers exist to you practicing safer behaviors?," "If you wanted to, could you change your safety behaviors?," followed by the probing question, "If not, why?" We also broadly assessed participants' ability to overcome identified barriers through the question, "How can you reduce the barriers we just discussed to adopt safer behaviors?" More specifically, after these broader questions were discussed we asked, "If other people see you driving your motorcycle safer, what will they think?," which is a question based on peer influence as a common barrier identified in the literature.

Perceived benefits of driving a motorcycle safer also were probed during the interviews. Examples of scale items previously used to assess perceived benefits include, "If my partner insists on practicing safer sex, this means she or he really cares about me," (Mattson, 1999, p. 247) and "I think it is my obligation to keep myself safe for the people who care about me by wearing a helmet when I ride," and "In the event of an accident, a helmet would protect my head" (Ross et al., 2010, p. 32). Again, we started this section of the interview with broader questions to gauge participants' recognition of perceived benefits and moved to more specific questions. Example questions from the interview guide include, "How safe do you feel when you ride your motorcycle?" "Do you want to start being safer when you ride your motorcycle?" followed by the probing question, "Why or why not?"

This section of the interview allowed us to have an open conversation with participants about their perceived barriers to and perceived benefits of being safer while driving their motorcycle, at the same time using a pragmatic standpoint to allow participants to be realistic about their current behaviors and potential to change those behaviors in the future.

Immediacy Informing Perceived Susceptibility and Perceived Severity Interview Questions

The next section of the interview introduced the HRT tenet immediacy/goal setting, which also served as guidance for the interview questions that strived to assess participants' perceived susceptibility to motorcycle accidents and injuries and the perceived severity of those accidents and injuries. The introduction to this section is depicted in Research Project in Practice Illustration Figure 4.5. You will notice in the introduction to participants for this section of the interview we continue to be nonjudgmental and realistic toward participants' current behavior choices. However, we probe what may influence them to make short-term or long-term changes in the future, in an effort to capitalize on these opportunities when targeting this audience to reduce immediate harm in the future.

An example follows that involves the design of interview questions to address perceived susceptibility and severity, guided by the immediacy/goal setting tenet of HRT. Ross et al. (2010) quantitatively identified the impact of short trips and long trips on bicyclists' safety behaviors. However,

Research in Practice Illustration

Immediacy/Goal Setting

Mental note for the researcher: Allow participants the flexibility to discuss any short-term goals they've set or behaviors choices made to reduce susceptibility to harm while driving a motorcycle and/or their ability to develop goals in the future.

Use of tenet in practice: Probing perceived susceptibility and perceived severity

"Now that we have talked about your general view toward motorcycle safety, and the benefits and barriers of practicing safer behaviors, I would like to discuss how you view your likelihood of experiencing a motorcycle accident or injury. I would like to explore what situations have caused or may cause any short-term or long-term changes to your safety behaviors, recognizing that you may not have a desire to alter any behaviors right now."

Figure 4.5 Research in Practice Illustration.

besides just assessing the impact of trip length on safety behaviors, we went a step further during the interview and utilized the HRT tenet immediacy/goal setting to probe whether or not participants recognized and were open to developing short-term safety goals. The section of the interview guide that addressed perceived susceptibility/severity included the questions: "How often do you go on long trips? Short trips?," "In what ways, if any, does the length of your trip determine what safety behaviors you practice?," "Explain why you think it is easier or harder to practice safer behaviors on particular trips," and "How does this affect your safety behaviors both close to home and further from home?" These questions encouraged participants to discuss their safety behaviors on short trips and long trips and the difference in these behaviors, while providing an opportunity to discuss short-term goals to reduce harm when driving a motorcycle.

Empowerment Informing Self-efficacy Interview Questions

The next section of the interview guide utilized the HRT tenet empowerment to probe participants' self-efficacy to adopting safer behaviors while driving a motorcycle. The introduction to this segment is provided in Research Project in Practice Illustration Figure 4.6. During this section of the interview we were trying to assess what, if anything, increased participants' confidence to safely drive their motorcycle.

Specifically, the HRT tenet empowerment supports the concept that the more choices individuals have in progressing toward a healthier lifestyle, the more likely they will choose an option they can adhere to, subsequently increasing confidence and ability to maintain the healthier behavior (Reid, 2002). Therefore, questions assessed participants' confidence in implementing safety choices by asking questions including: "Do you feel confident in your ability to safely ride a motorcycle?," "Explain a time when you could not perform a particular maneuver on the road?," and "How did it make you

Research in Practice Illustration

Empowerment
Mental note for the researcher: Allow participants to share any and all options they have to be safer, what choices they have made in the past, and what motivated them to adopt these behaviors.

Use of tenet in practice: Probing self-efficacy
"Now we are going to discuss your ability to alter your motorcycle safety behaviors. Specifically, I'd like you to explain the choices you feel exist to being safer on your motorcycle and your ability to embrace some of these options in the future."

Figure 4.6 Research in Practice Illustration.

feel?" Besides addressing participants' personal confidence to react to risky situations, we also asked participants if there were any safety behaviors they practiced previously but do not anymore, and probed why their safety behaviors increased or decreased over time. Finally, we asked participants what safety behaviors they would recommend to novice motorcyclists and what steps a novice motorcyclist should take to learn more about motorcycle safety. This allowed us to assess what safety choices were imperative to provide to new, at-risk motorcyclists to start building their self-efficacy to practice safer behaviors and eventually, help other motorcyclists modify their safety behaviors during motorcycle rides.

Community Collaboration Informing Formative Research and Audience Analysis

The last section of the interview guide incorporated the HRT tenet community collaboration to facilitate the necessary formative research with an emphasis on the demographic characteristics of the target audience, and how to create enabling environments to support safer behaviors. The community aspect is necessary to consider and include during all phases of a health campaign or intervention, including those guided by theory. Therefore, cooperation with and from the community is essential in fostering enabling environments for individuals whether it is through policy or removing structural barriers that encumber behavior change (Rhodes & Hendrich, 2010; WHO, 1986). This section of the interview inquired of participants what collaborations they deemed essential to reduce barriers and improve their surrounding environment in reference to safety behaviors. The introduction to this section of the interview is provided in Research Project in Practice Illustration Figure 4.7.

Consistent with literature about the importance of the external environment and information about the socio-demographic characteristics of an audience, we developed narrow questions to help further segment motorcyclists as a target audience. First, we asked motorcyclists whether or not collaboration with other stakeholders was important to improve motorcycle safety efforts. Participants were able to provide specific stakeholders and potential partners in their local communities. In addition, we asked participants what they think is missing from current campaign materials and safety messages and what they recommend be included in future promotional materials. Then, we asked if there were specific motorcycling individuals or groups who needed more support and how collaboration could help target these groups. Questions in this segment of the interview included: "What types of motorcyclists (e.g., gender, age, behaviors, etc.) do motorcycle safety community efforts need to target?," "Who should we partner with to target these motorcyclists?,"

Research in Practice Illustration

Community collaboration
Mental note for the researcher: Encourage participants to share how they think community-based motorcycle safety efforts should collaborate with motorcyclists to improve motorcyclists' surrounding environment and persuade safety behaviors.

Use of tenet in practice: Formative research and audience analysis
"I would like to end by discussing how community-based motorcycle safety efforts can better target motorcyclists and persuade them to practice safer behaviors. Specifically, I would like to know what people or groups may be influential during communication with motorcyclists. I'd also like you share any external barriers that makes it difficult for you to be safer."

Figure 4.7 Research in Practice Illustration.

"What exists in the environment that prevents you from being safer while driving your motorcycle?" and "What improvements can be made to your current environment to facilitate safer behaviors?" These questions helped us focus on the individual, group, and community aspects of motorcycle safety and culminated the interview.

Summary of Developing a Harm Reduction Interview Protocol

This section of the chapter provided an explanation of how research questions were generated from a harm reduction perspective while eliciting participants' attitudes and opinions about the RHBM components including motorcycle safety cues to action, perceived benefits of and barriers to practicing motorcycle safety, perceived susceptibility and severity to being injured in a motorcycle accident, self-efficacy to practice safety behaviors, and community influence regarding motorcycle safety. Although preliminary research is important to understand the health and safety issue enough to probe participants, the way in which questions were developed, using the metatheoretical tenets of harm reduction to educe the components of the theory, is a new approach to framing research questions and subsequently interview questions.

In addition, integrating harm reduction terminology at the beginning of each interview section helped engage participants in the metatheory. The research study in practice illustrations show how we utilized the section introductions to create a less abstract and more action-oriented discussion of theoretical components during the interview. These introductions, guided by harm reduction metatheory, encouraged participants to openly share their experiences. Below, we provide a checklist to help create an action-oriented discussion with participants.

Applying harm reduction metatheoretical tenets during an interview:

- Gently probe participants to share their risky health and safety behaviors, while maintaining neutral probes and non-verbals toward participants and their responses.
- Dialogue about and focus on health and safety behaviors participants think are realistic for them to achieve at the current point in time, regardless of how small the behavior change may be for them.
- Gauge participants' readiness to change behaviors, with an emphasis on behaviors they can change immediately to reduce potential harm in the near future.
- Encourage participants to identify choices they have to become safer and healthier over time and dialogue about those choices until they determine a choice(s) that best fits both their internal readiness to change and external environment that can help facilitate a change in behavior.
- Treat participants as experts to learn more about the target audience and what groups should be involved to create more enabling environments and partnerships to reduce harm among target audience members.

Next, we discuss how we incorporated the use of a metatheory to analyze the results.

ANALYZING THE RESULTS

During your previous experiences analyzing and coding qualitative data inductive, deductive, or both approaches may have guided your analyses. You also may have used theory to guide your analysis. In this section, we discuss a new approach to data analysis and detail how the results of our motorcycle safety study were analyzed with respect to the proposed harm reduction metatheory.

According to Boyatzis (1998), *theory-driven code development* is the most frequently used approach in social science research for coding qualitative information. Utilizing a deductive, theory-driven approach to identify *themes* allows codes to emerge from the data and be compared with the evolving theory or metatheory (Glaser, 1992; Glaser & Strauss, 1967; Lindlof & Taylor, 2002; Strauss, 1987). This analytic approach was necessary to answer our research questions. Using this analysis method, "the researcher begins with his or her theory of what occurs and then formulates the signals, indicators, or evidence that would support this theory. The elements of the code are derived from the hypotheses or elements of the theory" (p. 33). In our research project, a proposed metatheory guided a theory.

Because we had knowledge of the overarching tenets in the harm reduction metatheoretical framework and identified potential connections before analysis, we analyzed the data deductively (Yin, 2011). However, upon completion of the deductive analysis an inductive approach was used with the perspective of harm reduction in mind, to ensure we did not overlook results based on the pre-determined framework. Interweaving qualitative studies with both inductive and deductive analysis, as in our research project, is not uncommon and often provides a more nuanced understanding of the data (Yin, 2011). First, we stress the importance of organizing your data before the analysis.

Using Harm Reduction Metatheory to Organize and Analyze Data

Organizing Data

Before the data was coded, each interview transcript was saved as a separate data file for thematic analysis and coding. We added a column on the right side of each data file to organize the electronic codes. Then we identified the five HRT tenets (i.e., humanistic value, pragmatism, immediacy/goal setting, empowerment, and community collaboration) in the data files. If a tenet was recognized in the discourse, it was listed in the column to the right that corresponded with that interview section. Once each data file was organized with respect to the metatheoretical framework, we began coding each data file. Before we discuss the steps we utilized in our analysis, we provide an overview of the qualitative coding process, from a grounded theory perspective.

Coding in Qualitative Research

First, when making sense of qualitative data, *grounded theory* starts with studying, scrutinizing, and defining the data to understand what it might mean (Charmaz, 2006). Coding, or defining what the data are about, is the first analytic step in this process. Strauss and Corbin (1998) called this process *open coding* and Charmaz (2002) referred to it as *initial coding*. Coding involves "naming segments of data with a label that simultaneously categorizes, summarizes, and accounts for each piece of data" (Charmaz, 2006, p. 43). In this first step, coding often is done by reading the text and coding line by line or incident by incident to identify potentially useful concepts (Bernard & Ryan, 2010; Charmaz, 2006). Since these initial codes are preliminary, it is important to remain open and if necessary, improve the fit of the codes to the data. The process of remaining open to the data involves continuous checking of codes or theorizing and defragmenting the text, which occurs after initial coding, during the focused coding and checking of the data (Bernard & Ryan, 2010).

Next, during theory-driven coding, we look for emerging themes from the participants' communication or expression of the elements of the proposed metatheory. During theory-driven coding, it is important to integrate examples of concepts and consider how the examples might be related to broader, more inclusive concepts, called categories. This method of categorizing involves the constant comparison method, which Glaser and Strauss (1967) argued is important in developing theory. Therefore, after initial, open coding, constant comparison, also called *theoretical* or *axial coding*, categories further emerge from the data and can be compared with the evolving theory or metatheory (Glaser, 1992; Glaser & Strauss, 1967; Lindlof & Taylor, 2002; Strauss, 1987). The *constant comparative method* can be used to isolate and refine themes, reflect on each theme, and examine whether it is similar to another theme that appeared previously, which stimulates the production of new themes (Bernard & Ryan, 2010). Moving from initial coding to focused coding to theoretical coding when data is compared allows us to pay special attention to the context, interaction, consequences, and other aspects that may influence the social processes being studied (Lindlof & Taylor, 2002). In our research project, a grounded theory approach and in particular, performing thematic analysis, coding, and constant comparison of the data, allowed for consideration of how harm reduction may function as a metatheory and guide the RHBM in influencing perceived motorcycle safety behaviors.

Finally, as the coded categories emerge, it is possible to begin linking categories together around a central category (Glaser & Strauss, 1967). During this process, the constant comparative method is used (Glaser, 1992; Glaser & Strauss, 1967; Lindlof & Taylor, 2002; Strauss, 1987) in addition to negative case analysis. *Negative case analysis* occurs when the researcher searches for cases that do not confirm the models or theoretical constructs (Lincoln & Guba, 1985). Basically, *grounded theory analysis* generates a model about whatever phenomenon the researcher is studying, while determining whether the model hangs together as interviews are conducted and analyzed (Bernard & Ryan, 2010). Now that we reviewed types of coding, we outline the steps used to code the harm reduction data in our study.

Coding Harm Reduction Interview Data

Based on the literature and definitions presented for the five HRT tenets, themes were identified and coded within each interview. Informed by Boyatzis's (1998) and Charmaz's (2006) instructions for developing theory-driven codes, we engaged in several steps provided in Research Project in Practice Illustration Figure 4.8. The illustration shows how we used the proposed metatheory to organize and analyze the data with respect to the RHBM.

In this section we discussed qualitative analysis and explained how our data set was analyzed, with an emphasis on theoretical inference. Our analysis of

Research in Practice Illustration
Example of Using Metatheory to Code Data

1. **Initial coding** occurred in which seven data files were analyzed both line by line and incident by incident to deductively derive codes.
2. After initial coding provided analytic direction, **focused coding** occurred in order to synthesize and further explain the data. Data files were reviewed to ensure fit within the initial codes developed previously and to further elaborate the code.
3. After focused coding, **theoretical coding** occurred in which each transcript was coded for the presence or absence of each of the five HRT tenets in possible behavior change when the components of the RHBM were used to engage participants in conversations. The theoretical codes further specified possible relationships between the categories developed during the focused coding stage.
4. Based on the initial, focused, and theoretical coding, a preliminary codebook was developed. Content of each data file was then reviewed to ensure fit within the code and to further elaborate the code.
5. This process was conducted for each tenet of HRT across each interview. Theoretical coding for each tenet sought to discover possible relationships between HRT and the RHBM, integrating the proposed metatheory with the theory.
6. Reliability of the coder and the code was determined.
7. Codes that emerged in the deductive analysis process were used to address the research questions, which asked in what ways HRT, in tandem with the RHBM, could guide conversational interviews with motorcyclists about their safety behaviors, particularly focusing on how the tenets of HRT emerged in these conversations.
8. Once all of the codes were finalized and defined with their respective themes a codebook was created.

Figure 4.8 Research in Practice Illustration: Example of Using Metatheory to Code Data.

data incorporated the use of metatheory to help organize and code the data files in an effort to address the research questions.

SUMMARY

In this chapter we continued to discuss our process of metatheory building in qualitative research methodology. After reading this chapter you should understand how we incorporated harm reduction metatheory to develop theory-driven research questions, an interview protocol, and analyze the data collected from in-depth interviews. Although we used motorcycle safety as a research illustration throughout this chapter, you can use literature and metatheory that complements your health or safety issue to inform your research questions, interview protocol, and data analysis. The next chapter highlights some of the results deduced from using harm reduction metatheory to inform qualitative interview methodology.

REFERENCES

Berg, B. L. (2004). *Qualitative research methods for the social sciences* (5th Ed.), Boston: Allyn and Bacon.

Bernard, H. R., & Ryan, G. W. (2010). *Analyzing qualitative data: Systematic approaches.* Thousand Oaks, CA: Sage Publications.
Boyatzis, R. E. (1998). *Transforming qualitative information: Thematic analysis and code development.* Thousand Oaks, London: Sage Publications.
Burawoy, M. (1991). *Ethnography unbound: Power and resistance in the modern metropolis.* Berkeley: University of California Press.
Charmaz, K. (2006). *Constructing grounded theory: A practical guide through qualitative analysis.* Thousand Oaks, CA: Sage Publications.
Charmaz, K. (2002). Qualitative interviewing and grounded theory analysis. In J.F. Gubrium and J.A. Holstein (Eds.), *Handbook of Interview Research* (pp. 675–694). Thousand Oaks, CA: Sage Publications.
Corbin, J., & Strauss, A. (2008). *Basics of qualitative research* (3rd Ed.). Thousand Oaks, CA: Sage.
Edwards, M. G. (2010). *Organisational transformation for sustainability: An integral metatheory.* New York: Taylor & Francis Group.
Glaser, B. (1992). *Basics of grounded theory analysis.* Mill Valley, CA: Sociology Press.
Glaser, B. G. & Strauss, A. L. (1967). *Discovery of grounded theory: Strategies for qualitative research.* Chicago, IL: Aldine.
Hermanowicz, J. C. (2002). The great interview: 25 strategies for studying people in bed. *Qualitative Sociology, 25*(4), 479–499.
Johnson, J. M., & Rowlands, T. (2012). The interpersonal dynamics of in-depth interviewing. In J.F. Gubrium, J.A. Holstein, A.B. Mavasti, & K.D. McKinney (Eds.). *The SAGE handbook of interview research: The complexity of the craft* (pp. 99–113). Thousand Oaks, CA: Sage.
King, N., & Horrocks, C. (2010). *Interviews in Qualitative Research.* Thousand Oaks, CA: Sage.
Lincoln, Y. S., & Guba, E. G. (1985). *Naturalistic inquiry.* Beverly Hills, CA: Sage.
Lindlof, T. R. & Taylor, B. C. (2002). *Qualitative communication research methods* (2nd Ed.). Thousand Oaks, CA: Sage.
Lofland, J., Snow, D., Anderson, L., & Lofland, L. H. (2006). *Analyzing social settings: A guide to qualitative observation and analysis* (4th Ed.). Canada: Wadsworth.
Mattson, M. (1999). Toward a reconcepualization of communication cues to action in the Health Belief Model: HIV testing counseling. *Communication Monographs, 66*, 240–263.
Mattson, M., & Basnyat, I. (2008). Infusing HIV test counseling practice with harm reduction theory: An integrated model for voluntary counseling and testing. In T. Edgar, S. Noar, & V. Freimuth (Eds.). *Communication perspectives for HIV/AIDS in the 21st century* (pp. 137–167). New York, NY: Lawrence Erlbaum Associates.
Marlatt, G. A. (1998). *Harm reduction: Pragmatic strategies for managing high-risk behaviors.* New York, NY: The Guilford Press.
Patton, M. Q. (2002). *Qualitative research and evaluation methods* (3rd Ed.). Thousand Oaks, CA: Sage.

Reid, R. J. (2002). Harm reduction and injection drug use: Pragmatic lessons from a public health model. *Health and Social Work, 27*(3), 223–226.

Rhodes, T., & Hedrich, D. (2010). Harm reduction and the mainstream. In T. Rhodes and D. Hedrich (10th Ed.), *European Monitoring Centre for Drugs and Drug Addiction Monographs: Harm reduction evidence, impacts, and challenges* (pp. 19–33).

Ross, T. P., Ross, L. T., Rahman, A., & Cataldo, S. (2010). The bicycle helmet attitudes scale: Using the health belief model to predict helmet use among undergraduates. *Journal of American College Health,* 59, 29–36.

Rubin, H. J., & Rubin, I. S. (2012). *Qualitative interviewing: The art of hearing data.* (4th Ed.). Thousand Oaks, CA: Sage.

Rubin, H. J., & Rubin, I. S. (2011). *Qualitative interviewing: The art of hearing data* (3rd ed). Thousand Oaks, CA: Sage.

Spradley, J. P. (1979). *The ethnographic interview.* New York, NY: Holt, Rinehart, and Winston.

Stage, C. W., & Mattson, M. (2003). Ethnographic interviewing as contextualized conversation. In R.P. Clair *Expressions of ethnography: Novel approaches to qualitative methods* (pp. 97–105). Albany: State University of New York.

Strauss, A. (1987). *Qualitative analysis for social scientists.* Cambridge, England: Cambridge University Press.

Strauss, A., & Corbin, J. (1998). *Basics of qualitative research: Grounded theory procedures and techniques* (2nd Ed.). Thousand Oaks, CA: Sage Publications.

Stronach, B. (2003). Alcohol and harm reduction. In E. Buning, M. Gorgullo, A.G. Melcop, and P. O'Hare (Eds.), *Alcohol and harm education: an innovative approach for countries in transition* (pp. 27–34). Amsterdam, ICAHRE.

Tanno, D. V., & Jandt, F. (1994). Redefining the "other" in multicultural research. *Howard Journal of Communication, 5,* 36–45.

Watzlawick, P. (1984). *The invented reality: How do we know what we know? Contributions to constructivism.* New York: W. W. Norton.

Wengraf, T. (2001). *Qualitative research interviewing: Biographic narrative and semi-structured methods.* Thousand Oaks, CA: Sage.

World Health Organization, Health and Welfare Canada, Canadian Public Health Association (1986). Ottawa Charter for Health Promotion, WHO, Copenhagen.

Yin, R. K. (2011). *Qualitative research from start to finish.* New York, NY: Guilford Press.

Chapter 5

Qualitative Analysis Informed by Harm Reduction Metatheory

Implications for Motorcycle Safety

In the previous chapter we continued to discuss our proposed harm reduction metatheory and how this metatheory can be studied through qualitative research methodology. Specifically, we showcased how we incorporated harm reduction tenets with another health behavior theory to better understand motorcycle safety attitudes and behaviors. Besides providing guidance about ways to integrate harm reduction into health and safety research, we also showcased how a metatheory can be incorporated to develop theory-driven research questions, an interview protocol, and analyze the data collected from in-depth interviews. This chapter extends our discussion of the utility of harm reduction as a metatheory into the realm of evaluation by highlighting some of the results deduced from using harm reduction metatheory to inform qualitative interview methodology. This chapter is guided by the following objectives:

- A review of sampling in qualitative research
- Integrating harm reduction metatheory into the write-up of results
- Implications for motorcycle safety from using a harm reduction metatheoretical framework
- Participants' use of harm reduction metatheory to inform the researcher

Before reporting the results of our research project, we address the topic of sampling in qualitative research and highlight the sample of at-risk motorcyclists we recruited and interviewed.

SAMPLING IN QUALITATIVE RESEARCH

When conceptualizing a research project, sampling strategies need to be considered and written into the final results of the study (Denzin & Lincoln, 2011).

In qualitative research, people are referred to as *sampling units* that are recruited to help answer the research question(s) (Lindlof & Taylor, 2002). Unlike with quantitative samples, we cannot make statistical generalizations from qualitative samples. However, because qualitative samples can be used to make analytical inferences and transferability of findings to address research questions (Miles & Huberman, 1994), the importance of recruiting an unbiased sample and collecting data until saturation is reached should not be underestimated. According to Firestone (1993), if conducted correctly qualitative sampling can provide the opportunity to understand new or existing theory and allow researchers to make inferences about the larger population of interest to the project.

Several types of sampling exist. Common sampling strategies include purposeful sampling, theory-based sampling, convenience sampling, and snowball sampling (for typology of sampling strategies see Miles & Huberman, 1994, Figure 2.6). However, two types of sampling in qualitative research are particularly common: theoretical sampling and purposive sampling. *Theoretical sampling* finds examples of theoretical constructs with the expectation that the data collected can aide in the generation and expansion of theory (Denzin & Lincoln, 2011; Glaser & Strauss, 1967; Kuzel, 1992; Pattson, 1990). Purposive sampling is utilized when the research topic is informed by preexisting data on which research questions were based. Regardless of the type of sampling procedure utilized in your research project, there are some similarities that exist across sampling strategies. A meta-analysis of the literature pointed out some of these parallels (Curtis, Gesler, Smith, & Washburn, 2000). Some of the key points of parallel included that qualitative samples often are small but intensely studied, conceptually driven, reflexive and detailed about basis for case selection, and designed for analytic generalizations rather than statistical generalizations (p. 1002). In addition, Miles and Huberman (1994, p. 34) proposed six characteristics of qualitative sampling strategies:

Features of Qualitative Samples

- Be relevant to the conceptual framework and the research questions.
- Generate rich information about the phenomena being studied.
- Produce believable explanations and descriptions of the research topic (this relates to reliability of the data).
- Produce transferability of findings.
- Be conducted in an ethical manner.
- Contain a feasible recruiting plan in terms of participant accessibility.

One of the sampling strategies we utilized for our research project about motorcycle safety is known as purposive sampling. *Purposive sampling* occurs when samples are chosen with a specific intention (Yin, 2011).

When selecting participants using purposive sampling, it is important to obtain a variety of information and perspectives pertaining to the research topic, meaning that participants, who may offer differing views, need to be enlisted (Kuzel, 1992). Utilizing purposive sampling methods and recruiting a wide range of cases is one way to help avoid bias in your research project (Yin, 2011).

Maximum variation sampling, a type of purposive sampling, is a common form of recruitment in qualitative research in which the researcher attempts to find participants with a wide range of characteristics and experiences (Lindlof & Taylor, 2002). Then, among these diverse backgrounds, the researcher tries to identify noteworthy, common patterns (Kuzel, 1992; Patton, 1990). This sampling technique aims to "discover the diversity or range of the phenomena of interest and provides a useful antidote to error and bias that emanate from singular research roles or role relationships by pushing the researcher to consider ways of looking beyond the most convenient contexts or those to which his role grants him primary access" (Lofland et al., 2006, p. 93).

Besides purposive sampling, we also referenced *convenience sampling* in our project, which often is preferred because it utilizes cases that are easily available and accessible (Yin, 2011). Researchers also use *snowball sampling* to identify potential cases from research participants and others who make suggestions of additional people who may have rich information to share with the researchers (Lindlof & Taylor, 2002; Patton, 1990).

We continue our discussion of sampling in qualitative research by returning to our research project and detailing how we recruited the sample of at-risk motorcyclists for our study.

Harm Reduction Motorcycle Safety Research Sample

We used a maximum sampling variation strategy, purposeful sampling, to recruit participants because it is an appropriate technique to learn about variation across a set of cases (Lofland et al., 2006). Although other types of purposeful sampling exist (e.g., random purposeful, stratified purposeful), this type of maximum variation sampling allowed us to "study a representative subsection of a precisely defined population in order to make inferences about the whole population" (Arber, 1993, p. 38). This sampling technique provided an advantage because it allowed us to recruit a wide range of cases, including motorcyclists who were younger, older, male, female, novice, intermediate, and experienced, all operating a variety of motorcycles. This range of cases facilitated a comprehensive understanding of motorcyclists' subgroup patterns (Patton, 2002). Therefore, this sampling technique was useful for the target audience of motorcyclists, who have individual habits and experiences while they collectively ride motorcycles.

Participants in our study, which was designed to assess the feasibility of the proposed harm reduction metatheory, were motorcyclists who practiced higher-risk behaviors while driving a motorcycle. The same qualifiers were applied to each participant. *Risky motorcycling behaviors* were identified from a survey that is conducted by the Motorcycle Safety Campaign on Purdue University's campus and community. This survey assesses risks motorcyclists engage in before or during motorcycle rides. All participants identified themselves as an at-risk motorcyclist based on the following qualifications:

- Regularly does not wear a helmet while driving a motorcycle
- Regularly wears minimal or no safety gear while driving a motorcycle
- Regularly speeds while driving a motorcycle
- Regularly consumes alcohol before driving a motorcycle
- Has been in at least one near-miss motorcycle crash or has been in a motorcycle crash

If motorcyclists reported engaging in at least one of these five qualifying behaviors, they were eligible to participate in an interview. Besides the qualifiers, the only other condition necessary for participation was that the motorcyclist be a resident of Indiana. Currently, Indiana does not have a law requiring adults riding a motorcycle to wear a helmet. Participants from states that do have a law requiring adults riding a motorcycle to wear a helmet may have revealed very different safety attitudes and behaviors.

Thirty-seven motorcyclists participated in an interview. Of the 37 motorcyclists who participated in the study, twenty-nine ($n = 29$) were male and eight ($n = 8$) were female. The participants ranged in age from 18 to 70 ($M = 40.5$ years). The average number of years participants had been riding a motorcycle was 17.5, with a range of six months to 54 years. Participants from the sample were residents of 13 different cities within nine counties throughout Indiana. Table 5.1 further details the demographics of the sample.

Data from motorcyclists were collected until theoretical saturation was achieved. *Theoretical saturation* is achieved when "we cease to be surprised by what we observe or we notice that our concepts and propositions

Table 5.1 Participant Demographics

Demographic	*n*	*n*
Gender	Female = **8**	Male = **29**
Age	≤30 = **13**	≥31 = **24**
Years Riding	0–10 = **18**	≥11 = **19**
Motorcycle Type	Harley-Davidson (or similar type) = **19**	Crotch rocket (or similar type) = **18**

are not disconfirmed as we continue to add new data" (Lindlof & Taylor, 2002, p. 129). Besides being a matter of no new data, however, saturation also denotes the development of themes, including variations, theory building, and identifying relationships between concepts (Corbin & Strauss, 2008). *Saturation* helps determine the sample size for a study because "sampling is terminated when no new information is forthcoming from new sampled units; thus redundancy is the primary criterion" (Lincoln & Guba, 1985, p. 202). The researcher determines when saturation is achieved based on the ability to return to the data and find redundancy in themes and examples that are repeated (Corbin & Strauss, 2008). Now that you know more about the sample for our research project, we will briefly discuss the process of reporting the results from a harm reduction qualitative data analysis.

A REVIEW OF WRITING RESULTS OF A QUALITATIVE RESEARCH PROJECT

So far we discussed several phases of instigating a qualitative research project to enhance the utility of HRT, in particular. The longest phase of a qualitative research project often comes after data analysis, when it is time to present your interpretation of the data in writing. Your analysis of the data may be impeccable but if you cannot present sections of your data to tell a story, it will be difficult to advance your responses to your research questions. Because there are not many examples of reporting harm reduction qualitative data, and no examples that report harm reduction data from a metatheoretical lens, we present useful tips for reporting results and then present some of the results of our harm reduction motorcycle safety qualitative analysis to elucidate these tips. Our focus is on writing results in a way that can connect qualitative data, theory, and harm reduction metatheory. However, depending on your research questions, your writing may have a different focus and thus other literature may provide more specific direction for reporting your results. First, we provide a brief review of writing results for qualitative research projects.

After analyzing the data from your interviews, you will most likely find yourself surrounded by numerous quotes from participants. It may be hard to choose which quotes to include in a final report of your study. However, keep in mind that data not used in your report still served a crucial purpose—validating the results of your study. In addition, it is possible that you may return to the data and use it in a later report or publication. In the meantime, however, Lindlof and Taylor (2002) suggested selecting data points that "clearly reflect the nature and scope of your claims; that is, data should clearly embody the phenomenon that forms the objective of the claim"

(p. 296). Accordingly, when reporting the results of our research study, we emphasize the ways in which the tenets of HRT functioned as a metatheory throughout the interviews.

In addition, it is important to report data points from a variety of participants, especially if you interviewed participants at various times, places, and of different demographics. This rich and varied representation of the data helps further validate and express your interpretations of the data (Katz, 2001). Katz also suggested including revealing and colorful data to show what may not be obvious to others. You will notice in the reporting of our results that we utilize quotes from almost all of our participants, regardless of the vocabulary they used during the interview, in part to depict aspects of the motorcycling culture that other people do not always experience or understand. By revealing some of the more vivid responses, readers are able to better understand concerns that motorcyclists have about their own safety and reasons why they may have developed risky driving patterns. As a result, we can better express and aid others in understanding the phenomena being studied.

Now that you know some ways of choosing what data you want to report, the next issue is presenting the data. Several researchers have provided strategies to organize and present data from a qualitative research project. The most common strategy of reporting results is to present results in codes and themes and sometimes subthemes that emerged during the data analysis (Lindlof & Taylor, 2002). Miles and Huberman (1994) suggested organizing and displaying the data in diagrams or another visual depiction in an effort to make it easier for readers to see these themes and patterns. In our case, we utilized a spreadsheet to visually organize the data by code and theme. In addition, we color-coded each participant to ensure participant representation across the codes and themes. We utilized this spreadsheet to help us identify themes within a particular research question but then subsequently, these data sheets helped us see connections among the five tenets of HRT and how these overarching tenets served as guidance throughout the whole interview. In addition, separate versions of these data sheets were cleaned and edited (refer to Haas, 2012) so readers could further reference topics that were discussed during the debriefing of the results.

Once the data is organized, there are several ways in which you can present the data in writing. Lofland et al. (2006) advised writing an outline to help organize your ideas, with the understanding that your final product may vastly differ from your original intentions. In our case, we were trying to determine the relationship(s) between the data we collected and the proposed harm reduction metatheory. According to Lindlof (2001), the writing must join the analysis of the data to the theory, which in turn, produces conclusions and implications of the research. Lindlof continued to describe this process of "analytic synthesis," in which we must return to the research questions that guided the study and support how the data informs and strengthens the theory (p. 91). Therefore, you will see in our presentation of the data the ways in which motorcyclists' responses supported the application of the five tenets of HRT as overarching, metatheoretical tenets that could guide qualitative interviews while strengthening theoretical application. Examples of how we reported the results and the impact of the results on the application of HRT as a metatheory are reported in the next section.

RESULTS FROM QUALITATIVE DATA ANALYSIS INFORMED BY HARM REDUCTION METATHEORY

In this section, we show how concepts and themes surrounding motorcycle safety are related to harm reduction as a metatheoretical framework. In Chapter 4 you read how we engaged participants in the metatheory during the interview. We were able to engage each harm reduction tenet to converse with participants. Specifically, humanistic value informed cues to action, pragmatism informed perceived benefits and barriers, immediacy/goal setting informed perceived susceptibility and severity, empowerment informed self-efficacy, and community collaboration informed formative research and audience analysis to encourage dialogue about environmental barriers and influential communicators.

After using a particular tenet of harm reduction to introduce the purpose of each interview section, participants openly discussed their personal reasons and justifications for changing or maintaining their personal safety behaviors while driving a motorcycle. The dialogue that occurred during the interviews illustrated that engaging harm reduction tenets during conversations with participants encouraged us to listen to motorcyclists to understand why and how they practice risky motorcycling behaviors. Below, we report the results from RQ1a–RQ1e to illustrate how a proposed metatheoretical tenet of harm reduction can inform a component of the Reconceptualized Health Belief Model (*RHBM*) in qualitative research methodology. You will see how we reported some results of this qualitative study, both in terms of supporting the generation of harm reduction as a metatheory and enhancing the use of the components of RHBM in health and safety research. Because there is not enough space to discuss all of the results for each research question and the codes and themes that emerged within each research question, we provide interview excerpts, to showcase how harm reduction functioned as a metatheory and how the results provide a more positive tone around harm reduction in future research projects.

Harm Reduction Humanistic Value as a Metatheoretical Tenet

Research Question 1a asked in what ways the HRT tenet humanistic value informs the RHBM component cues to action to encourage motorcyclists to discuss their current safety behaviors while driving a motorcycle (for a list of the research questions refer to Research in Practice Illustration 4.1). Appendix A shows the codes and themes that emerged during this portion of the interviews. Throughout this segment of the interview, risky behaviors that motorcyclists engaged in were recognized, not criticized, and probed to help us learn more about the risky behaviors and if any cues, including interpersonal communication, mass media communication, or policies, ever prompted participants to question their personal safety choices and assess if a change in behavior was necessary.

Several cues to action were discussed, some having more influence in raising participants' awareness to think about and later initiate a change in their personal safety behaviors. Specifically, participants discussed their family, non-motorcyclists, and fellow motorcyclists as cues that caused them to reflect on personal safety behaviors. Participants also stated that media, helmet laws, and knowing someone who was almost killed in a motorcycle crash prompted some form of behavior change. Six codes and several themes emerged during our discussion with at-risk motorcyclists. Following we highlight some ways that the tenet humanistic value informed participants' specific cues to practice both safer and riskier behaviors, with a focus on family and friends of motorcyclists who both drive and do not drive a motorcycle as the cue to action.

Non-critical Communication from Motorcyclist Family Members as a Safety Cue

Family members who also drive motorcycles were referenced throughout the interviews as being influential and, in most cases, a positive cue to action for participants to practice safer behaviors. Many participants reported that a majority of their family members ride a motorcycle and subsequently indicated that they became a motorcyclist because their family member, often a father, brother, or uncle, was a motorcyclist. Examples are provided in the following interview excerpts, indicating first that family participation in motorcycling may be a factor in next of kin becoming a motorcyclist and then subsequently, support from family members had a positive impact on safety behaviors when participants started riding a motorcycle.

> Participant 29 Excerpt: "I've just always been attracted to it. Ya know it's a really, you could argue that it's a family thing, that both my brothers and my father, we all rode, or they all rode and I always wanted a motorcycle."

> Participant 23 Excerpt: "Yeah, I mean my mom when she talks to me about it I'm like okay mom, I understand but it's not as serious as my dad's [advice] would be because he's ridden and he's . . . actually he rode that bike too so he knows how to handle it more and actually drive it and what to look out for and stuff like that."

> Participant 35 Excerpt: ". . . every time they're [parents] always telling me, just reminding me to watch out for other drivers, watch out for sand pockets on turns, and anything like that. And just to always watch your blind spots and everybody else."

These excerpts indicate that having a motorcyclist in the family can be a positive source of support because these individuals recognize the challenges involved with riding a motorcycle and maintaining personal safety while on the road.

Although not all participants indicated that their family members who ride a motorcycle had as great an impact as those participants who cited taking a motorcycle safety course and wearing a helmet in response to family influence, a majority of participants made some of their decisions based on advice from family. For example, one participant stated that since his brother wears boots, it is probably a good idea to start wearing boots while riding his motorcycle (Participant 11). Overall, based on the responses coded within this theme it became apparent that family members who ride a motorcycle have the opportunity to serve as a nonjudgmental source who can provide expert advice to other motorcyclists in their family. Next we highlight examples in reference to the various ways that critical communication of fellow motorcyclists can cue riskier behaviors.

Critical Communication from Fellow Motorcyclists as a Cue to Risky Driving

Using humanistic value to inform participants' cues to action, the fellow motorcyclist, who was not a family member, emerged as a source who influenced personal safety choices. Although family members modeled and encouraged safer behaviors for their kin to follow, fellow motorcyclists did not always promote safer behaviors for others to follow and instead, cued riskier behaviors through peer pressure and negative judgments of the motorcyclist, or by being a passive bystander in a dangerous situation. Examples of these risky cues to action are summarized in the selected themes that follow.

The first of these themes is keeping up with the group mentality. Participants discussed peer pressure from other motorcyclists and continued to say that they succumb to peer pressure, pressure others, or try to avoid the group-riding environment altogether so they do not encounter an uncomfortable situation. The following excerpts showcase the motorcycling cultures within various motorcycling groups and the pressure that exists among peers who ride motorcycles together. Because of the presence of peer pressure in the motorcycling culture, changing behaviors was deemed an unrealistic barrier to overcome by several participants.

> Participant 3 Excerpt: "So initially when I'm flying down, well with the wheelie up like guys are doing because you know you have to do that or you're not a guy. You're just a punk, you're scared, you don't wanna be a chicken. It's just a whole mentality. You know I mean it sounds stupid and I'm telling you right now . . . me telling you about it . . . I feel like, 'Dang he's stupid, what would he do that for?' But at the same time ya know, you have to do it. I know it sounds stupid. It's like a fraternity. You have to do it because you wanna . . . you wanna be in the group. Ya know there are always choices but then again there's not. It's peer pressure. Ya know even if you're an adult it's just as bad as when you're a kid. Ya know, truly it is. Probably more so."

> Participant 12 Excerpt:
> P12: Most people I ride with don't wear a helmet.
> E: Okay. So if you started to wear a helmet would they um, give you a hard time?
> P12: Yes.
> E: What would they say?
> P12: (Pausing/smirking) (10.0).
> E: You can be honest.
> P12: They'd call me a pussy.
> E: Okay.
> P12: They'd tell me to give up my man card.
> E: Okay.
> P12: Cause the people I bike with, we're like the outlaws, the Hells Angels. We usually don't wear helmets.

However, some participants felt confident enough to let the group go ahead with their riskier behaviors while they hung back. This coping tactic was shared particularly by female participants who rode motorcycles. For example, one female participant continued to ride with groups but specifically stopped riding in male-dominant groups because of the peer pressure males put on females to keep up during group rides. She stated, "Males do because they get a rush from it. Um your perception and speed changes so they like that rush. We're not trying to have that rush" (Participant 1).

Another related theme within this code regarding negative peer influence emerged from participants describing the group in which they ride as practicing the same behaviors together, regardless of whether the behaviors are safe or risky, although the behaviors usually are riskier rather than safer. For instance, one participant said, "But just riding around town and out in the country, I like the no helmet thing. And that's, that's the way my buddies are, all the same thing." (Participant 28). This example illustrates the response received from older, more experienced motorcyclists including the following: "Everyone was naked. We discussed about the helmets and uh no one liked them and uh I think we were all just too young to realize it" (Participant 27). This participant indicated that although they all talked about helmets together, no one initiated the behavior to start wearing a helmet and in response, no one wore a helmet. Participants also described risky behaviors engaged in as a group other than wearing a helmet. One participant, who described himself as a regular drinker during motorcycle rides, said "They're, they're wild, they're outta control. They drink, they ya know, whatever you can think of is what they do" (Participant 30).

Lastly, another similar theme surfaced that indicated passive support for risky behaviors motorcyclists practice when participants commented that everyone who rides a motorcycle knows the risks involved with riding and it is not anyone else's role to say something about the choices that other motorcyclists make. Instead, choices should be left to the discretion of each individual motorcyclist. As a result of motorcyclists believing in personal choice, motorcyclists may choose not to share their opinion with a fellow rider. Participants continued to say that the motorcycling culture promotes freedom of choice, such as, "We live in a free country so you're free to act in any way you want as long as you're not hurting anyone else" (Participant 3). Similarly, Participant 13 said, "There's a law out there that says 'let those who ride decide,'" emphasizing the aspect of individual choice.

Participants indicated that everyone who rides a motorcycle should know the risks involved and therefore, safety does not really need to be discussed. For example, one participant said, "No it's all understood. So you don't really talk about it ya know we understand that it's a risk but we still take it" (Participant 6). Therefore, since motorcyclists should know the risks involved in motorcycling and they are given the right to choose a majority of their safety behaviors, participants concluded by saying anything that happens to a motorcyclist is their fault because of the choices they made given the risks of riding a motorcycle. The following interview excerpt serves as an example.

> Participant 23 Excerpt: "I've heard so many stories about people wearing no gear and riding and stuff like that. I guess it's just up to that person. What they wanna wear that day; if they get into an accident I guess it's their fault then for not wearing the right stuff. So it's their opinion and what they wanna wear."

This same thought process was expressed by participants throughout the interviews, including Participant 8 who said, ". . . Well the less you wear if something happens that's kinda your own fault."

Throughout this section we discussed the influence fellow motorcyclists have on safety behaviors. There were two predominant reasons provided during the interviews regarding why motorcyclists listen to the advice of fellow motorcyclists. This is where participants began using the concept of humanistic value to offer feedback to us for promoting behavior change among this target audience. First, participants indicated that fellow motorcyclists who gave advice were usually older and more experienced riders. Participants stated that, because of their experience and, in some cases, flawless motorcycling record, they trusted and respected the advice. The following example depicts this notion.

> Participant 30 Excerpt: "I'm always rebellious but when it comes to the people that I talk to, they are people that have ridden for a long time. Longer than me, so I listen to them. Cause they're still alive. It's either luck or skill and I'm not gonna take my chances, I'll listen."

This participant stated that he usually is rebellious when other people try to provide him with motorcycle riding tips and motorcycle safety tips. However, when he started discussing the advice that his fellow, more experienced motorcyclists, provide the dynamic changed. He cited luck or skill as the reason why those motorcyclists are still alive and just in case it was by skill, he was going to listen to their advice. Therefore, motorcyclists who are considered experienced, or even intermediate, may be able to positively influence another motorcyclist's safety behaviors more readily than a non-motorcyclist, risky motorcyclist, or novice motorcyclist. This group of motorcyclists plays an important role in intervening to reduce the negative consequences some motorcyclists may experience during risky motorcycle rides.

However, just being an experienced motorcyclist does not automatically mean advice will be welcomed and followed by others. The second reason mentioned among participants for listening to a fellow motorcyclist was due to the way the advice was provided. Participants indicated that if another person was rude or critical when talking to them, they probably would not listen. The following interview excerpt provides one example of this response.

> Participant 7 Excerpt: "The Harley owners group really stresses the helmets and the safety gear at every meeting. Even though it's not a law in Indiana they required it or asked everybody to wear helmets. We have a safety director and he might come up and say something to us. Ya know like, 'I see you don't have your helmet today', or ya know but that, like I said, was years ago. Now we wear them all the time. Years ago they did make a mention of it when we didn't have it."

Participant 7 indicated that the safety director would often say something to the motorcyclists who were not wearing a helmet. And although he did not always require a helmet, since it is a personal choice and that may have caused some motorcyclists to completely reject the advice, the director at least cued the motorcyclists to think about that specific behavior and perhaps contemplate whether or not they should wear a helmet for the ride that day.

In this summary of results that utilized the tenet humanistic value as metatheoretical guidance, we found that the way fellow motorcyclists communicate with motorcyclists can serve as a positive or negative cue to adopt safer behaviors. For additional codes and respective themes, refer to Appendix A, which showcases the relationship between the metatheoretical tenet humanistic value and the theoretical component cues to action. In the next section, we utilize several of the themes that emerged to showcase the potential of humanistic value as a metatheoretical tenet in qualitative research methodology.

Humanistic Value as a Metatheoretical Tenet in Qualitative Harm Reduction Research

The importance of humanistic value was brought up repeatedly as participants discussed motorcycle safety cues to action they receive. Achieving saturation among participants who stated that they are safer due to the influence of other motorcyclists, or that they are the ones who influence other motorcyclists to be safer, indicates the cyclical nature of cues to action in harm reduction health and safety research and the importance of intervening and noncritically communicating with risky individuals to initiate changes in personal safety behaviors.

Although several types of cues to action were discussed during the interviews, we feature two to demonstrate how humanistic value informed this portion of the interviews. First, family members who ride motorcycles had a strong influence on other motorcyclists' safety behaviors. This influence is most likely because participants described their family members as being experienced, credible, and supportive. These motorcyclists/family members acknowledge that the motorcyclist is engaging in a risky behavior and rather than criticizing, they try to offer supportive advice.

Fellow motorcyclists also can influence motorcyclists' safety behaviors. For example, participants described the effect a crash of another motorcyclist had on their desire to change safety behaviors. Participants stated that other motorcyclists simply described the in-depth content of what happened during their crashes and that was enough to make them second-guess their current behaviors. The person who was in a crash did not lecture the participant to start wearing a helmet, probably because this individual, like many motorcyclists, respect motorcyclists' rights to make their own decisions, as the tenet humanistic value indicates (Mattson & Basnyat, 2008). Instead, the crash victim respected the participant while discussing their personal experiences as a result of engaging in risky driving behaviors. However, the results that surfaced during this portion of the interviews indicated that more often than not, fellow motorcyclists remain silent and allow fellow motorcyclists to make their own decisions, or pressure motorcyclists to engage in riskier behaviors than they would if riding alone. To counter this, not judging a fellow motorcyclist for their decision to be safer, or even encouraging safer behaviors while driving their motorcycle, is important for facilitating and maintaining safer behaviors among this target population.

Participants often mentioned that they do not adhere to the advice of certain people or media messages because of how that message or advice is provided. When asked how they respond to the advice other people provided, participants often said that it depends how people talk to them. They continued to say that if the advice or message is negative, judgmental, not supportive, or critical of them and their behaviors, they won't think twice about what the person or message said. This action especially was illustrated when discussing the influence of non-motorcyclists and safety messages in the media. Participants indicated that presenting safety advice in a nonjudgmental, noncritical way, just as the HRT tenet humanistic value advises, is an important consideration when cueing other motorcyclists to think about their personal safety behaviors.

Overall, the results of our research project indicate that when communicating with motorcyclists, being respectful of the motorcyclists' current behavior choices is critical and humanistic value can be used to guide accurate, welcomed cues to action for motorcyclists. Humanistic value can serve as initial recognition of the risky driving behaviors that motorcyclists may participate in on the road. Instead of criticizing these risky behaviors, however, results demonstrate that developing encouraging, respectful cues to action that strive to raise awareness about safety choices and behaviors may be well received by risky motorcyclists.

To see all of the codes and themes that emerged during this portion of the interview, refer to Appendix A. These additional patterns also support the notion that cues to action, regardless of communication type and medium, can be more targeted when guided by the harm reduction tenet humanistic value. Next, we offer some results from the next research question.

Harm Reduction Pragmatism as a Metatheoretical Tenet

In our project, Research Question 1b asked in what ways the HRT metatheoretical tenet pragmatism informs the RHBM component perceived benefits and perceived barriers to encourage motorcyclists to discuss their current safety behaviors while driving a motorcycle. Throughout this portion of the interview participants were probed to discuss perceived barriers to practicing safer behaviors while driving a motorcycle in addition to personal, perceived benefits of practicing safer behaviors while driving a motorcycle. Throughout the discussion of perceived barriers to and perceived benefits of practicing safer behaviors, being realistic about what participants have more and less control over in order to reduce their risks while driving a motorcycle was recognized. This recognition of realistic behavior change, depending on the barriers a motorcyclist experiences while driving a motorcycle, helped us probe and learn more about what participants perceived having control over when it comes to assessing and changing their safety behaviors.

Throughout the interviews, several perceived barriers to and perceived benefits of safety behaviors were discussed, some having more of an influence on participants' ability to initiate and potentially sustain a change in their personal safety behaviors. Specifically, participants discussed their perceived barriers to wearing safety gear, perceived barriers to driving defensively and maintaining personal safety on the road, and their previous and/or current age as a perceived barrier to being safer while driving a motorcycle. Motorcyclists also indicated that they continue to take chances while driving a motorcycle or are complacent with their current, risky behaviors because they do not perceive barriers on the roadways to negatively impact their safety. Finally, participants discussed the perceived benefits that exist as a result of safer motorcycling behaviors. Seven patterns emerged within the pragmatism guiding perceived barriers and perceived benefits discourse. Appendix B includes the seven codes and their themes, a definition, and example from an interview to provide a more in-depth description of each code and respective theme. We highlight a couple of the patterns that emerged during the interviews, with an emphasis on the functionality of pragmatism as a metatheoretical tenet in qualitative harm reduction research. We start by discussing a pattern that emerged regarding participants owning but not wearing their safety gear during motorcycle rides.

Owning but Not Wearing Safety Gear

Participants discussed several reasons and barriers that contribute to them wearing minimal or no safety gear, or being riskier in general, while driving a motorcycle. First, participants identified who they ride their motorcycle with as a contributing factor to whether or not they wear safety gear. This theme was consistent with a general code that emerged within the humanistic value guiding cues to action discourse. Participants continued to describe the pressure of living up to the mystique of being a motorcyclist by riding in groups and not wearing safety gear as a part of that group's expectation. Throughout the interviews participants commonly stated that when riding with a group "you try showin' off" (Participant 23). Other participants' experiences are reported in the following excerpts.

> Participant 29 Excerpt: ". . . a part of peer pressure is living up to the mystique of riding motorcycles. And they think that a helmet doesn't fit into the live to ride, ride to live sort of mentality. I've spoken to my sister repeatedly. I've said, 'listen, you need to wear a helmet ya know, why don't you wear a helmet?' and um and that's how I got on the subject with her that she said, 'well none of my friends do.'"

> Participant 20 Excerpt: "I've had some of them tell me that I ride a little slow. Oh yeah. Because when you ride in a group and you got somebody that's going 70 at the front and you got somebody who wants to do 60 at the back, but they have to do 65 or 70 to stay with the pack. I mean that's just the way it works. Or you ride by yourself."

Feedback during this section of the interview overlapped with some of the patterns that emerged in Research Question 1a about fellow motorcyclists' influence. Participants continued to mention the role peer pressure from other motorcyclists has on the risky behaviors they engage in while driving a motorcycle. Participants indicated that members of a group tend to push each other beyond their abilities. The following interview excerpt provides an example.

> Participant 24 Excerpt: "Well I think peer pressure is one of the biggest things, when they're in with the wrong group. Particularly when you're mixing alcohol I think that's a lot of peer pressure. And speeding or riding above their abilities is peer pressure; trying to keep up with somebody who's obviously a lot better than you are."

Since the role of peer pressure and the influence of other motorcyclists were mentioned again within the pragmatism discourse, it is evident that the impact motorcyclists have on each other's behaviors is strong and, in some cases, can negatively impact safety behaviors, as this theme demonstrates.

Another theme within this section of the interview, the cool factor, further supported this point. The cool factor emerged during interviews when participants indicated that safety gear is not cool or fashionable enough to wear while riding a motorcycle, making it less desirable to wear. A majority of participants brought up looking cool as a significant barrier to wearing safety gear. For example, Participant 33 said it is all about "Being cool. As silly as that sounds I really think that's one of the things that causes people to be risky." Similarly, Participant 22 said, "It's about what the, what the helmet looks like. If somebody thinks it looks stupid or it's not cool, they're not gonna wear it. That's mainly what it is." Other participants' comments follow.

> Participant 34 Excerpt: "Uh the number one barrier would be that they just don't think it's cool. Ya know they're riding a motorcycle to be free and they like to feel that wind in their face and through their hair. Some of us don't have hair. Um but honestly I think it's more of uh ya know, I'm doing this, I'm a rebel type deal. I just think some people are ya know, what's the phrase . . . too cool for school. So they're, they're just gonna be that rebel."

> Participant 31 Excerpt: "I think the biggest one is just because they don't think it's cool I guess or something. I know that sounds kinda cliché but um I honestly think that's the biggest one they just, they see a lot of the more popular people who do own motorcycles and they typically don't wear helmets. They try to fit in with the bigger crowd and they just kind of throw the safety part out of the window."

Even participants that did wear a helmet or other safety gear specifically referenced their helmet as cool, making it easier to wear. For example, one motorcyclist said, "I ride more with groups and nobody wears a helmet. I'm the only one who wears a helmet. It doesn't bother me a bit. I have skulls on my helmet so I'm fine" (Participant 30).

Some participants went on to state that it may be possible to overcome this barrier by developing and promoting more stylish safety gear. For example, one participant made the following suggestion:

> Participant 21 Excerpt: "I mean it doesn't look as cool to wear all the safety gear. Although to be honest lately a lot of the safety gear as become a lot more stylish and I think that helps. People aren't gonna wear it if it looks like you're wearing PPE from a factory or something ya know if you're wearing some really ugly stuff. But as the safety gear becomes more stylish I think that more people will wear it."

This theme demonstrates the impact that being cool and fitting in with the general motorcycling culture has on safety behaviors. However, some participants indicated that if safety gear was more fashionable and perhaps marketed as cooler and more stylish, it may be easier for the benefits of wearing safety gear to outweigh the barriers, making wearing safety gear a realistic goal for motorcyclists to practice while driving a motorcycle. Another overarching code we highlight is motorcyclists' voluntarily making risky choices while driving their motorcycle, due to their perceptions of low susceptibility to crashes and invincibility on the road.

Taking a Chance

Another pattern within the pragmatism guiding perceived barriers and perceived benefits discourse was participants knowingly taking certain risks while driving their motorcycles. Participants often rationalized their participation in these risky behaviors by saying that it is fun, and in some cases, worth the risk. This code was characterized by four themes.

One theme that emerged within this respective code was drinking and riding. This theme emerged as participants either described their current drinking behaviors while driving a motorcycle or the negative consequences that occurred as a result of drinking while driving their motorcycle. Most participants acknowledged that the benefits involved with drinking and driving a motorcycle are minimal and that, because the risks of drinking and driving a motorcycle are so great, they try to keep their consumption to a minimum.

> Participant 36 Excerpt: "Oh drinking. Not to the point where you're drunk but still. If you've had even a few beers it's gonna affect, ya know affect your reaction time and stuff like that. We've all been there. I try not to do it but sometimes it happens."

> Participant 27 Excerpt: "Stopping for a couple beers with a few guys and not thinking that a couple beers would make any difference. Ya know just one or two, just changes it. There's something there. And I, I own a boat and I never drink on it, ever. And I see people on boats drink all the time. Stuff happens too fast on boats and it happens too fast on motorcycles. So I learned that and uh, went over some railroad tracks at maybe 60 where I should've gone over at maybe 20 and ya know literally flew over them. And ya know on a motorcycle you can leave the ground all the time ya know. You don't on Harley's as much but on smaller, fast bikes like I had at the time, you leave the ground easy. And uh that was really dumb."

> Participant 3 Excerpt: "You know that it's wrong and you do it anyway, like ya know F-it. Driving too fast or maybe you've had more than one drink at a cookout and you're like, ya know what I'm fine, gimme another beer, sober me up. That's my favorite sayin', 'Gimme another shot, sober me up.'"

Because drinking often occurs in a group and can be fun, participants said that they tend to go beyond their limit. These participants continued to mention alcohol consumption as a barrier to riding their motorcycle safely that they do not have complete control over, since peer pressure to drink is prominent in the motorcycling culture. Although, participants did not view alcohol consumption as a barrier they could realistically overcome, they did discuss their ability to drive defensively to overcome external barriers (e.g., drivers of other vehicles). We present this data next.

Driving Defensively as Key to Being and Feeling Safe

This code, driving defensively as key to being and feeling safe, emerged after participants discussed how they define motorcycle safety (sample questions about this topic were provided in the previous chapter). As participants identified what behaviors are inclusive of motorcycle safety, common barriers to maintaining safety on the road were discussed. Participants identified driving defensively as a way to overcome safety barriers, especially when avoiding a collision with a car or truck. In one of these themes, participants noted the importance of being aware of their surroundings at all times. The following interview excerpts illustrate this point.

> Participant 34 Excerpt: "Uh when I ride I always ride on the defensive ya know. A lot of times they say ride on the offensive. But I'm always looking out for other people to see what they're gonna do because you don't know if they've seen you or not. So I always pretend that they don't see me so I can ya know, or if I see a car coming across the road I'll slow down until I know that I can get by them before they pull out."

> Participant 28 Excerpt: "Driving uh defensively. That to me is the biggest. You gotta, you gotta think that the, when you're pulling out on the road you gotta think that the car doesn't see you. That's the way I try to ride. I just act as if well he's not seeing me and if I have to sit there and wait for him to go by or whatever it takes, that's what I do."

> Participant 15 Excerpt: "If you're going by a side street and you see a car pulling up you look at that car and if they don't make eye contact with you, that's a, that's a serious safety issue. When you're at an intersection and you've got the opportunity to make a right-hand turn and they don't see you, that's a safety issue. That right there, that's where I've also seen, I've seen, I've seen two people run right through, right through an intersection, not even slow down at the intersection, and turn. And one of them, one of them immediately got in a crash. The other one made it through but it's still one of these things that if you're on a motorcycle you need to be aware all the time, also in driving a car or truck."

Participants stated that constant awareness is necessary because drivers of cars or trucks often do not see them. For this reason, they cited drivers of other vehicles as a barrier that they cannot control while riding their motorcycle. However, something they can control is being aware of drivers of cars and trucks and if necessary, reacting to their inattention. If some of these prevention measures fail and a crash occurs, motorcyclists also referenced the importance of equipping their motorcycle and their bodies with protective gear in order to preserve their safety. Lastly, we highlight some of the benefits, or lack thereof that participants referenced about driving their motorcycles safer.

Benefits of Safe Motorcycling

This code included participants' views about the benefits that exist to practicing safer behaviors on a motorcycle. Motorcyclists cited internal, external, or no obvious benefits to practicing safer behaviors. We highlight their feedback about no obvious benefits of practicing safety behaviors. Participants indicated that it is difficult to appreciate the benefits of safer riding because the experience is not exciting. Specifically, participants said that when motorcyclists are safer they often do not get into crashes and other people do not know who they are because they cannot see their face through the gear. Participants indicated that, because being safer takes some of the excitement out of riding, they do not necessarily consider safer behaviors a benefit. These responses were similar to those of sensation seekers who enjoy taking risks; primarily because they believe nothing will happen as a result of those risky behaviors (Zuckerman, 1994). In the following excerpt, a participant described this idea.

> Participant 28 Excerpt: "You don't see the benefits of it because it, ya know you don't, you don't think about it. If you don't get in an accident you're going, 'Well, this is kinda boring'. But you don't think of the fact that, 'Well I'm being safe therefore I'm not in a wreck'. So I think it's something you don't see but it's, it's just part of the game ya know."

Another participant commented that for a lot of motorcyclists it is more important to be recognized than to be safer. For that reason this motorcyclist said, "So I think probably like 10% of motorcyclists see the safety or the positive to wearing safety gear" (Participant 32). Therefore, regardless of how many benefits motorcyclists may recognize as a result of being safer, the results also indicate that being safe takes some of the excitement out of driving a motorcycle, which may affect some motorcyclists' safety choices. Now that we highlighted some of the codes and respective themes that emerged within this section of the interviews, we summarize how the HRT tenet pragmatism served as an overarching tenet that better informed the perceived barriers and benefits participants described as contributing to how they operate their motorcycle.

Pragmatism as a Metatheoretical Tenet in Qualitative Harm Reduction Research

Motorcyclists consistently discussed risky behaviors they practice while driving a motorcycle and what behaviors may be possible to change in the future. Mainly, the results emphasized the importance of being realistic toward motorcyclists about their ability to change certain behaviors. Results also indicated that a gap exists regarding what safety behaviors motorcyclists believe they can change and what safety behaviors motorcyclists believe they cannot change. Specifically, the results demonstrated that motorcyclists view the barriers and benefits of safe motorcycling separately. In response, it is necessary to integrate barriers and benefits into a cost-benefit analysis as emphasized in the RHBM. Perhaps pragmatism can facilitate this integration of benefits and barriers to assist behavior change.

When discussing perceived barriers and perceived benefits from a pragmatism standpoint, participants openly acknowledged and discussed their risky motorcycling behaviors. However, the results revealed a pattern of more perceived barriers to driving a motorcycle safer than perceived benefits of driving a motorcycle safer. Some barriers that were identified to driving a motorcycle safer included the weather conditions, gear being uncomfortable or not stylish, being influenced by other motorcyclists, and not having control over choices drivers of other vehicles make while driving. Participants continually acknowledged that because several barriers to being safer are not within their control, they partake in harm-reducing actions such as being aware of their surroundings, following traffic laws, and checking their motorcycle. These results showed that motorcyclists are realistic about the barriers beyond their control and are willing to take harm-reducing actions to combat some of those external barriers.

However, the safer behaviors that are directly within these participants' control are the behavior changes they did not want to make. This resistance to personal behavior change may be because motorcyclists do not perceive enough benefits to changing their behaviors or they think that behavior change is not realistic. Barriers that motorcyclists have direct control over in order to reduce personal harm while driving a motorcycle include speeding less and taking turns slower, not consuming alcohol or consuming less alcohol while riding their motorcycle, ignoring the judgmental comments from other motorcyclists, exploring safety gear that is more comfortable, avoiding riding in bad weather, and not allowing age, or thrill-seeking desires to dictate behavior choices. Although motorcyclists have almost complete control over these behaviors, participants indicated that they continue taking chances and engage in these behaviors because they are fun and they do not believe anything bad will happen as a result of the risky choices. Generally, results demonstrated that motorcyclists acknowledge and believe that drivers of other vehicles or the environment are more likely to cause them to crash than their risky riding behaviors.

This barrier is perhaps the greatest barrier that needs to be addressed for this target audience to begin changing some of their personal safety behaviors. This issue is perplexing because typically individuals engage in safer behaviors because they believe these behaviors will decrease their vulnerability and threat to harm (Brown et al., 1991). Participants indicated that it is important to be aware of drivers of other vehicles to reduce potential harm. However, the interviews with motorcyclists also indicated that they do not see themselves as a perceived barrier to safety and thus, there are no benefits to changing their personal behaviors (e.g., drinking less alcohol, speeding less, wearing personal protective equipment). This lack of acknowledgment of their personal behaviors as a barrier to maintaining safety may be because they acknowledge more benefits of risky riding (e.g., fun) and not enough benefits of being safer. Also, it is possible that motorcyclists do not think personal behavior change is realistic for them to achieve, which indicates when pragmatism may be useful to guide the RHBM.

Pragmatism emphasizes the notion of realistic, nonjudgmental approaches to unveil barriers that motorcyclists perceive to practicing safer behaviors. The results from RQ1a revealed the need to develop and disseminate nonjudgmental messages to initiate behavior change. Participants indicated that if a message was critical, they would not listen to the advice. Therefore, it may be that the judgmental messages motorcyclists perceive toward their own safety behaviors cause them to ignore these messages and not think about their own safety behaviors as a threat to themselves. Instead, motorcyclists spent a majority of the interview discussing the barriers that other people pose to them, often in a critical tone. It may be easier for motorcyclists to focus on the negative influence other people have on their safety behaviors than work to address some of their own behaviors. In addition, since participants referenced several risky behaviors that they practice, it may be overwhelming to think about changing all of these behaviors. Perhaps working with motorcyclists to be realistic about what they can or cannot address at the present time would be helpful. Emphasizing harm-reducing behaviors instead of abstinence behaviors (e.g., drinking one beer versus eight while riding) may not be as overwhelming.

Interviews with motorcyclists accentuated that realistic behavior change, as promoted by the HRT tenet pragmatism, is important. In addition, by using this HRT tenet to guide interviews, it was discovered that when it comes to personal behavior change motorcyclists typically perceive the benefits of safer riding and the barriers to safer riding as functioning separately, rather than together, to help influence behavior change. In perceiving these two components as functioning separately, it is difficult for motorcyclists to recognize that the benefits of being safer may outweigh the barriers to safer riding, which in this case, are their own behaviors on a motorcycle.

For example, a motorcyclist may consistently not wear safety gear, such as a helmet, because it is not stylish. Or, other motorcyclists may influence them not to wear the gear. Motorcyclists may not see this behavior as risky but a nonjudgmental cue to action may cause them to contemplate behavior change. Being pragmatic with motorcyclists and suggesting that perhaps they can start with a helmet instead of a full set of gear may not be as overwhelming for this audience. However, at this point, motorcyclists may only consider the barriers (e.g., it does not look cool, it does not fit right, my friends will make fun of me) and then separately consider the benefits (e.g., better protection and more confidence while riding my motorcycle). Examining these factors separately, motorcyclists may be more inclined to side with their friends and not risk being made fun of during a group ride. However, if messages realistically address both the barriers to and the benefits of wearing a helmet, it may be easier for motorcyclists to weigh the benefits and barriers together, and comply with the recommended behavior of wearing a helmet. Therefore, allowing these two components of the RHBM to function together, as intended, guided by a realistic, gradual approach to behavior change, may facilitate safer behaviors on the road.

Overall, results from the interviews suggest that pragmatism can be used to guide realistic, nonjudgmental messages and advice for motorcyclists to more accurately perceive the barriers to and benefits of safer motorcycling. Employing pragmatism can help to not overwhelm motorcyclists about their behavior choices and instead encourage them to be realistic about their risky behaviors and their ability to reduce those behaviors over time. Specifically, focusing on just one harm-reducing behavior instead of several may be a starting point. The results demonstrate that motorcyclists' harm-reducing behaviors are already in practice when it comes to avoiding mistakes made by drivers of cars or trucks, but not when it comes to avoiding mistakes and mishaps as a result of their own risky behaviors on a motorcycle. Therefore, the role of pragmatism in acknowledging personal behaviors and initiating behavior changes that are realistic may be helpful for motorcyclists and other target audiences in future projects.

While reading this section, you may have conceptualized some realistic behavior changes for other target audiences. Perhaps this section may help guide practical communication with these audiences in the future. Next, we summarize some of our results from the next research question.

Harm Reduction Immediacy as a Metatheoretical Tenet

Research Question 1c asked in what ways the HRT tenet immediacy and goal setting informs the RHBM component perceived susceptibility and perceived severity to encourage motorcyclists to discuss their current safety behaviors while driving a motorcycle. For your reference, Appendix C shows all the codes and themes that emerged during the interviews, including definitions and examples. Throughout this portion of the interview, participants were encouraged to discuss their perceived susceptibility to motorcycle crashes and injuries and subsequently, any short-term or long-term changes to their safety behaviors or changes they wanted to make as a result of feeling more susceptible to crashes and injuries.

First, participants discussed risky behaviors, such as excessive speeding and high alcohol consumption that they typically engage in while driving a motorcycle and why they partake in these risky behaviors. Consequently, participants discussed their perceived susceptibility to crashes and perceived severity of those crashes based on their current behaviors. Typically, participants discussed either their own crash and/or close-call crash as a cue that increased their perceived susceptibility to crashes. They also referenced seeing or hearing about a motorcycle crash as something that increased both their perceived susceptibility to and perceived severity of motorcycle crashes. Subsequently, participants were probed to discuss what short-term behavior changes they made or could make to reduce the possibility of getting injured while driving a motorcycle. While employing the immediacy and goal setting tenet of HRT, participants discussed a series of compromises they make to lower their susceptibility to crashes. Consequently, eight codes emerged throughout this portion of the interviews. We feature a couple of these codes and their respective themes to exemplify how the HRT tenet immediacy and goal setting enhanced the RHBM components perceived susceptibility and perceived severity, starting with participants' perceived susceptibility to crashes.

Risk of Crashes

During this portion of the interviews participants discussed their perceived susceptibility to crashes and whether or not these perceptions cue them to change their safety behaviors. These themes were reflected in participants' accounts when discussing whether or not they thought about motorcycle crashes and if so, what impact those thoughts had on their safety behaviors. The themes within this particular code indicated that overall, motorcyclists do not worry about their risk of a crash, but acknowledge the possibility. In the following excerpts, participants acknowledge the possibility of getting into a crash, particularly their risk of crashes with another vehicle.

> Participant 15 Excerpt: "Every time you get on a scooter. I do that every time I get in my truck. If you don't think about that on a motorcycle you're a moron. And that's where personally, that's what I think. You, you almost have to keep that on your mind. You have to be aware of everybody else. It's not up to them to be aware of you."

> Participant 21 Excerpt: "Yeah like every time, the whole time I'm on the bike. Like, it just goes hand-in-hand with being conscious of uh your surroundings. As

soon as I pull to the end of my street and pull out on the busy street it, ya know it's like, 'Should I pull out, do I have enough time, or should I just be safer and wait?' I usually wait, I don't ya know pull out. I don't know why but getting hit from behind, because I'd be totally out of control, is a fuckin' huge fear of mine."

Participant 31 Excerpt: "My two instructors said 'You're going to get in an accident, like at some point in your life you're going to get in an accident, it's impossible to avoid.' And so I, I guess I'm kind of hoping, well that was my one so I'm good now. Um but I definitely feel like there's a possibility of um at some point a car won't see me and will pull out in front of me and maybe I won't have enough time to react or I won't have space to react."

In response to their higher perceived risk of a collision involving another vehicle, participants try to maintain awareness to avoid the possibility of a crash with another driver. However, participants also emphasized that every motorcyclist will experience a crash at some point during their tenure as a motorcyclist and because a crash is inevitable, they may as well keep riding and have fun. So, even though susceptibility to crashes is acknowledged, in most cases, participants took crashes and the consequences of the crashes in stride, as illustrated in the following excerpts.

Participant 21 Excerpt: "I mean lots of my friends have been in accidents. Every, everybody's been down at some point, whether it was their fault or it was just on dirt bikes or ya know whatever. Everybody's been down. Everybody who rides I think that I know has been down in some capacity."

Participant 20 Excerpt: "Nothing you can really do about it. You just hit a certain patch and down you go. Even the most experienced riders in the world go down on gravel."

Participants perceived their susceptibility to having a crash to not only be high, but inevitable. Despite their susceptibility to crashes being high, participants continue to participate in risky behaviors, saying that they could get hurt just as easily by driving a car or performing another daily activity. The following excerpts provide examples.

Participant 2 Excerpt: "So uh it's just a risk you take. I mean we take a risk getting up every day and going to work. We take risks everyday getting up and some people like jogging. That's a risk. Ya know you never, you read in the paper a lot of times that so and so went jogging and they came home and dropped dead or were hit by a car ya know. It's just something that we, I guess can't control entirely. We can put things in place to help minimize the risk. Um unfortunately sometimes as humans we ignore those things."

Participant 35 Excerpt: "It very easily could happen but I very easily could go the rest of my life without being in one, I guess. If, as long as you have the

> right training and use the right safety gear and take the right precautions I don't, I think it's just as dangerous as riding in a car or on a plane or something."

However, participants did not mention trying to reduce their risks of crashes and injuries while participating in motorcycling throughout the interviews, indicating the importance of the HRT tenet immediacy to help cue motorcyclists' perceived susceptibility while driving a motorcycle.

Although participants did not reference many cues as impacting their perceived susceptibility to crashes and injuries, one event that did temporarily impact perceptions of invincibility on the road were the occurrence of motorcycle crashes among family and friends, a personal motorcycle crash, or close-call crash while driving a motorcycle, as outlined next.

Personal Crash or Close-Call Crash

Participants discussed crashes or close-call crashes they experienced. Although several participants referenced getting right back on their motorcycle, a majority of participants indicated that after a close-call crash, they realized they were not invincible. In response, they started minimizing the risky behavior that comprised their safety in the close call or started practicing safer behaviors in case they ever were involved in a crash. Similarly, participants who were actually in a crash indicated that they started to minimize some of their riskier behaviors while driving a motorcycle, even if those behavior changes were short-lived. The crashes that participants described were generally a result of their risky driving behaviors and not someone else's fault, demonstrating the importance of pragmatism being used in conjunction with immediacy and goal setting to help motorcyclists realize the rationale of changing behaviors within their control. Some of the participants' experiences and subsequent reactions to those experiences are reported in the following excerpts.

> Participant 31 Excerpt: "I guess I was still tired because I thought I was at the next signal and so I got in the right lane to go straight through it. Um so like the first signal or the left lane was the straight and the right lane was the turn right. But then the next one it switches to the left lane turning and the right lane is going straight. So I was in the right lane and then I realized, 'oh wait no I need to go straight here.' So I shifted over but that was a mistake because then the car that was stopped at the stoplight was too close to me and so I was going too quick and um when I hit the brakes then I, I had to hit em' pretty hard so my, I squeezed the back pedal and I spun, or swerved I guess like this (gesturing) and then um I have running boards so it's just like long boards that you can rest your feet on. And one of those hit into the back bumper of the car ahead of me and cracked it. So I tried to avoid it [the rain] already but in that case like I was going to work and so I needed to, because otherwise it's just too far to walk."

Participant 27 Excerpt: "I hardly rode at all then, like a couple miles a year, like back out here. Ya know out in the country, no more highways. Yeah cause I realized that you couldn't be defensive enough. You could never anticipate that in a million years and yet, it, it happened and that was not even an accident, that's just ya know like insanity, like it's hard to describe. And that was as close to an accident as you could have. But Natalie was just an infant, maybe a month old, and she would've been . . . and that's when I . . . that was the one. Yeah. It happened so fast. It made me aware that, that, that it didn't matter, that your reflexes weren't gonna help ya."

Participant 7 Excerpt: "But I started feeling conscious of and worried about deer. And we did cut back on the number of hours we spent on our bikes. We definitely did. We don't ride near as much as we used to. I mean, we still ride regularly but I mean we would go overnights and all that. We didn't see any more after that but that was the first day. We were like 'oh man.' It does take a little bit out of the sport after you experience or have seen something like that. It just, like I said we don't do it as much as we did."

Participant 29 Excerpt: "Two years ago I was riding to work (5.0). Yeah two years ago I was riding to work and um I was sitting. I was sitting at the turn lane where there's a green arrow. And so um I, I was the only one at the light and, what did I do? I was trying to adjust the button on my jean jacket and I looked down. And so I was fixing the button on my jean jacket and then when I looked up there was a green arrow. So my feet are both flat on the ground, while I was adjusting my jean jacket, and so when I looked up and saw there was a green light I went to put my hands on the motorcycle, on the handlebars, and when I did, this great big giant pickup truck, one of your bigger pickup trucks, um came and rear ended me. Now I definitely uh I don't sit at lights anymore ya know. If the light is red I still don't, I don't mess around. Ya know if there's a problem with my jacket or my gear or whatever, or if my cell phone rings, I'm not gonna touch it. I'm gonna go to a safe spot on the side of the road or in a parking lot to deal with that because yeah, I'm really aware and worried because you don't know if somebody's on the cell phone and they're just gonna bump you or it coulda been worse, easily."

Experiencing or almost experiencing a crash served as a wake-up call for most participants, who indicated subsequently changing at least one behavior while driving their motorcycle whether it was avoiding driving at night, in the rain, on highways, or simply being more aware that crashes can happen. However, drivers of cars and trucks were responsible for some crashes experienced by participants, as noted in other excerpts throughout the chapter. Other participants described their main reaction to these crashes as swerving to avoid a collision, making those crashes a single-vehicle accident. Their responses, such as the following excerpt, also indicate the importance of constantly being aware and having the ability to quickly react if encountering a dangerous situation.

> Participant 21 Excerpt: "I was on 26 heading toward Kokomo and um, some senile old farmer pulled out on a farm road that wasn't even a road, straight out onto the highway at like half a mile per hour, and uh right in front of me. I was going highway speed. And uh I had to make the decision I mean, I was gonna hit him for sure and I had to make the decision to, I mean do nothing and hit him and possibly die slamming into the side of his truck or the decision I made was to uh stop on the rear brake, lock the rear tire, lay the bike down, and try to get away from him. So I slid on my side. So yeah I stomped on the rear brake, laid the bike down, and tried to kick away from the bike as I'm sliding and uh, the bike ended up smashing into the side of his truck, I ended up rolling, rolling into the ditch. Um it knocked me unconscious, gave me a . . . I did have a helmet on and a leather jacket and jeans. And uh it gave me a contusion on my hip, um looked the size of my other two butt cheeks. And um my leather jacket, you could see through it, where it grounded into the road. Um my helmet was cracked in half. So uh another car pulled up and uh the guy got out, woke me up, was like, 'Are you okay?' and I'm like, 'No, I think I'm hurt.'"

Not all participants experienced a personal crash but all knew someone who had been in a crash. Similarly, hearing about a crash influenced participants' feelings of invincibility and reminded them that, despite their novice or veteran motorcycling status, a crash can happen to anyone. Some responses that informed this theme follow.

> Participant 9 Excerpt: "We had a guy at work pass away a couple years ago because uh a lady did a U-turn on 49 here and uh he hit the side of her van, I think. Um another guy at work hit a deer. He's alright though. So yeah I guess a lot of those things you never think is going to happen to you but you gotta keep in mind that it can."

> Participant 25 Excerpt: "I almost had, I was driving my Harley out on Colorado Street toward 30 and there was a little girl on a bicycle and uh I was going south and she was headed north. And she, she turned right in front of me ya know. She was going that way, I'm going this way, and she just turned right in front of me. So I made a dirt bike out of my Harley Davidson. But, there was no accident. But I was, I was very upset. Well first, your first thought, your first reaction is, the little girl on the bicycle. My main concern is her. My biggest concern was not to hit her. And do whatever I had to do to avoid her. That was my biggest concern."

> Participant 11 Excerpt: "Um, I just think about it all the time when I hear about stuff like that. It's like, 'wow that could've been me' and it's just kinda scary. I dunno. Yeah there's this kid at work at this job I just had, and uh he rode and I only knew him for like, he only worked on the weekends. So I only worked with him like three times. But uh he had someone on the back of his bike and got in an accident and I think he gave her his helmet and then he actually died. It's pretty crazy. I mean, ya know after that I'll wear a helmet all the time for sure."

In reaction to the various types of crashes described during this section of the interviews, participants reported some immediate changes in their behavior, indicating that crashes are a cue that influences perceptions of susceptibility. Motorcyclists communicated that after a crash their perceived susceptibility was high and in response they immediately changed their behaviors. However, after some time lapsed and their perception of susceptibility decreased, so did their safer behaviors. Participants indicated that their increased susceptibility to crashes often was temporary and they eventually reverted back to their riskier motorcycling behaviors including excessive speeding and alcohol consumption, riding without gear, and riding in adverse conditions. This was illustrated by Participant 30 when he said, "It definitely makes me . . . it, it makes me feel more susceptible but then you know how feelings just leave?"

Naturally Driving Risky

Participants often described risky motorcycling behaviors as natural reflexes, making those behaviors seem relatively harmless. Some of their descriptions of naturally driving riskier are reported next, in addition to some conscious decisions these motorcyclists make to help reduce the likelihood of negative consequences because of those risky behaviors.

> Participant 2 Excerpt: "And that's probably the danger of the bike that I have. It's easier to do that. You don't think about that. It's uh sorta a reaction, it's sorta a habit. It's something that just happens."

> Participant 6 Excerpt: "Um for the most part we don't wear helmets. They have em' ya know they put em' on from time to time ya know if you're really gonna go fast or somethin' like that or feel you're gonna do some risky driving and then you put on a helmet. But if you're just cruisin' and things like that then you don't wear a helmet."

> Participant 30 Excerpt: "Once you hit like 70 you're dead. I mean and 70 is mostly the posted speed limit on most highways. So even with a helmet, 70 mph, you get in an accident at 70 mph you're not comin' out of it. So even the speed limit is risky. So I, I just speed on the straightaway's with not a lot of cars around. I mean, and I don't consider it risky because there's not much that could screw me up. I mean, there is, I'm not saying there's nothing but there's not a lot that could screw that up."

> Participant 17 Excerpt: "Honestly for me no because I'm, I'm, well I'm a fairly experienced drinker and I limit myself to three beers. So I don't see that as being a risky behavior because I'm having a max of three beers within a five hour time span."

> Participant 8 Excerpt: "I will sometimes wear different gear depending on the length of the trip and depending what roads we're gonna take. Um if I know

we're gonna be going on like 94 or ya know some other really uh heavy traffic area or something like that even if it's hot out I will still wear like the leather jacket versus just a t-shirt."

Although participants reported it being easy to naturally progress into riskier driving situations, they also reported a small series of compromises, which is a start toward gradually changing personal safety behaviors (for additional examples see Appendix C). However, the results show that these smaller changes need to be sustained and additional safety behaviors targeted as well. A summary and implications for utilizing harm reduction and immediacy and goal setting at the metatheoretical level are presented in the following section.

Immediacy as a Metatheoretical Tenet in Qualitative Harm Reduction Research

The notion of immediate, short-term changes to safety behaviors were often mentioned as participants discussed situations that influenced their susceptibility to motorcycle crashes and their perceived severity of those crashes. The results indicated that motorcyclists are comfortable making immediate changes in their motorcycling behaviors. However, because their heightened perceptions of susceptibility and severity often were short-lived, they soon reverted back to their previous, riskier behaviors. However, the results were encouraging because some events, including a personal motorcycle crash or close-call crash, or seeing or hearing about a motorcycle crash, served as strong cues for participants to immediately change safety behaviors while driving a motorcycle. The response from participants to develop a series of compromises in order to be safer while riding their motorcycle demonstrates the idea of prioritizing goals and developing coping strategies in order to reduce harm and susceptibility (Mattson & Basnyat, 2008). Therefore, motorcyclists understand the importance of and are capable of developing and implementing short-term strategies to reduce harm while driving a motorcycle. Despite this, the results revealed a few other areas that need further consideration.

First, although encouraging that some cues to action are strong enough to initiate immediate behavior changes, it would be safer for motorcyclists and drivers of other vehicles if a crash or close call did not have to occur to prompt behavior changes. The results demonstrated that the strongest motivation to immediate behavior change is if a motorcyclist experiences a crash or knows someone who experienced a crash. Other than experiencing personal crashes or learning about the crashes of family and friends, participants did not indicate feeling highly susceptible to crashes or injuries.

It is difficult to provide short-term goals for the target audience of motorcyclists if they do not perceive a sense of urgency or need to change any behaviors. The results indicate that it is necessary to determine what cues, events, and communication strategies can encourage motorcyclists and provide a sense of urgency to change their safety behaviors. In other words, what besides a crash can challenge motorcyclists' feelings of invincibility on the road? For instance, in addressing Research Question 1a, participants suggested being real with health messages and showing the gruesome outcomes of a crash. Perhaps more graphic messages would increase motorcyclists' perceived severity of crashes and sustain behavior changes for a longer period of time, without personally seeing or hearing about someone being involved in a motorcycle crash.

Second, although participants indicated changing safety behaviors immediately after a crash, they admitted that these changes were short-lived. For example, participants said that, after they heard about a friend's crash they wore their helmet the next day while driving a motorcycle. However, as time went by they eventually stopped wearing their helmet. Similarly, participants indicated that they modify their riding behaviors in several situations that they believe are riskier. For example, they change their behaviors in order to maintain safety in adverse weather conditions or while riding at night. However, these changes also are temporary and these participants do not intend to sustain these changes when riding conditions are more favorable. Although participants immediately react to crashes with specific behavior changes, the perception of susceptibility is not enduring and neither is the behavior change.

Therefore, a primary challenge that emerged as a result of the interviews is sustaining short-term safety strategies adopted by motorcyclists. The results indicated that motorcyclists are capable of developing and implementing short-term strategies to reduce their perceived susceptibility and severity of a crash. In addition, participants did not mention a series of strategies or goals they pursue if their perceived susceptibility to and severity of a crash is high. Instead, they tended to initiate one temporary behavior change. If this one behavior was sustained, the individual could begin modifying another behavior to reduce potential harms while driving a motorcycle. Working to develop both short-term and long-term goals for motorcyclists to practice in response to their increased perceptions of susceptibility and severity may help them continue pursuing safer riding behaviors.

Overall, the results indicated that motorcyclists currently allow their perceived susceptibility to crashes and perceived severity of those crashes to guide their immediate behavior changes. Motorcyclists quickly change one behavior in response to a sense of vulnerability. The sense of vulnerability is short-lived however, and because motorcyclists quickly change a behavior, perhaps without thinking about all of the benefits it could provide, often they just as quickly revert back to previous, riskier behaviors. Although this immediate behavior change is better than no behavior change, perhaps motorcyclists do not have enough time to process and understand how their previous risky behaviors were influencing their ability to be safer on the road. The HRT tenet immediacy may assist motorcyclists in more closely assessing their current safety behaviors. Helping motorcyclists consider their behaviors on a continuum and perhaps aiming to change their safety behaviors over time may be useful. It is important to capitalize on any behavior that may make a motorcyclist feel susceptible to a crash.

These results suggested that health and safety practitioners might not capitalize enough on cues to action for motorcyclists. As noted previously, perhaps communication messages could accurately and without judgment, illustrate the consequences of motorcyclists' risky driving behaviors such as speeding and excessive alcohol consumption. For example, if a Poker Run is advertised in the newspaper, the ad could include information about the importance of helmets or not consuming too much alcohol during the event. Perhaps strategically placed safety messaging would increase motorcyclists' perceptions of susceptibility and subsequently encourage behavior change. Therefore, through the HRT tenet immediacy and goal setting motorcyclists could be cued for sustained behavior change prior to someone being injured or killed in a crash. The role of immediacy and goal setting in acknowledging and initiating personal behavior changes may be particularly helpful when it comes to sustaining those behaviors over time. Hopefully our dialogue about participant responses within this section helped illustrate how immediacy can function to guide a specific theoretical component in harm reduction health and safety research. The next section summarizes results for the HRT tenet empowerment informing the RHBM component self-efficacy during the in-depth interviews.

Harm Reduction Empowerment as a Metatheoretical Tenet

Research Question 1d asked in what ways the HRT tenet empowerment informs the RHBM component self-efficacy to encourage motorcyclists to discuss their current safety behaviors while driving a motorcycle. Appendix D includes the codes and themes that emerged during the interviews. Throughout this portion of the interviews, participants were able to discuss choices they made to increase their confidence and skills while driving a motorcycle. Discussing personal choices participants made or may make in the future helped us learn what motivates motorcyclists to question and change personal safety behaviors, in addition to what external influences may empower motorcyclists to make behavior choices. During the interviews, participants continued to discuss safety choices they made throughout their time as a motorcyclist. Four codes emerged as participants discussed ways they took responsibility to initiate safer behaviors, while also recognizing their environmental constraints such as road conditions and drivers of other vehicles. Participants discussed their personal changes as realistic, short-term behaviors that were easier to initiate. Specifically, they shared accounts of how they became a safer motorcyclist over time, including starting with smaller behavior changes to build their confidence while driving a motorcycle. We reflect on some of the codes and respective themes that emerged during this section of the interviews, with a focus on the importance of empowerment in probing participants' self-efficacy to safely drive their motorcycle. As you read the results, you may think of ways to empower other target audiences that may be helpful in your own harm reduction research.

Becoming a Safer Motorcyclist

When discussing different safety choices they made over the years, participants described how those choices influenced their confidence and ability to safely operate their motorcycle. By changing a few small behaviors over the years, participants proudly communicated that they are safer and feel confident in their ability to react quickly and avoid dangerous situations.

One theme emerged as participants described personal safety behaviors they currently perform that they did not practice as a novice motorcyclist. This finding is not surprising because participants indicated throughout the interviews that when they were younger they felt invulnerable to crashes and injuries but as they got older they started to practice safer behaviors to combat some of their new feelings of vulnerability. Participants indicated that becoming safer is something that just happens over time, perhaps as they realize all of the safety options they have while riding their motorcycles. For example, Participant 7 stated, "I was less likely to use safety precautions before when I was an early rider. It was all about being cool, ya know. Now it's totally different. I can't think of anything that I could do much safer. I read all the books."

Participants discussed various choices they made to ensure that their motorcycle would be as safe as possible, including installing loud exhaust pipes, bright headlights, and sidebars in case of a crash. Because participants chose to install these extra safety features on their motorcycle, they felt more confident in their own safety while driving their motorcycle in addition to these features being precautions to avoid serious injury. Following are some excerpts that supported the development of this theme.

> Participant 9 Excerpt: "Um I guess since I've had a couple motorcycles, one thing is that a lot of the closer calls I've had were actually on my quieter motorcycle. The fact that this one has decently loud pipes and everything makes people seem to know you're there when the other one was just, well about as

> quiet as a car basically. They wouldn't see you, wouldn't hear you, more likely to cut you off. So uh as far as making people aware of where I am I feel safer on that one . . . on the loud one."

> Participant 16 Excerpt: "Ya know sometimes it's also just the other cars. A lot of times people say they don't see us . . . but like on my bike you can definitely hear me. I got loud pipes on it. I got a lot of lights."

> Participant 6 Excerpt: "Like someone will turn, that's the main thing like someone will turn and you will be there. Like a lot of times they don't see you, that's why it's good to have loud pipes so at least they can hear you coming."

These comments demonstrated that making their motorcycle safer provides motorcyclists a certain peace of mind when driving on the road. Particularly, participants felt that with more equipment on their motorcycles, drivers of cars or trucks can better hear and see them on the roadways. Also, participants felt safer on their motorcycle because the equipment they installed can minimize injuries in a collision. Participants attributed these choices part of becoming a better, smarter motorcyclist.

In addition, participants communicated that as they became more experienced riding it was easier to maintain their composure and react quickly when confronted with a possible collision than it was when they first starting driving a motorcycle. Participants indicated that when they did not feel confident in their motorcycling skills, they panicked during many hazardous situations that they encountered, putting them at greater risk of being in a crash. Over time, as participants fine-tuned their motorcycling skills and became more confident in their decisions, they stated that it was easier to react to these hazardous situations and remain calm. Participants told of previous situations during which they had to avoid panicking. Over time, as efficacy increased, so did their ability to maintain personal safety. The following excerpts illustrate this point.

> Participant 21 Excerpt: "I mean you notice things uh, like, like I said before when you're a more experienced rider, your, your panic mode goes to the proper thing to do instead of the freakin' out. Ya know, I've watched the inexperienced rider friends of mine, especially with the rockets, everybody thinks they're a master rider because they're young. Um I had a friend of mine do a wheelie on the highway behind a car and it was like one of the first times he pulled off a long wheelie and he completely froze up and ran into the car in front of him while he was on the wheelie. Because he just panicked and didn't know what to do . . . just froze. Now there's a lot less of that. Now that I'm a more experienced rider, I think my instinct usually goes to more proper behavior."

> Participant 15 Excerpt: "Triage. You don't really think about anything you just do what you know you've done. It's one of these things . . . how many times

have you had someone pull out in front of you and you swerve so you don't crash? You don't think, you react. You react and that's where experience will guide your reaction."

Generally participants asserted that the more experience they gain on their motorcycle the less they panic in an unsafe situation. In additional themes within this code about becoming a safer motorcyclist, participants discussed the importance of choosing a motorcycle that fits their body, taking time to familiarize themselves with the motorcycle, practicing riding, or taking a motorcycle safety course to increase confidence when potentially dangerous situations are encountered on the road. Some examples from these themes are provided in the following excerpts.

Participant 28 Excerpt: "I started out, like I said I started out with smaller dirt bikes, rode those and then we went up to 650cc, a Triumph. And then I had a 1000 Kawasaki and now I have the Honda. So I kinda progressed to the bigger bikes. And the bigger bikes are easier to ride, I think. I think they're . . . that Goldwing is like riding on a carpet almost. It's pretty cool. It was all a learning thing. We just started out with small bikes and then kinda learned those and then built up from there."

Participant 22 Excerpt: "When you first start out you don't know what's gonna happen with the motorcycle. As you get better you learn your own bike. It's kind of personal to your own vehicle. You jump on somebody else's bike that you don't know you're probably gonna wreck it. I'm just saying. You'll be a lot safer. I mean if you know what your bike can do, handling it and all that you should be alright."

Participant 11 Excerpt: "I knew that if I could do the stupid things I had to do for that [motorcycle] test that I could probably do it on the highway cause some of the things on the test were super hard."

Throughout the interviews participants reiterated the relationships between experience, confidence, and safety. Specifically, knowing that they can make better choices to avoid a crash helped participants feel more confident in their riding abilities. Appendix D shows the variety of choices participants made to be safer, indicating that each motorcyclist has a varying level of comfort and adaptability in response to behavior change, hence the importance of empowering motorcyclists to choose an option that they are at ease with and more likely to sustain over time. Additional codes within this section of the interview focused on empowering the younger generation of motorcyclists to start practicing safety behaviors earlier and to empower motorcyclists to discuss how to safely operate a car or truck around motorcyclists with drivers of those other vehicles. These codes and some respective themes are briefly illustrated in the subsequent sections.

Emphasizing Safety for Youth

Participants stressed that targeting youth is one of the best ways to empower safer decision-making at an early age and sustain those decisions throughout life. Many participants felt that a larger emphasis on youth bicycle safety exists today and has had a positive impact on individuals' abilities to practice safer behaviors. As the following excerpts illustrate, it is more difficult to change the older generation, but it is possible to impact the younger generation who have not yet solidified all their safety choices.

> Participant 28 Excerpt: "I think we are headed that way as far as people accepting uh wearing safety protection. Um the old schooler's are probably not gonna go along with it but the younger generation seems like they're, they're pickin' up on it. So I think we're headed in the right direction as far as safety."

Other participants noted that, because they did not have a safety mentor when they were growing up, they wanted to serve as that resource for their family and friends, while these individuals were still impressionable. An example of this sentiment is provided in the following excerpt.

> Participant 1 Excerpt: "But when I bring him into that [my nephew], when I do, I will put more safety features in place for him, which I didn't do. The schools and things that teach him the safety and the riding. We go watch little kids racing and stuff and they have on the pads and stuff. So that is a culture that I will introduce to him that was not introduced to me."

These participants expressed that safety is becoming more prevalent on both an individual and societal level. They also stressed the desire to teach adolescents in their family the importance of safety that they never learned. Further they indicated that the emphasis placed on safety for two wheels is more prevalent in society than it was decades ago, which may help promote and sustain safer behaviors in the future. Finally, we discuss the emphasis participants placed on empowering drivers of cars and trucks to safely maneuver amidst motorcyclists.

Empowering Motorcyclists and Drivers of Other Vehicles to Share the Road

During this portion of the interview another pattern emerged when participants discussed what affects their confidence when driving a motorcycle. Participants continued to reference their personal behaviors and choices as superior to other drivers, including motorcyclists. Within this discussion, the motorcyclists interviewed made no reference to changing their personal behaviors. Instead, they continued to say that everyone else needs to be safer and watch for motorcyclists. Although participants continually stated throughout the interviews that drivers of cars or trucks need to be targeted by safety initiatives, such as health campaigns, their responses also demonstrated that motorcyclists need to be involved in efforts to make the roads safer. It is possible that providing motorcyclists with the tools to adapt some of their behaviors in addition to having rational discussions with drivers of cars and trucks will facilitate some of these changes toward safety. Examples from two themes that emerged within this code follow.

> Participant 15 Excerpt: "There are just so many people that are not aware of that. That's why we see people read a book when they're driving, texting; I get so mad when I see that [the texting]. I can multi-task, a lot of people can't. But uh when you're texting when you're driving I got an issue with that."

> Participant 14 Excerpt: "I mean ya, I mean it's a safety issue obviously but I mean if (4.0) if people would just respect the bikers and not pull out in front of them. And people on mopeds, uh someone almost rear-ended me on a moped the other day. On Creasy traffic stuck in fuckin, stuck in traffic. And he was just weaving in and out and I'm like, 'that's how you get fuckin killed on a bike.' Regardless of if it's a fucking motorcycle, uh moped, whatever. Like you have got to be cautious with that shit and he wasn't at all. And I mean the safety issue is a big problem . . . it is."

In addition, when participants were probed to discuss if they feel in control of their motorcycle and confident in their skills to react to a precarious situation, motorcyclists continued to describe their angry responses to drivers of cars and trucks who almost caused a crash with them. Most motorcyclists simply said something like, "Here we go, dumbass people not paying attention" (Interview 33). Others went more in-depth about their follow-up behaviors toward the driver of a car or truck, such as in the following excerpt.

> Participant 16 Excerpt: "Oh well when they do that I pull up behind them and let them have a piece of my mind. I pull up in front of them. I mean I get around them and get in front of them and see if they wanna stop. Hopefully they'll realize enough to never cut me off again."

This feedback demonstrates how motorcyclists may react toward other drivers on the road. These reactions toward other drivers indicate that motorcyclists also need to be involved in efforts to make the roads safer. When participants continued to discuss their confrontations with other drivers, however, they often said that the confrontation did not help because the other drivers usually did not know what they did wrong in the situation. Therefore, motorcyclists' insistence on targeting drivers of cars and trucks for safety is also necessary. This suggests the strategy of collaboration to initiate and sustain a safer environment for all travelers traversing the roads, and is further addressed in the section during the discussion of Research Question 1e. Next, we provide a summary of how utilizing empowerment as a metatheoretical tenet guided these in-depth interviews and helped us probe participants about their efficacy to safely drive a motorcycle both as novices and seasoned riders.

Empowerment as a Metatheoretical Tenet in Qualitative Harm Reduction Research

Research Question 1d asked in what ways the HRT tenet empowerment can inform the RHBM component self-efficacy to encourage motorcyclists to discuss their current safety behaviors while driving a motorcycle. The importance of empowerment was consistently supported as participants discussed choices they made to become a safer motorcyclist. Initially the results indicated that motorcyclists appreciate having a variety of safety choices they can perform while driving a motorcycle. Specifically, participants mentioned learning a range of alternatives to be safer while driving their motorcycle during a motorcycle safety course. In addition, the results demonstrated that when motorcyclists make their own choices regarding what safety behavior(s) they want to change and consistently perform, they feel more confident operating their motorcycle. For example, although motorcyclists can utilize several different strategies to avoid a crash, experience over time may allow them to better assess their surroundings and feel confident to quickly change lanes instead of laying the motorcycle down.

Throughout the interviews, participants discussed ways they took responsibility to initiate safer behaviors while driving their motorcycle. During these discussions however, motorcyclists also acknowledged the role of the environment in creating specific barriers that increase their risk for crashes. Understanding the influence the environment has on safety behaviors is important when addressing the HRT tenet empowerment because individuals need to understand what behaviors are within their control and they can take responsibility to address (Rhodes, 2002). For example, several participants decided to install louder exhaust pipes on their motorcycle to be safer around cars and trucks. In this situation, participants took responsibility to make their motorcycle safer as a result of other drivers not noticing them on the road. Some of the other decisions participants reported making over time to minimize their chances of a crash included installing other pieces of equipment on their motorcycle, starting with a smaller motorcycle, and practicing with the motorcycle in secluded areas.

These results indicate that perhaps communication messages through interventions or campaigns should target motorcyclists to start with smaller, simpler behavior choices they can make on their motorcycle to be safer.

Obviously not wearing a helmet or other safety gear and drinking alcohol are all high-risk behaviors when driving motorcycle. However, these behaviors also have more barriers to overcome in order to practice and sustain these behaviors over time. Perhaps motorcyclists' self-efficacy would increase if they were given the option to take a safety course, buy a smaller motorcycle, and learn how to make that motorcycle safer. Once some of these simpler safety choices are mastered, motorcyclists may feel empowered to move on to more complex safety behaviors such as wearing a helmet and other safety gear. Perhaps additional communication needs to occur with motorcyclists that encompasses several safety options. This additional discourse would promote a harm reduction approach for motorcyclists, recognizing the numerous choices involved to make themselves and their motorcycles safer. Once motorcyclists perform some of these behaviors, they may consider and adopt additional behavior changes over time (Bandura, 1977).

A portion of the results also suggested that if younger motorcyclists are empowered early, it may be easier for them to make and sustain safer choices for an extended period of time. Participants discussed the ways that the safety culture has changed, mainly by encouraging youth to wear safety gear on other two-wheeled vehicles. By socializing children with these behaviors, it may make their safety choices as a motorcyclist more automatic or easier. Since they wore helmets as children, this group may feel encouraged to continue this behavior through adulthood. Also, discussing safety at a young age may help these individuals know how to respond to peer pressure within a motorcycling group. These results show the importance of educating children about their safety options, instead of waiting until they are adults when behavior change may be more challenging and less realistic.

Finally, the results indicated that more of an egalitarian partnership needs to exist between motorcyclists and drivers of cars and trucks. During the interviews, participants continually criticized the safety choices and behaviors made by drivers of cars and trucks and other drivers of two-wheeled vehicles. Perhaps if motorcyclists calmly and rationally dialogued with drivers of other vehicles and discussed what these drivers can do to be safer around motorcycles, these drivers' self-efficacy to perform these safety behaviors on the road they share with motorcycles may increase. For example, when a motorcyclist is having a conversation with a driver of a car or truck about motorcycles, instead of arguing that other drivers do not look for or pay attention to motorcyclists, the motorcyclist can provide information about what part of the lane they occupy so they can avoid oil on the middle of the road. Because motorcyclists drive on the sides of lanes, they can ask other drivers to always turn their head and check in their blind spots for motorcycles. Motorcyclists need to capitalize on the opportunity to provide drivers of cars and trucks with strategies to be safer around motorcycles. Empowering motorcyclists to practice this role with drivers was a need revealed in the interviews and is one small behavior change they can make in order for the roads to be safer for everyone.

Overall, the results illustrated that it is important for motorcyclists to have a plethora of choices when negotiating how they can be safer but still have fun while driving a motorcycle. Empowerment can serve as a tool to provide several small and large safety choices for motorcyclists. As motorcyclists successfully achieve smaller behavior changes, their self-efficacy to practice the larger safety behaviors may increase. In addition, motorcyclists can serve as a resource to empower drivers of other vehicles to practice safer behaviors around motorcyclists. The next section discusses the results of RQ1e.

Harm Reduction Community Collaboration as a Metatheoretical Tenet

Research Question 1e asked in what ways the HRT tenet community collaboration informs the formative research and audience analysis during a harm reduction approach to encourage motorcyclists to discuss their current safety behaviors while driving a motorcycle. Appendix E shows the codes and themes that emerged during this section of the interviews. In this portion of the interview participants were probed to discuss whether they considered collaboration important to enhance motorcycle safety messages and resources, who the key stakeholders would be in such collaborations, and who these stakeholders should work together with to make the roads safer for motorcyclists. These issues and questions are typical of what a health and safety researcher or practitioner would address in the formative research process when beginning or assessing a specific target audience regarding a health issue (Kosmoski et al., 2007; Mattson, Haas, Gillig, & Kosmoski, 2011). Therefore, motorcyclists guided the researcher through key areas motorcycle safety efforts should focus on when beginning or correcting intervention efforts, including communication messages.

Throughout these discussions, participants recognized the barriers that exist in the surrounding environment to maintain their safety while also acknowledging that risky motorcyclists need to be targeted through health and safety efforts as well. In order for these environmental barriers to be addressed and to reach the risky motorcyclists, participants valued the idea of collaborating with a variety of people. Motorcyclists referenced several groups that need to be involved to help improve safety on the roads.

From discussing how community collaboration could enhance motorcycle safety messages and resources, four codes emerged. We highlight some of the patterns that surfaced from this portion of the interviews in the following sections. The first code that we summarize is the importance of collaboration with key stakeholders and community members.

Collaboration is Essential to Raise Awareness

One pattern that emerged was the value of collaboration. Although some participants stated collaborating may be difficult, they also asserted that it is essential to increase community awareness around motorcycle safety in order to promote sharing the roadways with two-wheeled vehicles. In addition, participants felt collaboration with particular groups was necessary to infiltrate the motorcycling culture. Motorcycling culture was depicted throughout the results of this project as a culture influenced by peer pressure that can sometimes facilitate riskier driving behaviors. Excerpts that illustrate these themes are provided in the following sections.

Primarily, participants said that collaboration is essential to help raise awareness about the presence of motorcycles in local communities. These participants referenced the lack of safety information in their respective community and thought collaboration could help promote safety. They indicated that because drivers of cars and trucks do not receive enough education about motorcycles, more venues need to promote and advertise motorcycle safety messages. Examples of what participants said about increasing efforts to communicate with drivers of cars and trucks about motorcycle safety follow.

> Participant 12 Excerpt: "Not about the riders themselves, but about getting more, getting more in the student education about motorcycle riders and what they choose to do as riders. Cause motorcycle safety is more about the people that aren't riding than the people that are riding because you, as a four-wheeler, forget that you have a box around you and when you do whatever you do you don't think about the person that's out on the bike that doesn't have that. So I would educate the general public about the riders. That's the best rider safety you can get, is getting people that are involved in riding to educate."

> Participant 34 Excerpt: "Ya know maybe if they had commercials out. I would say a good percentage of the motorcycle accidents that happen are caused by motorists that aren't paying attention and don't see them. They're looking for cars; they're not looking for motorcycles. So um ya know the bumper stickers they have that say 'watch out for motorcycles,' uh maybe if they had billboards or even did commercials just to remind others ya know that there are motorcycles out there. I mean most motorcycle accidents aren't caused by the motorcyclist; it's caused by somebody coming out because they didn't see them."

According to participants, infiltrating safety messages that target drivers of other vehicles into the community may help remind people that they play a role in motorcycle safety and have a responsibility to pay attention to motorcyclists on the road. The following excerpts provide examples.

> Participant 2 Excerpt: "It's an important message to get out there. I think even, I know it sounds funny but even those little yellow bumper stickers, ya know, 'be aware, motorcycles are everywhere.' That's important. I mean especially for young drivers in cars even, they have to understand that there's more than just their vehicle on the road. It's, it's a respect thing between everybody on the road. Um and just knowing and seeing, 'okay, there are motorcycles out here, there are bicycles out here.' It's just a reminder of what's out there."

> Participant 18 Excerpt: "Even if other groups are directly involved with motorcycling um, uh anyone who is a driver on the road is gonna come in contact with motorcyclists and it will just help to make all drivers more aware that there are bikes on the road and to not tailgate them and to watch. Ya know, look twice before you pull out, that kinda thing."

> Participant 23 Excerpt: "I guess probably the best thing would be like trying to start to introduce it more into the permit tests and stuff like that. So like kids who are learning how to drive understand that there are certain things with bikes that are different than with cars, so they aren't assuming that everything's just the same and that everything rides the same."

However, besides using collaboration to target drivers of cars and trucks, participants were just as cognizant that collaboration was needed with specific stakeholders to penetrate and influence the motorcycling culture to be more safety oriented. Participants often commented that the motorcycling culture promotes unsafe, riskier motorcycling behaviors instead of safer motorcycling behaviors. Although they acknowledged that it may be difficult to promote this change, participants supported the idea of enhancing the safety culture within motorcycling groups, as the example that follows indicates.

> Participant 3 Excerpt: "The culture doesn't change. I mean ya know we're talkin about cultures, especially a Harley rider culture. Ya know it's just, it's just the whole live to ride, ride to live thing. Harley riders are just full of testosterone so I mean it's a culture, it's a culture. Are you a man or are you ya know, come on. I tease my . . . you're gonna talk to [Interviewee 4]. [Interviewee 4] doesn't ride a Harley, he rides a Triumph. So Triumph's are looked at as ya know, ya know . . . man up, step up, get a Harley. Every time he would start his motorcycle, if he ever starts it by me it would sound like a lawn mower to me. Like he was cutting the grass ya know. And to you it might sound funny but to a guy it's like ya know, it's a macho thing."

As the next example suggests, participants referenced the difficulties of changing behavior and sustaining behavior changes among groups of motorcyclists to enhance a culture of safety.

Participant 2 Excerpt: "I think the message is important. Now the effectiveness, it's the same as the railroad crossing safety campaigns. You still see people go around the gates. You still, ya know it still happens. Um you're never gonna have a fail, a fail proof way to force everybody to follow some common safety practices. Um Michigan, they have a helmet law, but you still see guys here and there without a helmet. Ya know they enforce it hard too. You're always gonna have something to be unsafe with."

Despite the barriers that exist to consistently involving motorcyclists in safety initiatives, participants recognized the importance of trying to target them through safety messages and interventions. If done effectively, some participants believed that collaboration and continued enforcement of safety messages would start to change the safety traditions cultivated by risky motorcyclists, even if it takes a long time. In addition, participants provided specific groups and individuals that have the power to begin addressing and changing the motorcycle safety culture. This mentioning of key stakeholders instigated another theme within Research Question 1e that we highlight in the next section.

Who's Got the Power

As was asserted through the previous discussion, the motorcycle culture needs to change in order for safety behaviors to change and be maintained. Participants provided a variety of outlets they perceived as powerful in influencing motorcyclists to change their safety behaviors. During these discussions, five themes emerged: motorcycle clubs, organizations, and dealers, American Bikers Aimed Toward Education (ABATE, a not-for-profit, safety, educational, charitable and advocacy motorcyclist organization), the Bureau of Motor Vehicles (BMV), law enforcement, and local venues and event rides. Following, we list a few excerpts of participants' support for involving these groups, to demonstrate how they consider collaboration with these entities as ways to improve the health and safety of motorcyclists.

Participant 5 Excerpt: "Well you can collaborate with different groups ya know like ABATE and a couple of them are advocacy programs. Um which generally that's pretty well known. Um but get in with the different clubs is how to do it. There are more than just the big bad scary biker clubs. They're just groups of guys that want to hang out and ride."

Participant 13 Excerpt: "Uh I think ABATE does a real good job. Because anybody who wants to learn to ride they just go to abate.com and ya know sign up and you can go ride anytime you want. Ya know the cost is cheap, they provide the motorcycles, they provide the gear, they provide the helmets. And you're gonna learn how to ride and you're certified. Ya know that way you're safe because you learned how to ride."

> Participant 35 Excerpt: "Um I think maybe the biggest one would probably be the uh like the state patrol on the motorcycles. I know they don't have very many of them anymore. I know a lot of them are not doing it anymore or just switching to actual uh cars. But I think uh actually getting with them and making a solid program with them would be a pretty good asset."

> Participant 15 Excerpt: "But it's about uh other local rides that you have. Uh ABATE is not there, it's not there when you have a lot memorial rides for people that have died ya know. And that's where they should bring to mind the fact that it's more than let's ride. Let's think about what we're doing. Someone just got killed. He was riding drunk. Why are you doing that on two wheels, that's stupid."

> Participant 36 Excerpt: "Ya know maybe the police department, the fire department, ya know some of the EMT people. It probably wouldn't hurt to get them, to kinda make people aware ya know here's what we've seen, this is what happens, and make it real graphic for em' so they really think twice."

> Participant 20 Excerpt: "I like that idea over where they done at Purdue, with the signs and stuff. I think that's a good idea. I think it's a really good idea. Just put out signs that say watch, like for the cars."

Besides discussing the importance of collaborating with the appropriate people and organizations, participants also delved further into the target audience of motorcyclists, indicating that different subgroups exist among motorcyclists and that they may need to be approached differently to promote behavior change. Participants' feedback during this section of the interview was particularly helpful in terms of audience segmentation.

Targeting Motorcycling Subgroups

All of the participants had an opinion about who was riskier while driving their motorcycle and tried to address why and how particular groups of motorcyclists need to be targeted to change their safety behaviors. Particularly, younger (e.g., crotch-rocket) motorcyclists and older (e.g., Harley) motorcyclists were discussed. We display some feedback we received about each group in the following sections.

Younger (Crotch Rocket) Motorcyclists. Participants identified younger motorcyclists who drive crotch rockets as a risky group who need more attention for two reasons. First, because they are younger they have less experience driving a motorcycle, putting them at higher risk for having a crash. Second, these motorcyclists tend to drive at high-risk speeds and are more willing to perform daring stunts (i.e., wheelies) while driving their crotch rocket, also putting them at a higher risk for having a crash. The following excerpts illustrate these points.

> Participant 27 Excerpt: "Certainly the younger crotch rocketed ones. I mean those bikes are made to be crazy. There's only one reason to own those. So I would say yeah as a demographic the ones that are buying that. I mean a real young kid can't buy one [a Harley] because they cost so much but that, that younger group buys crotch rockets."

> Participant 30 Excerpt: "Let's get away from Harleys and talk about the young kids on the crotch rockets. Those are the ones that are idiots. Those are the ones that go 100 mph with no helmet, short sleeves, and shorts. Those are the ones between 18 and 24. Those are the ones that need to be sat down and smacked around."

> Participant 12 Excerpt: "Crotch rockets . . . sport bikes. They, they've seen way, way too many movies about uh riders who ride their wheelies down the road. Who do . . . they create too many risks. So that would be the group that I'd talk about. They're just too risky, they ride at high rates of speed for a short distance. They don't pay attention to what's in front of them."

> Participant 2 Excerpt: "Right now I think that your café style bikes . . . um crotch rockets some people call them. Um I think that some of those guys are trying those crazy stunts. You see them trying to speed, do stunts, on major roadways with people all around. They think that highways are a performance arena and it's not. And I think that is what bothers me the most. I didn't do those kinds of things. I didn't do the wheelies or the ya know in the middle of the road with 50 cars around me. I knew better."

Comments about safety behaviors of the older demographic of motorcyclists are discussed in the next section.

Older (Harley) Motorcyclists. Participants identified the older group of motorcyclists as needing more attention for two reasons. First, although these motorcyclists have more experience and know more about driving a motorcycle, that experience also results in stubbornness. Because these older motorcyclists are set in their ways, they are less likely to change their behaviors. The following excerpts illustrate these points.

> Participant 29 Excerpt: "I think the Harley riders, they should, they should wear shirts with sleeves. They should wear a helmet and yet they don't, they don't. However, those guys have racked up enough time on their bikes to where they probably can ride a little bit better. I don't know if I would have that kind of reaction."

> Participant 27 Excerpt: "And then um I think the older riders are dangerous too because they're slower-witted, their muscles are gone, their balance is going, their minds are slower, there's no doubt about it that that's dangerous. I mean whether anyone wants to talk about it it's gotta be physiologically fact."

> Participant 23 Excerpt: "I guess well it'd be more risky I guess, like cause they say the same thing with cars. Like, the most risky people are the ones that are just starting out or the really old ones because old ones have tons of experience but they don't have any reaction time. Or the young ones who have no experience but have a lot of reaction time. So I guess it goes the same thing for bikes . . . maybe you are more likely to crash in the beginning or end."

Participants cited collaborating with the groups referenced previously as a starting point to educate and influence behavior change. Another code that emerged within this section of the interviews was collaboration with stakeholders and policymakers to make the environment safer for motorcyclists.

Clean-Up

Finally, participants discussed some hazards as barriers to maintaining their safety while driving a motorcycle. They indicated that collaboration with local cities could help address some of these hazards to make the roads safer. Mainly, they discussed road hazards and weather-related hazards. Examples are provided in the following excerpts.

> Participant 34 Excerpt: "The only thing I would say is ya know when gravel gets in the road. Um for instance out on Main Street here they put gravel on the side of the road and if a car goes into that gravel it kicks it into the road. So that I don't like, especially going around corners."

> Participant 36 Excerpt: "Oh just uh they were, it was at night and they were working on the road I was on. And they had paved one side and not the other so there was a lip in the middle and you couldn't see it at night. I didn't realize it and when I went through the curb I drifted into the middle of the road and hit that burl and it upset the bike and I had a girlfriend on the back and it threw her off and threw me over the handlebars."

> Participant 31 Excerpt: "And then I would say roundabouts are kind of new. Although I don't dislike them but they do seem like uh, it seems like cars already in the roundabout are not paying attention to people who might not be paying attention to them and just pulling in without looking. Um and so it seems like both drivers might not be looking and that could result in them easily having a collision."

> Participant 35 Excerpt: "Um I think the most difficult would probably be after, after the winter in the spring when everything's starting to melt off but the spring rains haven't quite come in yet. Because um, in my county they actually use a lot of, they use a lot of sand and salt mixture and that for some reason just likes to stick on the road for a very long time. And whenever the spring rains do come then the oil from the road comes up. So I mean I think the transition between the rains in the spring from the winter is probably the roughest time."

In addition, participants said that because of cold weather, motorcycling season is only half of the year in Indiana. One participant said, "Well I think the biggest thing around here is that ya know motorcycles are only out like half the year because of ya know they're only in season half the year. So when people get used to them being around then ya know . . . they're not" (Interview 4). In the following excerpt, the participant referenced the difference between motorcycle awareness in Indiana and a state like Florida, where people are more used to sharing the roads with motorcycles all year.

> Participant 27 Excerpt: "I mean we're literally a four-month season and I'm sure that ya know California and Arizona and Florida and southern bikers are more experienced. I'm sure of it. And I'll bet that the, the um car ya know operators are also more experienced with them around. Ya know when we go to Florida we see way more bikes and it's just more obvious and I think that that's important."

Because of the shortened motorcycling season in Indiana, motorcyclists stressed the need to collaborate and raise more awareness at the beginning of each motorcycling season.

Community Collaboration as a Metatheoretical Tenet in Qualitative Harm Reduction Research

The importance of collaboration as a tool to increase awareness and behavior change was brought up repeatedly as participants discussed key stakeholders to involve in collaborative initiatives and who to target on the roadways. The results indicated that collaboration could be challenging for motorcycle safety community efforts, but motorcyclists still believe it is necessary to initiate changes in safety behaviors.

Participants continued to acknowledge their risky behaviors while driving a motorcycle and shared what particular subgroups need to be targeted in motorcycle safety messages and community initiatives. However, throughout these discussions motorcyclists also recognized barriers that exist in their surrounding environment that influence their safety behaviors. According to the World Health Organization (WHO, 1986), creating environments conducive to individuals practicing harm-reducing behaviors is crucial. Therefore, collaboration with the community is necessary to help construct enabling environments for motorcyclists to change their safety behaviors (Rhodes & Hendrich, 2010; WHO, 1986). Participants recognized this need as they stated their support for collaborating with a variety of organizations such as ABATE, the BMV, and institutions of higher education, to co-create a safer environment for motorcyclists.

Participants' feedback supported the notion of community collaboration facilitating all components in the RHBM with regards to motorcycle safety. For example, participants identified organizations and venues they perceived as being influential in changing behaviors. These organizations and venues would be strong partners for motorcycle safety initiatives within the community by helping initiate more targeted cues to action among motorcyclists. Working with Harley dealerships or the BMV to distribute nonjudgmental, realistic cues to action may be beneficial.

In addition, participants often mention road hazards as a barrier to maintaining personal safety. Collaboration in the community could help minimize some of these environmental barriers and help protect motorcyclists from increased susceptibility to crashes while driving their motorcycle. Participants referenced some specific ways collaboration with community organizations could help address and accomplish other components of the RHBM, such as cues to action and perceived barriers. This feedback indicates that identifying and utilizing credible community-based settings to promote motorcycle safety messages and resources may be useful.

Participants also provided input about different subgroups of motorcyclists. For health and safety practitioners, formative research about the target audience is important. Participants' feedback about younger motorcyclists who drive crotch rockets as a risky subgroup was consistent with previous research about the motorcycling population, including that age mediates the perceived barriers and perceived susceptibility to having a crash in addition to the perceived benefit of having more fun on the road (Elliot et al., 2003). However, participants also specified several reasons that older, more experienced motorcyclists need to be targeted for safety behaviors. In addition, participants supported motorcycle safety education at a young age while adolescents are still impressionable. The variety of subgroups that motorcyclists identified shows that consistent audience analysis within the community is crucial.

All and all, the results from these interviews emphasize that fostering collaborations is an important component to fully address motorcycle safety. The discourse also demonstrates that collaborations with individuals and groups that motorcyclists perceive to be experts in motorcycling can provide guidance throughout the rest of the proposed, integrative model of HRT guiding the RHBM. It is possible that working with some of these powerful stakeholders can help initiate stronger cues to action, reduce perceived barriers to safety on the road, and produce materials that raise awareness about motorcycle safety.

In this section, we utilized excerpts from interviews with at-risk motorcyclists to demonstrate how a tenet of HRT could guide the RHBM and inform the interviews. Next we summarize the results from Research Question 1.

METATHEORETICAL UTILITY OF HARM REDUCTION TENETS

Research Question 1 asked in what ways HRT, in tandem with the Reconceptualized Health Belief Model (RHBM), can guide conversational interviews with motorcyclists about their safety behaviors while driving a motorcycle. Within participants' accounts, they discussed what ways humanistic value can guide cues to action, what ways pragmatism can guide perceived benefits of and perceived barriers to driving a motorcycle safer, what ways immediacy and goal setting can guide perceived susceptibility to and perceived severity of motorcycle crashes and injuries, what ways empowerment can guide self-efficacy to practice and sustain motorcycle safety behaviors, and what ways community collaboration can facilitate the formative research conducted in a harm reduction approach to guide the RHBM. Within the interviews several codes and themes emerged that support a variety of ways HRT can guide the RHBM in first, understanding motorcyclists' safety choices and second, encouraging a shift in practicing and sustaining safer behaviors while driving their motorcycle. We hope the excerpts illustrated how the metatheory was used to guide the interviews and in turn, strengthen the theoretical constructs of the RHBM.

In the previous chapter, we explained how the metatheoretical tenets of HRT were used to help us interact with interview participants. The interview excerpts provided in this chapter demonstrated how participants responded to the use of metatheory guiding the interview (see Table 5.2; column 1). However, analysis of the results also revealed that participants simultaneously used the tenets of HRT to engage the researchers and offer feedback about ways to target motorcyclists and improve traffic safety (see Table 5.2; column 2). The next section elaborates on this occurrence during the interviews.

Participants' Engagement of Metatheory Informing the Researchers

The results supported the use of a harm reduction tenet informing a component of the RHBM. You may have noticed when reading participants' responses through the interview excerpts that they consistently offered feedback that suggested how a tenet of harm reduction could be applied to influence other motorcyclists to change their risky behaviors and provide guidance for communicating with other at-risk motorcyclists about motorcycle safety. Changing the way the tenets of HRT functioned in this research project and using them as metatheoretical guidance allowed us to realize and understand the different ways each tenet could guide a theoretical component and uncover barriers to behavior change.

Table 5.2 Participant Response to a Metatheoretical Framework during Interviews

Metatheory Framework	*Participant Reaction to Metatheoretical Framework*	*Implications for Issue in Practice*
Humanistic Value	Responded positively to people within same subgroup and who do not judge behaviors.	Tailor cues to action to be less critical toward target audience in future messages.
Pragmatism	Willing to acknowledge the barriers within their control, even if they cannot identify more benefits of changing a particular behavior.	Identify realistic barriers for audience to overcome followed by benefits of targeted behaviors.
Immediacy/Goal Setting	Willing and able to make immediate changes when susceptibility is high, even if perceived severity remains low.	Encourage short-term goals to build self-efficacy for additional, sustainable behavior change in the future.
Empowerment	Participants able to identify several small choices made in the past, increasing confidence to initiate additional behavior changes.	Provide audience the opportunity to start with smaller behaviors and empower them to mentor others in their same sub-group to change behaviors.
Community Collaboration	Participants pinpoint collaboration as necessary because there are a variety of subgroups within the target audience that need to be addressed by different stakeholders.	Use feedback from the target audience to identify potential partners and approach them with a strategic plan to reduce barriers and promote an enabling environment.

First, we were able to utilize the concept of each tenet to converse with participants. Participants candidly discussed their personal reasons and justifications for changing or maintaining their personal safety behaviors while driving a motorcycle. However, during the interviews, participants also consistently offered feedback for how the tenets of HRT could be applied to influence other motorcyclists to change their risky behaviors. In the next section, we provide examples of how participants utilized the HRT metatheoretical tenets to offer feedback about creating effective motorcycle safety messages.

Participants' Emphasis on Nonjudgmental Cues to Action

In our effort to address Research Question 1a we maintained a nonjudgmental relationship with the participants. After acknowledging that motorcyclists often engage in risky behaviors and that this interview is an opportunity to learn about those risky behaviors, we proceeded to ask questions about cues to action for motorcyclists. Introducing the interview in this way allowed participants to feel more at ease to freely share their own experiences. Then, as the interview progressed, participants continued to reference the importance of other people treating them in a respectful manner and not judging their risky motorcycling behaviors. For an example of this, refer to Research Project in Practice Illustration Figure 5.1.

In this sense, the tenet humanistic value was an interpersonal tool to dialogue with individuals so they could openly discuss their health and safety behaviors. Interestingly, motorcyclists stated that a common reason they do not adhere to motorcycle safety messages or advice from others is because the communication surrounding their behaviors is too negative and critical. To respond to this concern, participants recommended how future messages need to target certain groups of motorcyclists. Consequently, humanistic value serving as an initial, or overarching tenet of the interviews allowed for deeper probing and understanding of participants' personal safety choices and ways to enhance future communication with the larger group.

Participant Emphasis on Realistic Behavior Change

To address Research Question 1b we probed participants to identify their perceived barriers to and perceived benefits of driving a motorcycle safer, with a focus on what barriers are realistic to overcome. Communicating with participants that we understand some barriers are outside their control allowed participants to be more candid about their safety behaviors, including why particular barriers were difficult for them to overcome. Then, as the interview progressed, participants continued to reference the importance of overcoming particular barriers that even they were having difficulties with (e.g., driving a motorcycle at high speeds or while under the influence of alcohol) as well. Participants continued to reference ways we, as researchers and health practitioners, could try to reduce the negative consequences of these behaviors and eventually, the risky behaviors themselves.

Research in Practice Illustration

Participant using harm reduction tenet to inform motorcycle safety cues to action
"Well I guess it depends on how it's presented. Ya know like after I got done riding and someone said, 'Hey I saw you doing this' or 'I, I seen that you stopped too suddenly when we were riding as a group and you need to, need to have more of a space between us.' Yeah positive reinforcement." (Participant 26)

Figure 5.1 Research in Practice Illustration.

Research in Practice Illustration

Participants using pragmatism tenet to inform perceived barriers to motorcycle safety
"And maybe um somehow without turning people off, but in cahoots with those Poker Runs, ya know maybe that would be a venue to be doing that ya know. It would have to be in the coolest way ya know, without turning people off. Bikers are just a different breed. They're there for the freedom so they don't wanna be legislated out of their freedom or whatever but just, common sense always has an audience, I think. Ya know and if you're able to do it in the right way the message would get through. That would be a good format." (Participant 27)

"Make it not bar to bar. Make it be like an ice cream stand (haha) or to a restaurant stop to stop. Or a park. It doesn't have to be bar to bar to bar but that's the draw. That's what people come for. And, I just...it's just not my cup of tea. I go because it's usually a good cause and it makes money for something good but I'd rather have it go someplace else." (Participant 7)

Figure 5.2 Research in Practice Illustration.

Research Project in Practice Illustration Figure 5.2 exemplifies, from participants' perspectives, how to address the heavy drinking that occurs at Poker Run events without abolishing those events, making behavior change more realistic for motorcyclists.

Ultimately, the tenet pragmatism provided an interpersonal tool to dialogue with participants so they could openly discuss what challenges they encounter to being safer. But at the same time, motorcyclists stated that a common reason they do not adhere to safety behaviors is based on the perception of not having control over these particular barriers. This caused participants to recommend how future initiatives need to address some of these barriers including making the external environment more motorcyclist friendly, continuing to educate drivers of cars and trucks, and being creative in minimizing the factors that make risky motorcycling so appealing and prevalent, such as Poker Runs. In this sense, pragmatism serving as an overarching tenet for the interviews allowed a deeper understanding of personal safety choices and the ability to realistically change some of those choices in the future. As the examples we provided illustrate, participants were able to utilize tenets of the metatheory to inform the researchers about ways to better target and communicate with target audiences.

SUMMARY

In this chapter we discussed some common sampling methods in qualitative research, followed by the sampling procedures we used in our project. Then, we utilized the results from our research project to illustrate how harm reduction metatheory guided the RHBM, with an emphasis on how each tenet guided a portion of the interview methodology. Finally, we highlighted ways participants utilized the tenets of the metatheory to provide specific feedback related to targeting motorcyclists in the future. The next chapter discusses validity and reliability in qualitative research, with examples of how we adhered to research rigor while studying harm reduction as a metatheory.

REFERENCES

Arber, S. (1993). The research process. In N. Gilbert (Ed.), *Researching social life,* (pp. 32–50). London: Sage.

Bandura, A. (1977). Self-efficacy: Toward a unifying theory of behavioral change. *Psychological Review, 84,* 191–215.

Brown, L., DiClemente, R., & Reynolds, L. (1991). HIV prevention for adolescents: The utility of the Health Belief Model. *AIDS Education and Prevention, 3*, 50–59.

Corbin, J., & Strauss, A. (2008). *Basics of qualitative research* (3rd Ed.). Thousand Oaks, CA: Sage.

Curtis, S., Gesler, W., Smith, G., & Washburn, S. (2000). Approaches to sampling and case selection in qualitative research: Examples in the geography of health. *Social Science & Medicine, 50,* 1001–1014.

Denzin, N. K., & Lincoln, Y. S. (2011). *The SAGE handbook of qualitative research.* (4th Ed.). Sage.

Elliot, M. A., Baughan, C. J., Broughton, J., Chinn, B., Grayson, G. B., Khoules, J., Smith, C. R., & Simpson, H. (2003). *Motorcycle safety: A scoping study.* [Report No. TRL581]. Transport Research Laboratory.

Firestone, W. (1993.) Alternative arguments for generalizing from data as applied to qualitative research. *Educational Researcher, 22*(4), 16–23.

Glaser, B., & Strauss, A. (1967). *Discovery of grounded theory: Strategies for qualitative research.* Aldine Publishing, New York.

Haas, E. J. (2012). *Toward harm reduction as a metatheory for health communication campaigns: An empirical study of harm reduction metatheory and the reconceptualized health belief model addressing motorcycle safety.* Unpublished doctoral dissertation. West Lafayette, IN: Purdue University.

Hammersley, M., & Atkinson, P. (1983). *Ethnography: Principles in practice.* London: Tavistock.

Katz, J. (2001). From how to why: On luminous description and causal inference in ethnography. *Ethnography, 2,* 443–473.

Kosmoski, C., Mattson, M., & Hall, J. (2007). Reconsidering motorcycle safety at Purdue: A case study integrating campaign theory and practice. *Cases in Public Health Communication & Marketing.* Available from http://www.casesjournal.org.

Kuzel, A. J. (1992). Sampling in qualitative inquiry. In B.F. Crabtree & W.L. Miller (3rd Ed.), *Doing qualitative research: Research Methods for Primary Care.* (pp. 31–44). Newbury Park, CA: Sage.

Lincoln, Y. S., & Guba, E. G. (1985). *Naturalistic inquiry.* Beverly Hills, CA: Sage.

Lindlof, T. R. (2001). The challenge of writing the qualitative study. In A. Alexander & W.J. Potter (Eds.), *How to publish your communication research: An insider's guide* (pp. 77–96). Thousand Oaks, CA: Sage.

Lindlof, T. R., & Taylor, B. C. (2002). *Qualitative communication research methods* (2nd Ed.). Thousand Oaks, CA: Sage Publications.

Lofland, J., Snow, D., Anderson, L., & Lofland, L. H. (2006). *Analyzing social settings: A guide to qualitative observation and analysis* (4th Ed.). Canada: Wadsworth.

Mattson, M., Haas, E., Gillig, T., & Kosmoski, C. (2011). Engaging motorcycle safety in a university community: Toward a health campaign pedagogy model for community advocacy. In M. Brann, *Contemporary issues in health communication: Theoretical and practical case studies* (pp. 185–197). Dubuque, IA: Kendall-Hunt.

Mattson, M., & Basnyat, I. (2008). Infusing HIV test counseling practice with harm reduction theory: An integrated model for voluntary counseling and testing. In T. Edgar, S. Noar, & V. Freimuth (eds.). *Communication perspectives for HIV/AIDS in the 21st century* (pp. 137–167). New York: Lawrence Erlbaum Associates.

Miles, M., & Huberman, A. (1994). *Qualitative data analysis.* London: Sage.

Patton, M. Q. (2002). *Qualitative research and evaluation methods* (3rd Ed.). Thousand Oaks, CA: Sage.

Patton, M. Q. (1990). *Qualitative research and evaluation methods* (2nd Ed.), Newbury Park, CA: Sage.

Rhodes, T. (2002). The "risk environment": A framework for understanding and reducing drug-related harm. *International Journal of Drug Policy, 13,* 85–94.

Yin, R. K. (2011). *Qualitative research from start to finish.* New York, NY: Guilford Press.

Zuckerman, M. (1994). *Behavioral expressions and biosocial bases of sensation seeking*. Cambridge: Cambridge University Press.

Chapter 6

Validity and Reflexivity in Harm Reduction Qualitative Research

In the previous chapter we utilized results from our research project to present a new, meta-framework for using harm reduction when analyzing, reporting, and applying the results of a qualitative research project. You read how participants responded to interview questions guided by harm reduction metatheory and how the participants applied those same harm reduction tenets while providing us with feedback for future work in health and safety initiatives to target motorcyclists and drivers of cars and trucks to change safety behaviors.

During the data collection, analysis, and reporting of results in qualitative research projects, validity and reflexivity need to be considered. In this chapter, we address the importance of these issues when considering any qualitative research project. However, we more so consider these issues with respect to harm reduction integration in qualitative, theoretical research. We cover general issues of validity and reflexivity but also provide specific discussions about the impact of harm reduction as a metatheory on our process of determining validity and practicing mindful reflexivity. The chapter is framed by the following objectives:

- Understanding the importance of validity in qualitative research
- Reviewing descriptive validity, interpretive validity, and theoretical validity
- Using verification strategies to determine validity
- Practicing researcher reflexivity during qualitative research
- Considering the role of harm reduction metatheory on researcher reflexivity

We begin with some general definitions of validity in qualitative research. Then we move toward more specific definitions of validity and strategies that can be used to determine validity throughout a qualitative research project that incorporates harm reduction tenets.

VALIDITY IN QUALITATIVE RESEARCH

According to Flick (2002), researchers in the social sciences are still trying to determine how to best assess qualitative research. Hammersley (1987) commonly is cited by qualitative researchers for his assessment of *validity*: "An account is valid if it represents accurately those features of the phenomena, that it is intended to describe, explain, or theorize" (p. 67). However, throughout the literature a variety of definitions occur. Kerlinger (1964) discussed validity as measuring what we think we are measuring. Lindlof and Taylor (2002) defined a valid study as one that "the instrument makes the distinctions that are intended" (p. 239). Campbell (1996) referred to validity as consistency in data that is achieved when the steps of the research are verified through examination of items such as raw data, data reduction products, and process notes. According to Berg (2004), validity is achieved when data are linked in terms of some explanatory schema. More simply, Silverman (2005) associated validity with another word for truth.

Although a universal definition of validity does not exist, you can glean from the previous definitions that a primary concern of researchers is that validity is taken into account when designing a study, that threats to validity are acknowledged throughout the study, and precautions are taken to guard against those threats so the data can be used to truthfully describe and explain the research questions. Since there is not an agreed-upon definition of validity, it is not surprising that researchers focus on different criteria for constituting validity and utilize various methods for addressing threats to validity.

For instance, many researchers have proposed their own concept(s) of validity such as quality, rigor, and trustworthiness (Strenbacka, 2001; Seale, 1999; Lincoln & Guba, 1985). Hammersley (1992) also argued that the validity of ethnographic research should be judged on the theory production, transferability, consistency with observation, novelty of claims, credibility, reflexivity, and development of theory that results from the project. More broadly, there are several types of validity to consider during a research project. Within each type of validity there are different strategies we can use to design and accomplish a reliable study. In the following sections, we discuss descriptive validity, interpretive validity, and theoretical validity. We also address some common threats to these three types of validity and examples of verification strategies we engaged in to ensure a valid study. We begin with descriptive validity.

Descriptive Validity

There are several types of validity. Of primary concern at the initial stages of data collection is *descriptive validity*, which questions the accuracy of the data being collected by the researcher (Maxwell, 1992; Winter, 2000). Descriptive validity is concerned with whether what the researcher recorded is what actually happened (Johnson, 1997). It is common for other researchers or readers to be concerned with the factual accuracy of the information observed, experienced, and described (Runciman, 1983; Winter, 2000). In the various definitions that follow, the main issue questioned in descriptive validity is the possible omission of data that was necessary to understand the information shared during the interview (Thomson, 2011). Several researchers associate descriptive validity with "truthfulness," "trustworthiness," or "credibility."

Yin (1994) defined trustworthiness of a qualitative study as a criterion to test the quality of the research design. When addressing issues of descriptive validity, Hammersley (1992) discussed the importance of establishing credibility, or trustworthiness, in the research study. He specified that, when reading the results, we must ask ourselves if the claims we are making are plausible, given our existing knowledge base in that area. He went on to say that, "If we do not have previously existing knowledge in this area, could we reasonably expect the new claims to be accurate, given what we know about the context in which the research was conducted?" (p. 70). Guba and Lincoln (1989) also used trustworthiness in their discussions about post-hoc assessments of qualitative research to determine whether studies maintained rigor throughout the project.

More specifically, Guba and Lincoln (1981) substituted reliability and validity with trustworthiness containing the following aspects: credibility, transferability, dependability and conformability of the data. This is similar to Maxwell's (1992) concerns about being able to produce descriptively similar data or accounts of the same events if replicated at a later time. Glaser and Strauss (1967) used the term "credibility" to capture the same concept of descriptive validity when they said the data must accurately reflect what the participant said or has done. There are several verification strategies that can be used throughout the duration of a project to determine descriptive validity while maintaining trueness to the data.

Verifying Descriptive Validity

Rather than focusing on the truthfulness of a research design at the end of the project, researchers have recently begun to argue for *verification strategies* throughout the process of the project. Specifically, Morse et al. (2002) stated that "While strategies of trustworthiness may be useful in attempting to evaluate rigor, they do not in themselves ensure rigor" (p. 9). These researchers defined verification as a process of checking and being certain during every step of the project. In other words, descriptive validity, or accuracy of the data, can be better ensured through systematic, sound data collection procedures, such as those we've described in previous chapters about developing research questions, designing research instruments to measure what we want to measure, collecting data until saturation is reached, systematically checking data, including the fit of the data to the conceptual model being studied, and maintaining a positive, yet neutral relationship with participants to illicit honest responses (Kvale, 1989; Morse et al., 2002). There are various types of verification strategies to ensure validity throughout the entirety of a project. We address some of these strategies throughout the chapter.

During qualitative data analysis there are multiple ways of making sense of reality. Hammersley (1992) referred to this truth as a "subtle realist" tradition. Other researchers described this process as "securing a close approximation of the empirical world" (Snow & Morrill, 1993, p. 10) that is trustworthy by others in terms of what really happened during the data collection and analysis process. One reason why descriptive validity is so difficult to verify is because many opposing truths can exist within the same account (Winter, 2000). Therefore, at the very least, it is important to be able to verify how you devised the codes, themes, and subthemes from the data you collected. This ensures that others know what you observed and experienced, and provides insight into factual events that occurred during the interviews.

Verification strategies that determine the descriptive validity of a study include recruiting a sample that is appropriate, utilizing participants who have knowledge about the research topic, and collecting and analyzing data simultaneously (Morse et al., 2002). We discussed our recruiting strategy in Chapter 5, which was a purposive sampling technique to recruit a wide range of cases that could speak to the issue of motorcycle safety (Patton, 2002). We also discussed our process of completing an interview and transcribing the data shortly thereafter, while simultaneously conducting additional interviews. The iterative process of conducting interviews, transcribing interviews, and comparing the data concurrently allowed us to see the interactions among the different participants, which served as a verification strategy for descriptive validity. In the next section, we provide a more in-depth example of documenting the rationale to verify descriptive validity during the analysis of data.

Documenting Rationale for Data Analysis Decisions

Morse et al. (2002) argued that, although memos and notes may show proof of decisions that we make throughout a research project, these notes often are not helpful to determining the quality of those decisions or the rationale behind those decisions. Similarly, Runciman (1983) noted the possibility of factual accuracy that can be missing when reporting study results. To avoid possible errors concerning data selection and interpretation, we support and recommend going beyond simple note-taking during data analysis and instead, making specific notes to verify why you made certain decisions while analyzing your data. This step is particularly important during the coding process of a qualitative research project, since you must develop and organize a plethora of data into a single codebook. It is likely that you will organize data into codes and then themes that overlap and not realize the intersections of these themes until later, so it is important to document why you collapsed two or more themes within a code, created an additional theme within a code, or removed or added a code.

For example, during our analysis of motorcyclists' interviews, we developed a preliminary codebook based on initial, focused, and theoretical coding. Then, the content of each data file was reviewed to ensure assigned themes fit within a code and to further elaborate the code, if necessary. During this phase of the data analysis process we could start to see redundancy in some of the codes and/or themes within interview sections. At this time, we created a document titled "Code Tables with Justification for Changes" that contained support and rationale for why we were collapsing two themes within a code or deleting a code/theme in which we did not achieve a satisfactory level of saturation. We believe this verification strategy, documenting the rationale for all data analysis decisions, helped us remain true to the data and communicate results accurately to our audiences. An example of this process is provided in Research Project in Practice Illustration Figure 6.1.

As you read in Figure 6.1, we originally had two themes about personal crashes/near crashes that referenced participants' responses to these incidents in the form of a wake-up call, followed by a change in behavior, even if that behavior change was simply being more conscious while driving their motorcycle. As you can see in our notes, we felt that there were several similarities in participants' responses to their near crashes. In the note we provided a rationale for why we wanted to combine these themes within the personal crash/near crash code. There were two other incidents of combining codes within a theme. We documented this process for the integration of each code and kept this justification file in a separate document to maintain the organization of our data. Maxwell (1992) and Winter (2000) argued that the selection of relevant data often is the biggest threat to descriptive validity. However, we believe this iterative process of analyzing the data demonstrated our responsiveness and flexibility toward the data and helped verify the descriptive validity of the study. Although we made choices that involved narrowing data, we justified these decisions and provided full disclosure throughout this process.

Now that we've discussed descriptive validity, threats to descriptive validity, and possible verification strategies, we address interpretive validity in the next section.

Research in Practice Illustration
Example of Documenting Rationale for Data Analysis Decisions
***Using Excerpt from Immediacy/Goal Setting Guiding Motorcycle Safety Perceived Susceptibility and Severity Codebook**

Code: Personal crash/near crash

Theme 1: Now do...this.
Examples supporting Theme 1:

- *"I definitely uh...I don't sit at lights anymore ya know. If the light is red I still don't, I don't mess around. Ya know if there's a problem with my jacket or my gear or whatever, or if my cell phone rings, I'm not gonna touch it. I'm gonna go to a safe spot on the side of the road or in a parking lot to deal with that because yeah, I'm really aware and worried because you don't know if somebody's on the cell phone and they're just gonna bump you or it coulda been worse, easily."* (Participant 29)
- *"I tried to avoid it already but in that case like I was going to work and so I needed to, because otherwise it's just too far to walk. Um I do consider walking it sometimes...like...or if I need to go to the store for groceries then okay I'll put it off for a day or something like that just because it was raining."* (Participant 31)
- *"Umm just more cautious about umm my surroundings more aware of what's on the road...the gravel...umm that's about it. I mean it just snuck up on me. I was probably a little bit too relaxed."* (Participant 6)
- *"But I started feeling conscious of and worried about deer. And we did cut back on the number of hours we spent on our bikes. We definitely did. We don't ride near as much as we used to. I mean, we still ride regularly but I mean we would go overnights and all that. We didn't see any more after that but that was the first day (haha). We were like oh man. It does...it does take a little bit out of the sport after you experience or have seen something like that. It just...like I said we don't do it as much as we did."* (Participant 7).

Theme 2: Wake-up call
Examples supporting Theme 2:

- *"When the semi truck pulled out in front of me it made me realize that other people are not aware of me. And that was, that was the second time that happened so yeah, very aware, you have to be very aware of everybody else. It's not necessarily about what you're doing it's about what they're doing."* (Participant 15)
- *"I feel safe until people around you start to make errors or stuff like that. Like once one happens I know like I start to get a little more wary because if they're following you or they cut you off then you gotta be more wary of what they're gonna be doing next. Or like riding at night with people cause a lot of times people don't really notice bikes and stuff like that."* (Participant 23)
- *"I would also say that now that I've been in an accident...um...I think that would only enhance or make me a better rider just because um I'm then more conscious of, of just all the, of all those factors, all those contributing factors."* (Participant 33)
- *"I hardly rode at all then. Like a couple miles a year, like back out here. Ya know out in the country, no more highway, no more nothing. Yeah cause I realized that you couldn't be defensive enough. You could never anticipate that in a million years and yet, it, it happened and that's not an accident, that's just ya know like insanity, like it's hard to describe."* (Participant 27)

Note about collapsing two themes within the code:

Emily Inquiry: I would like to combine the theme "Now do __" with the "Wake-up call" theme. In the "Now do __" theme, participants specifically dealt with changing a behavior that caused the crash or near crash. However, participants also noted the importance of them changing behaviors to just be more conscious, similar to that of a wake-up call, which was the point of focus in the subsequent theme. In the examples above, participants often noted their accident as a wake-up call and as a follow-up, they changed a particular behavior. So, these two themes often intersected into one, comprehensive response to a crash or near crash.

Marifran Response: OK. Be sure to document, with support, all the analysis decisions we're making. For example, when we collapse codes/themes, keep track of how we did this and why.

Figure 6.1 Research in Practice Illustration: Example of Documenting Rationale for Data Analysis Decisions.

Interpretive Validity

Descriptive validity focuses on truthful reporting of the results whereas *interpretive validity* focuses on accurately communicating participants' feedback about the phenomenon being studied (Johnson, 1997). According to Maxwell (1992), "interpretive validity is inherently a matter of inference from the words and actions of participants in situations studied" (p. 49). In other words, are we communicating participants' voice back to the community accurately when analyzing the data and reporting the results? Terms including "conformability" and "justifiability" have been used to decide whether interpretive validity was acknowledged in the data (Walsh, 2003). There are several verification strategies that have been used to acknowledge interpretive validity. One method often used by researchers is member checking or member validation. However, we argue that, when incorporating harm reduction into a qualitative research project, reflexivity is a more crucial technique to accurately expressing participants' voices while also minimizing researcher bias. We briefly address researcher bias as a concern to establishing interpretive validity before discussing member checking and reflexivity as possible verification strategies.

Acknowledging and Responding to Researcher Bias

A common barrier to establishing interpretive validity is researcher bias. *Researcher bias* often stems from researchers looking for what they want to find, making special note of the information they want to find, and reporting the information they wanted to find, while overlooking other important aspects from the data (Johnson, 1997). In Chapters 4 and 5 we described the steps we took to develop a reliable protocol and conduct a valid analysis. However, in most research projects, it is possible that the analysis of codes and themes to create each respective codebook was biased by the researchers' interpretations. However, these interpretations are an unavoidable element of data analysis (Winter, 2000).

One way to contest researcher bias, and maintain interpretive validity, is to keep an open mind during each interview and not ask leading questions of participants. In our chapter about research methods, you may remember that we utilized open-ended and probing questions to better capture and understand motorcyclists' experiences. In addition, the repetition of codes and themes throughout each codebook respective to a tenet of harm reduction also depicts the similar issues that emerged throughout the interviews, as you will learn in a subsequent section of this chapter. This repetition of codes and themes minimized interpretation bias because similar barriers to safety were mentioned repeatedly during each interview. Besides these rigorous practices for conducting an interview, researchers often engage in member checking to prevent researcher bias and ensure interpretive validity.

Member Checking

We realize discussing issues of validity can be a capricious endeavor among qualitative scholars and researchers. However, member checking is one method researchers have used to respond to common threats of interpretive validity (e.g., researcher bias and influences of the participants on the environment) (Maxwell, 1992). *Member checking*, or *member validation,* consists of bringing your research findings back to the environment in which the data was collected and allowing participants to peruse and deem the results to be accurate and valid accounts (Lincoln & Guba, 1985; Lofland & Taylor, 2002; Maxwell, 1992). Although this strategy has been widely used by researchers to check and/or verify their instincts regarding the data, several scholars argue that member checks, albeit useful for certain projects, are not a verification strategy to ensure interpretive validity (see Guba & Lincoln, 1981; Hammersley, 1992; Morse, 1998; Morse et al., 2002).

These critics warned against the tendency to define verification in terms of whether readers, participants, or potential users of the research judge the analysis to be *correct*. They further warned that doing so can be a threat to validity. Morse (1998) argued that since results have been synthesized, decontextualized, and abstracted across participants, there is no reason for individuals to recognize themselves or their particular experiences within the results of an analysis. In some cases, participants may not agree with or respect how their character is portrayed in your analysis, especially if your research topic is sensitive. Winter (2000) conveyed the example of interviewing a convicted rapist with a long history of sex crimes, who argues for his/her innocence, as someone you may have to portray as an innocent victim in a series of accusations. If participants do not agree with your interpretation of the data, what options do you, as a researcher, have? The researcher may have to adopt the alternative perspectives of the data, be more descriptive in the results, and/or provide extra content to address each participant's concerns (Morse et al., 2002).

Because of this apprehension toward member checks and due to the metatheoretical nature of the research questions proposed in our study, we did not engage in member validation. Our goal was to empirically assess harm reduction as a metatheory and not necessarily uncover new issues in motorcycle safety, although results also informed this area of research. For example, if we had engaged in member checking, participants may not have understood why similar codes and themes were presented across interview sections. They also may not have appreciated the codes that focused on negative safety behaviors including excessive speeding and driving a motorcycle while under the influence of alcohol.

However, we did meet with participants who requested to learn the results of the study. Their reactions during these meetings supported our inclination that our findings informing harm reduction as a metatheory may not have been understandable or deemed important to them, as motorcyclists. However, the five participants we met with to discuss the results of the study did not disagree with or question the overall results about motorcycle safety behaviors. Rather, they were curious as to how the overall results would be used in the future to inform motorcycle safety initiatives.

Even though we did not utilize member checking to corroborate our analysis, we believe that verification strategies are necessary and those strategies may vary depending on your research questions and participants. One verification strategy we engaged in to maintain interpretive validity was reflexivity. According to Johnson (1997), being reflexive is the best way to avoid researcher bias. Reflexivity is discussed in the next section.

Verifying Interpretive Validity through Reflexivity

In addition to reflexivity serving as a verification strategy to ensure interpretive validity, we believe this research tool deserves special attention because of the novel way we apply harm reduction as a metatheory using qualitative methodology. Some researchers have argued for more reflexive examples in qualitative research (Mauthner & Doucet, 2003), therefore, we wanted to include specific examples of how we engaged in reflexivity during our harm reduction metatheoretical analysis and reporting of results. It is our intent that these examples promote the use of reflexivity in future harm reduction health and safety projects. We also discuss the ways in which harm reduction metatheory enhanced reflexivity during the research project, providing further support to integrate the use of metatheory into qualitative research methodology.

Generally, *reflexivity* is a basic awareness of the data. Gilgun (2010) stated that we are reflexive when we are "aware of the multiple influences we have on research processes and how the research processes affect us" (p. 1). We begin our discussion of reflexivity in qualitative research with a focus on the role(s) of the researcher. To illustrate maintaining this level of awareness, we consider some ways in which we were reflexive throughout our project including how we accounted for our personal interests in the research topic and how we accounted for the experiences of our participants when reporting the results.

Disclosing Your Emotional Ties to the Research Topic

First, one way to practice reflexivity is to initially disclose any personal and professional ties to the research topic (Gilgun, 2010). It is important to disclose and understand any emotional responses to the participants that may occur, and how previous experiences may affect your interpretation of the data. Although reflexive practice calls for this mindful reflection, there are few tools offered in the literature to facilitate this activity during a research project (Mauthner & Doucet, 2003). However, there are several ways we disclosed personal and professional ties, including the disclosure in the Preface of this book, about our emotional connection to the topic of motorcycle safety.

When participants inquired about our purpose for interviewing motorcyclists and/or for focusing specifically on motorcycle safety, we provided a candid response. Although we discussed our personal experiences with participants, we did not divulge too many details about either motorcycle accident to avoid biasing participants' responses during the interview. For example, if we would have said that one of the accidents occurred in part because of the motorcyclist's high BAC, participants may not have been as forthcoming about their own experiences consuming alcohol while operating a motorcycle. Research Project in Practice Illustration Figure 6.2 provides an example of such an interaction at the beginning of an interview.

As you read, we only disclosed our personal connection to the issue of motorcycling when probed by the participant and we offered an abbreviated version of our connection. We also were careful not to place blame on the motorcyclist, a driver of another vehicle, or the environment so we would not bias responses regarding any of these topic areas in subsequent discussions with the participant. As you read, the participant identified with this motorcycle accident by discussing his own experience of a friend dying in a motorcycle accident. By disclosing this information to participants when probed, they also were given the opportunity to respond to our emotional connection to the issue and further clarify, if they felt necessary, some of their statements throughout the interview, to aide our interpretation of what they were saying about issues related to motorcycle accidents and campaign messages.

Research in Practice Illustration
Accounting for Personal Interests During the Interview

Participant 15: *How does someone who is not a motorcyclist become interested in the issue of motorcycle safety?*

Emily: *Well I had a family member die in a motorcycle accident several years ago. That made me pay more attention to motorcyclists and motorcycle safety. Then I came to Purdue, where a motorcycle campaign was already in place, which further developed my interest in the issue.*

Participant 15: *Oh okay. Yeah, I just had a friend die in a motorcycle accident, too, not too long ago. About six weeks ago. It was due to his total lack of discretion and I dunno, self-preservation. But that's how I learn to drive more defensively.*

Figure 6.2 Research in Practice Illustration: Accounting for Personal Interests During the Interview.

Another area of reflexivity that researchers need to be cognizant of to determine interpretive validity is portraying participants' authentic voice when reporting the results of the analysis.

Portraying Participants' Authentic Voice

It is important to account for the experiences of your participants and portray their authentic voice in your interpretation of the data. Brown and Gilligan (1992) suggested that several readings of the interview text aides a voice-centered analysis of the data. Then, while reading the interview text, researchers suggest responding emotionally and intellectually to the feedback provided by participants (Brown, 1994) and documenting your thoughts next to the data. This technique provides several benefits. For example, Mauthner and Doucet (2003) argued that writing your interpretations within the data files allows for an examination of how your interpretations may alter the participant's feedback. They went on to state that, "This reading is based on the assumption that locating ourselves socially, emotionally, and intellectually allows us to retain some grasp over the blurred boundary between the respondent's narrative and our interpretation" (p. 419) which is important in maintaining reflexivity. In addition, we argue that documenting your interpretations of the data within each interview transcript allows the opportunity to compare and contrast across the interview transcripts and examine how our response(s) to participants are similar or may have been different and if so, potential causes for these discrepancies in the data analysis process.

We heeded this reader-response advice by Mauthner and Doucet (2003) and wrote personal interpretations of the data within each interview transcript. These personal notes were referenced when coding the data and subsequently, writing the results from the analysis. The notes helped us establish connections between participants, giving groups of motorcyclists a more assertive voice in the results. In Research Project in Practice Illustrations Figure 6.3 and Figure 6.4, we provide examples of this process, with one column containing the raw data and some of our comments to the feedback in the right column.

Recording these personal comments had multiple benefits. For instance, these recordings helped us disclose and in some cases, vent some of our frustrations toward participants' motorcycle safety behaviors. Simultaneously, however, these comments also prompted a personal exploration of ways not being a motorcyclist may have influenced our interpretation of their feedback. For example, because one of us is not a motorcyclist and the other researcher is a former motorcyclist, our meetings about the interview data allowed space for us to be reflexive toward our interpretations of the data,

Research in Practice Illustration **Excerpt of Personal Interpretation of Data from Participant 1**	
P1: No because I got right back on…I had to go to school. I was in college and I was gonna get back on it. And my friends were like…you can't ride like that…and I'm like well I gotta get to school. So they got a friend to take me every day for a couple of weeks. Umm I mean it gave me no fear it's just ya know…I tend to now ya know hot or not, cause it's the whole thing…the motorcycle is just free…in the wind…it's open and if you take all those things for granted, the asphalt will kill you (haha). So regardless of how hot it is, and that's why I have different types of helmets just make sure you have tons of vents on your helmets. So, you know the more expensive they get…they have nice little vents all over the place. So ya know you just try to stay vented. Umm (5.0) and I had…like I think I told your mother I had a $500 helmet that…which I had off one time and it went, "dink…dink…dink…dink…dink," when I turned the corner. You know, tryin to do real cool like that with riding with the helmet on the back (haha). Don't ride your helmet. And I didn't like all the dinks. Now that was $500 and I couldn't get the "dinks" repaired and fixed so, I'd rather put it on my head and it made sense then but…I mean since it did the "dink, dink" I probably have never ridden without a helmet on my head.	Accident did not cause motorcyclist to question if she would ride again—didn't affect desire to ride. Did find gear that could use in hot weather. Still riding, but riding safer than before the accident. Didn't like that an expensive helmet got damaged on back of bike—would rather wear it than pay for new helmet.

Figure 6.3 Research in Practice Illustration: Excerpt of Personal Interpretation of Data from Participant 1.

Research in Practice Illustration **Excerpt of Personal Interpretation of Data from Participant 37**	
E: Alright how often do you ride your motorcycle after consuming alcohol? *P37: Too much (haha).* *E: Okay, so typically how much will you drink and ride?* *P37: Well when we're out there all day long you're probably talking five, six beers.* *E: Do you notice it impairing your riding at all?* *P37: No not in that situation no. You do it all day long so, no.* *E: And in general do you think that consuming alcohol and then riding is a risky behavior for motorcyclists?* *P37: Oh yeah. Anytime when you drink and drive it's risky.* *E: Okay why is that?* *P37: Well a lot of people can't handle that. So somebody will have six beers, like I would…but it might bother them a little bit more than it would me. Ya know it's hard to say.*	Alcohol embedded in culture—participant notes motorcyclists drinking all day while riding. He notes that anytime people drink it is risky, except him. He notes that he is the exception. If everyone feels this way how can we change behavior? Similar to previous interviews—individual believes that drinking is risky but not for them, only view everyone else as a threat to their safety.

Figure 6.4 Research in Practice Illustration: Excerpt of Personal Interpretation of Data from Participant 37.

by reading and discussing the content from different personal experiences. During these research meetings and conversations, in which we critiqued our research encounters with participants, we participated in a postmodern aspect of reflexivity (Finlay, 2002; Wallis, 2010). Referencing discussions from our meetings and using interpretation notes during the stages of data analysis helped us identify areas we needed to continually revisit in subsequent research meetings and even latter interviews with participants. As a result, we better understood and could appreciate the stories that were being shared with us. We were able to show our emotions, surprises, and concerns toward the responses during our analysis but then continue to represent the participants' feedback and accurately tell their stories. This process allowed for a more thorough data analysis and helped us articulate what participants communicated during each interview. Besides engaging in mindful reflexivity from a traditional research approach to qualitative methodology, we discovered that using harm reduction as a metatheory also facilitated our ability to accurately depict participants' experiences due to the emphasis that the tenets of harm reduction place on personal choice, nonjudgmental attitudes, and noncritical communication toward individuals. We forward this new aspect of reflexivity in the next section.

USING HARM REDUCTION METATHEORY TO ENGAGE AND PROVIDE PARTICIPANTS' ACCURATE VOICE DURING DATA COLLECTION

In a qualitative study "research design should be a reflexive process operating through every stage of the project" (Hammersley and Atkinson, 1995, p. 24). During this project, we believe the added integration of harm reduction as the metatheoretical level enhanced the value of reflexivity for the researcher and the participants during the interviews. According to some researchers, a reflexive approach specifically involves a metatheoretical understanding of the data and the use of a theoretical framework for how to understand the subject matter (Alvesson, 2002). To maintain this level of reflexivity during our harm reduction motorcycle safety research project, we needed to have a grasp of metatheory, the potential of HRT as a metatheory, and how it could guide a theory to better understand motorcycle safety behaviors. In doing so, harm reduction metatheory was a useful tool in helping us maintain reflexivity during this project. Below, we highlight examples from data collection to showcase the process of metatheorizing while maintaining reflexive integrity. You will see how using metatheory helped us accurately portray participants' narratives.

From a data collection standpoint, we maintained an attitude of openness toward the participants. Based on the introduction to the study and participants' responses to the qualifying questions, we had to determine whether or not participants were being honest about their motorcycling experiences throughout the interviews and gently probe them, if necessary. It was important to probe participants if we felt they were not sharing their experiences in entirety, to give them a fully authentic voice during the analysis and reporting of results. Noncritical probing was achieved through application of harm reduction. We utilized the tenets of HRT to engage theory, while discussing a specific safety behavior. For example, we probed participants about alcohol consumption behaviors while driving a motorcycle through the HRT tenets humanistic value, pragmatism, immediacy/goal setting, and community collaboration. Engaging participants about the same behavior through each of these tenets allowed them to respond more than one time about the behavior, continue opening up, and sharing stories.

This method of questioning, which utilized HRT as a metatheoretical framework to better understand motorcyclists' experiences, demonstrated reflexive pragmatism and an epistemological awareness (Alvesson, 2002). At the same time, we could confirm the data from participants was valid by cross-checking their stories across interview sections and probing, if we needed clarification. Several excerpts from Interview 3 are included in Research Project in Practice Illustration Figure 6.5. In this illustration, we provide excerpts from three different sections of the interview in which we probed the participant about his drinking and speeding behaviors. You will notice he is a little bit more reserved about his behaviors in the introductory qualifying section of the interview but then as the interview progressed, he became more comfortable and shared some unique stories. By probing similar issues through a different tenet of HRT (i.e., a different perspective), we were able to draw out more information from the participant, ensuring we could accurately communicate his experiences and our perceptions of the data were aligned with his perceptions as a motorcyclist.

This method of similar topic questioning, introduced from a different standpoint depending on the HRT tenet being utilized, was an important aspect of reflexivity during the data collection process. This approach provided us with a greater sense of awareness and if necessary, we modified the probes during the interview. In other words, using the harm reduction tenets allowed for flexibility, which is a vital component of being a reflexive researcher. Grady and Wallston (1988) asserted that flexibility allows us to examine a research project from different perspectives. We believe incorporating harm reduction metatheory into qualitative research may enhance the flexibility during a project and provide a more well-rounded depiction of the data.

Research in Practice Illustration
Using Harm Reduction Metatheory to Probe Participant 3

Interview Excerpt from Introductory Qualifying Section
E: Okay. Do you consume alcohol and then ride?
P3: Sometimes ya know like when I go out. But sometimes I don't though. So it just depends. And ya know what, having a motorcycle is like a 24-hour party. Because you see someone and it's like 'hey' and you get waved down and you pull over and ya know it's like 'hey what's goin on.'

Interview Excerpt from Perceived Barriers/Benefits (Pragmatism) Section
E: What is your personal definition of motorcycle safety?
P3: (6.0). Seriously? Motorcycle safety for me would be one, not to be under the influence of anything, obviously. I mean obviously you're a better rider when you're not under the influence of alcohol or drugs. Secondly, ya have to be smart in terms of speed. I mean I don't speed in the, in the cities ya know I won't fly through an intersection because that's how you get killed. But when I'm on the highway ya know look out because I'm goin' 100 or as fast as it goes. But as far as umm...ya know it's just common sense basically. You have to be smarter than the driver because they don't care. Ya know when you're in the car you have a false sense of invincibility. But when you're on that motorcycle and you see that concrete//right there//exactly ya know! (haha).
E: Um so then what are some of the intentional safety choices that you make while you ride?
P3: Well I would say one of them is watching your speed and not necessarily because someone could take you out but also because ya know you can get pulled over ya know and then ya know it's...police. They make a big deal about speeding ya know but they do the same thing themselves so they're really hypocrites ya know. I love when police say that they're good people and ya know...99% of them are good people but there's that 1% that's just ya know...(4.0) so just ya know try to be safe try to be uhh obviously coherent and conscious of what's going on around you because ya know people will hurt you and they don't care. And I hate to bring up women but women are always on their phone and they're always ya know...they are though, truly. It's scary because they'll take you out. (hahaha).
E: Point taken. So those are some of the conscious safety choices, what are some of the riskier choices that you make while you ride?//
P3: //That you know that it's wrong and you do it anyway, like ya know like F-it. Driving too fast or maybe you've had more than one drink at a cookout and you're like, ya know what I'm fine...gimme another beer...sober em' up. That's my favorite sayin, 'Gimme another shot, sober me up'. So ya know, doin that and actually, ya know it really just comes down to that I guess. Ya know there's a saying that your life is made up of all the decisions you make. And all the decisions are what makes your life what it is. But truly ya know if you make a bad decision you could end up legless, you could end up crippled, because ya know, it just takes one second and you're done. It could be me.

Interview Excerpt from Perceived Risk/Severity (Immediacy) Section
E: Okay umm so you said earlier that you will ride over the posted speed limit and speed. How much over the speed limit do you go?
P3: I mean ya know and to be honest with you I'll tell you a story. I was actually last summer...I was in (City 1) on (Avenue). I don't know if you're familiar with (City 1)?
E: No.
P3: No, you're from (County)?
E: Yeah.
P3: Oh okay. So I was in (City 1) and I was actually flying. I wasn't even...I was at a bar...I had like 3 beers but I was nowhere near intoxicated or anything like that. So I was driving ya know it was 3 in the morning...I hit the gas...(City 1) is right next to (City 2)...I'm from (City 2)...from the harbor. So I fly...I'm flying and then about...I look back and about a mile back from me I see lights. I'm like what the fuck. I was going maybe 90 in a 35. So I stop in (City 2) and a (City 1) cop pulls me over and was like, 'Do you know how fast you were going?'. And I'm like, 'I'm in (City 2) dude, you're a (City 1) cop'. And he's like, 'Well I pulled you over, whatever'. He writes me a ticket for speeding and he just put it, over...over the posted limit. I mean obviously anything over 15 mph is reckless. So you can actually go to jail, get your car towed for anything over 15 mph. So, to make a long story short...I...I have a lawyer. I called him up, gave him some money, the lawyer actually went in there and, and took the 95 in a 30 down to an illegal parking ticket, which is a 50 dollar fine. So really it wasn't about the speeding. And I know police officers care about safety but what it was really, really about was just the money. Ya know it wasn't about safety, or speeding, or the law. So ya know when they say ya know, posted speed limits, it's really tongue and cheek because obviously I don't think anybody really follows the speed limit. Ya know really

Figure 6.5 Research in Practice Illustration: Using Harm Reduction Metatheory to Probe Participant 3.

Now that we discussed the importance of portraying participants' authentic voice during data collection, the next section discusses theoretical validity during a qualitative research project. In this section we continue focusing on reflexivity as a verification strategy.

they don't...unless you're drunk and you're doing something you shouldn't be doing so you're driving like an old man or an old lady. Ya know but, nobody ever does.
E: Okay. As far as then, consuming alcohol and then riding is that something that umm, you do regularly or is it more maybe you consume one beer and then ride or do you ride intoxicated a lot?
P3: Ya know what...honestly the reason that I love riding is because it actually stops me from drinking because you know it's like, 'Hey ya know I'm on my bike I shouldn't drink'. But at the same time, motorcycle riding revolves around drinking because...you go here...you hang out at this bar...everybody's out...everybody's out, they're drinkin', they're doin' this, they're doin' that. They're smoking; whatever they're doing ya know what I mean? I go to the umm...Quaker Steak; they have bike night on Wednesdays. So we shoot up there on Wednesdays and ya know we're up there. Well, what's everyone doing up there? They're getting shit feathered...oh I'm sorry...they're drinkin', they're eatin' wings, ya know what I mean...they're hanging out. There's live bands there, everybody's drinking ya know, so...(4.0)...no it's not cool to drink obviously when you're on your motorcycle. But at the same time, it's the whole culture...that's what you're supposed to do. So if I'm drinking water people are like, 'Are you runnin' a marathon dude, or what? Where's the beer at?'. I'm dead serious...dead serious. You see people hammering back shots//uhh huh//. Ya know jagger bombs and everything ya know. Like today I'll go out and I'll end up at (bar) tonight...I go to (bar) on Fridays. So I'll be on my motorcycle. I might have a two or three beers ya know what I mean. But then as far as ya know when you get older...when you were younger...when I was younger I was more reckless. But as you get older you ya know...you realize don't do it because your whole summer will be sitting in a hospital bed...bandaged up like in the cartoons. Its bandages from head to toe.

Figure 6.5 ***Cont.***

Theoretical Validity

When acknowledging validity, always keep in mind the aspect of thinking theoretically (Morse et al., 2002). *Theoretical validity* focuses on the theoretical constructions that we bring to, or develop, during a research project (Maxwell, 1992). According to Thomson (2011), "What theoretical validity seeks to evaluate is the validity of the researcher's concepts and the theorized relationships among the concepts in context with the phenomena" (p. 79). In other words, the tenets, components, and patterns must fit to create and communicate a story. In our case, to establish theoretical validity, we had to present data that supported HRT as a metatheoretical framework. It was our responsibility, as researchers, to show how the theoretical, or metatheoretical, framework fit together (Auerbach & Silverstein, 2003). Keeping an open mind toward the data during the analysis helped us initially discover and later verify how the data came together to support the proposed framework.

Verifying Metatheoretical Validity through Reflexivity

To determine theoretical validity it was particularly important to maintain reflexivity toward the data during the theory-driven code development. Although metatheory and theory were used during the interviews, their concepts were loosely applied to not constrict participants' responses about their safety behaviors. However, it was important to bring harm reduction as the metatheoretical framework back into focus when analyzing the transcripts. As Alasuutari (1996) stated, "being theoretically informed means that one is reflexive toward the deceivingly self-evident reality one faces in and through the data, able to toy with different perspectives to it, and that one is open to new insights about every day life and society" (p. 375). In other words, it is common that two or more theories may be put "into creative tension" when describing and validating the data (Lindlof & Taylor, p. 238).

Accordingly, in our case, reflexivity continued to serve as a verification strategy to determine metatheoretical validity. From a data analysis standpoint, we were not only cognizant of participants' unique experiences, but we also had to be aware of how the metatheory was evolving during the analysis. Therefore, any concepts that could not be theoretically coded utilizing the five HRT tenets were set aside and examined later to see if a new tenet could be added to HRT. It was important to continue challenging the indicated interpretation and challenging ourselves with alternate views, which may, according to Alvesson and Skoldberg (2000), help arrive at the strongest or most interesting interpretation and/or offer alternative interpretations to report as findings. Although a new tenet was not added to HRT, thorough analysis of the data revealed the intersections between each of the five tenets and their cyclical importance to reducing individual and societal harm through behavioral modifications.

An example of how our data supported HRT as a metatheory guiding the Reconceptualized Health Belief Model (*RHBM*) is provided in the following Research Project in Practice Illustration. In order to see how the data collected fit the proposed framework, we had to maintain reflexivity during the metatheoretical analysis, and be able to evaluate and understand how the overarching tenets of the proposed metatheory could guide the components of a theory (Weinstein & Weinstein, 1992). Through our process of mindful reflexivity to verify the metatheoretical validity of harm reduction, several relationships emerged that helped us better understand the intricacies of motorcycle safety.

In the examples provided in the Research Project in Practice Illustration Figure 6.6, you see that within each component of the proposed metatheoretical framework, an issue about motorcycling culture and peer pressure within that culture emerged as an issue that hinders motorcyclists' ability to be safer. Using a tenet of HRT to probe a component of the RHBM, motorcyclists discussed within each section of the interview how peer motorcyclists often pressure their fellow riders to engage in riskier behaviors. However, as the interview progressed, motorcyclists said that by empowering youth to be safer and collaborating with key partners, we may be able to address some of the negative issues within motorcycling culture that were referenced earlier.

We only illustrated one theme within each component of the metatheoretical framework that was supported by the data. Additional themes and respective codes also referenced the impact of motorcycling culture on safety behaviors. Also, other aspects and behaviors related to motorcycle safety, including alcohol consumption, speed, and age, emerged throughout the

Research in Practice Illustration **Motorcycle Safety Data Verifying the Harm Reduction Metatheoretical Framework** **Motorcycle Safety Culture Emerging During Each Tenet of Harm Reduction Metatheory**		
Humanistic Value / Cues to Action **Code:** Fellow motorcyclists' influence **Theme:** Keeping up with group mentality	**Definition:** The motorcyclist discusses the role of group peer pressure in engaging in risky behaviors while riding a motorcycle. Some motorcyclists continue to give in to the peer pressure while others avoid group riding because of the peer pressure that is present.	**Example – Participant 24:** *"That's one reason that I don't ride in big groups. Because it is easy for the peer pressure to get you in an unsafe situation. Like one thing, like at a stop sign maybe four or five people go through, and three of them not stopping. If one of them goes through all the rest go through which is really unsafe, and illegal. But ya know its peer pressure. I think peer pressure's a big thing and that's one reason to stay away from big groups."*
Pragmatism / Perceived Barriers & Benefits **Code:** Yeah I own it, doesn't mean I wear it **Theme:** Who I'm with that day	**Definition:** The motorcyclist describes the importance of living up to the mystique of being a motorcyclist and riding in groups, and not wearing safety gear is a part of that expectation.	**Example – Participant 29:** *"...a part of peer pressure is living up to the mystique of riding motorcycles. And they think that a helmet doesn't fit into the live to ride, ride to live sort of mentality and so yeah. Because I've spoken to my sister repeatedly, I've said, "listen, you need to wear a helmet ya know, why don't you wear a helmet?" and um and that's how I got on the subject with her and she said, 'well none of my friends do'."*
Immediacy & Goal Setting / Perceived Susceptibility & Severity **Code:** Alcohol embedded in the motorcycling culture **Theme:** Yes it impairs my skills, but it's part of it	**Definition:** The motorcyclist conveys that consuming alcohol negatively impacts personal ability to ride a motorcycle safely but continues to participate in the behavior because it is expected in the motorcycling culture.	**Example – Participant 36:** *"Um it just kinda goes together...drinking and riding. And as a group mainly, like poker runs and stuff it's going from bar to bar to bar. Um I guess the key is to not overdo it but...no, no, no alcohol would be better than any alcohol. But it just kinda seems to go together, the riding, and the drinking (haha)."*
Empowerment / Self-efficacy **Code:** Shift in societal norms impacting youth's safety **Theme:** Emphasizing safety for youth	**Definition:** The motorcyclist conveys that a larger safety emphasis exists to help target youth behaviors on a motorcycle.	**Example – Participant 28:** *"I think we are headed that way as far as people accepting uh wearing safety protection. Um the old schoolers are probably not gonna go along with it but the younger generation seems like they're, they're pickin' up on it. So I think we're headed in the right direction as far as safety."*
Community Collaboration / Formative Audience Research **Code:** Collaboration is essential **Theme:** To get into the motorcycling culture	**Definition:** The motorcyclist indicates that collaboration with several groups may help infiltrate the embedded safety choices of the motorcycling culture.	**Example – Participant 3:** *"I don't think it would change just because the culture doesn't change. I mean ya know we're talkin about cultures, especially a Harley rider culture. Ya know it's just...it's just the whole live to ride, ride to live thing."*

Figure 6.6 Research in Practice Illustration: Motorcycle Safety Data Verifying the Harm Reduction Metatheoretical Framework; Motorcycle Safety Culture Emerging During each Tenet of Harm Reduction Metatheory.

interview sections. This saturation of data and cyclical nature of the framework supports the notion of metatheoretical validity. Determining metatheoretical validity allowed for a deeper understanding of motorcycle safety and metatheory in action by allowing us to learn where and how participants applied the tenets of HRT when referencing motorcycle safety.

Now that we discussed three common types of validity to be aware of during a research project, with emphasis on how we engaged in mindful reflexivity during the data analysis process, we expand the concept of reflexivity in the next section. We do this by focusing on ways in which the proposed harm reduction metatheory itself emerged as a reflexive tool in this qualitative research project.

HARM REDUCTION METATHEORY AS A REFLEXIVE TOOL IN QUALITATIVE RESEARCH

There are several ways of undertaking the process of metatheorizing but regardless of the process chosen, we must continue to critically reflect on the research problems presented at the beginning of the study (Lincoln & Guba, 2003), which brings us back to being reflexive researchers. Through our own process of being reflexive during our interviews with participants and analyzing and reporting the data we also discovered that harm reduction, as a metatheoretical framework, exemplified reflexive capabilities. We now consider reflexivity from a slightly different perspective, focusing on reflexivity from a metatheoretical standpoint, rather than the internal, mindful stance of the researcher that we have been discussing throughout this chapter.

According to Ritzer (1992), metatheorizing is distinguished by reflexive practice. From a metatheoretical perspective, being reflexive includes describing why the new metatheory was proposed (Lyotard, 1984). Originally, we proposed HRT as a metatheory to guide the integration of health behavior theories and research into health and safety practice. We adapted Edwards (2010) eight-phase process to conceptualize the metatheory after making an argument through the review of literature for why HRT may serve as a metatheory (see Haas, 2012). Therefore, according to Lyotard, conducting the literature review to support the proposed metatheory involved a process of reflexivity.

In addition, to maintain reflexivity during our metatheoretical analysis, it was important to evaluate and understand how the overarching tenets of the proposed harm reduction metatheory could guide the components of the proposed theory (Weinstein & Weinstein, 1992). The results from our analysis, detailed in Chapter 5, demonstrated that a tenet of harm reduction could guide a component of the RHBM. Although our research questions specifically addressed motorcycle safety behaviors, the results provided implications for communicating with other at-risk populations and utilizing other health behavior theories in the process.

For example, in RQ1b the HRT tenet pragmatism was queried as guiding the RHBM component perceived benefits and perceived barriers. Utilizing the metatheoretical tenet of pragmatism to inform this component of the theory helped uncover that motorcyclists do not perceive many benefits to being safer on their motorcycle and find some of the barriers difficult to overcome. These findings can be applied to several other health behaviors, including why individuals continue smoking, abusing alcohol, or other drugs, and do not wear condoms when engaging in sexual activities. We discussed the potential for harm reduction metatheory to inform other health and safety issues in Chapter 2 of this book, as another way to engage this new utility of HRT.

Our results in response to RQ1 revealed the ways that HRT could be integrated with and guide one health behavior theory (i.e., the RHBM). After analyzing the results of the interview data, the tenets of HRT seemed to be reflexive and broad enough to guide components of other health behavior theories as well. We discuss the reflexivity of the five tenets in directing other theories in the next section. Specifically, we focus on the Theory of Reasoned Action/Planned Behavior and the Transtheoretical/Stages of Change Model.

Theory of Reasoned Action/Theory of Planned Behavior

The Theory of Reasoned Action/Planned Behavior (*TRA/TPB*) is used in predicting a variety of at-will behaviors. Based on the results of our research project, we believe that HRT may also be able to guide components of TRA/TPB to facilitate behavior change. First, empowerment focuses on providing individuals with the skills, motivation, and confidence to change their behaviors, despite what other people may think (Logan & Marlatt, 2010). This tenet may be useful when guiding the TRA/TPB component normative influence, which is an individuals' belief about whether influential others think they should perform a target behavior (Fishbein & Ajzen, 1975). Empowering individuals by meeting them where they are at in regards to behavior change and motivating them may help guide the normative influence component of TRA/TPB. For example, in our study, the results in response to RQ1 indicated that motorcyclists do care about what their fellow motorcyclists think and consequently, they often give in to peer pressure to be riskier. However, as motorcyclists became more confident over time, peer pressure (a type of normative influence) does not have as much of an impact on their riskier behaviors. In addition, the results revealed that if motorcyclists' care more about the other person's opinion or the person is important to them (e.g., children), they are more motivated to practice safer behaviors. Therefore, empowerment may help facilitate the ways normative influence is discussed with individuals trying to change a particular behavior.

In addition, the tenets humanistic value, pragmatism, and immediacy may be useful in guiding the attitude component of the TRA/TPB. According to Fishbein and Ajzen (1975), attitudes are influenced by the worth of the anticipated outcome if the targeted behavior is performed. Although attitude is a broad component, being nonjudgmental toward individuals' risky behaviors may help alter their thoughts toward behavior change. In addition, being realistic about the particular behaviors individuals have control over and do not have control over, and setting goals to become safer over time, may cultivate a more accepting attitude toward behavior change. Attitude is affected by several factors, so it may take several tenets of HRT to facilitate a change in attitude. However, the reflexivity of these tenets indicates that the integration of HRT as metatheory, guiding another theory, may be possible.

Transtheoretical Model/Stages of Change Model

Another common health behavior theory is the Transtheoretical Model/ Stages of Change Model (*TTM/SCM*). Previous research utilized HRT and the TTM/SCM together to try and influence substance abuse or alcohol abuse. However, none of this research determined how HRT influences the processes of change (Connors, Donovan, & DiClemente, 2001), perhaps because HRT was not guiding the components of the TTM/SCM but instead functioning side-by-side with it while trying to persuade behavior change. However, the results in our study provide insight into how the tenets of HRT could provide guidance for the core constructs of the TTM/SCM.

For example, humanistic value could be considered in developing more accurate messaging for individuals in the precontemplation or contemplation stage when someone is intending to take action in the near future. Motorcyclists discussed the role humanistic value can have in their recognition of risky health behaviors and cue them to think about or change behaviors. Humanistic value can play the same role for these two core constructs in the TTM/SCM. The concept of pragmatism also can help individuals understand and realize that their behaviors are risky, bringing them from the contemplation to the preparation stage. Immediacy and goal setting can be utilized when individuals are in the preparation stages of changing their behaviors. Planning and developing short-term goals at the beginning stages may help develop a realistic timeline for individuals as they move into the action stage. Then, empowerment may be a useful strategy for guiding individuals' progression through the maintenance and termination stages of the TTM/SCM.

Participants said that providing motorcyclists with the tools they need to sustain behavior change was important, such as taking a driver training class or making their motorcycle safer to drive. Similarly, providing individuals with the tools they need to sustain other behavior changes is important as well. Finally, collaboration with key personnel and understanding the demographic makeup of a particular target audience can influence the core constructs of the TTM/SCM when trying to initiate and sustain behavior changes. Research Project in Practice Illustration Figure 6.7 includes a table that depicts how one metatheoretical tenet of HRT, empowerment, may inform

Research in Practice Illustration
Empowerment Informing Theoretical Components

Theoretical Component	Motorcycle Safety Example
RHBM Component: Self-efficacy	• Provide motorcyclists with several choices to be safer while driving a motorcycle. • Encourage small behavior changes to build confidence over time. • Focus on youth to eventually minimize the negative effects of peer pressure to engage in risky motorcycling behaviors.
TRA/TPB Component: Normative Influence	• Encourage motorcyclists to practice the safety behaviors they want, despite what peers may think. • Probe motorcyclists to discuss why certain groups influence their behaviors. • Provide motorcyclists with scripts to respond to negative communication from influential groups.
TTM/SCM: Components Maintenance & Termination	• Provide motorcyclists with tools they need to sustain behavior changes. With the adequate tools, they may feel more confident in changing additional behaviors, upon sustaining previous behavior changes. • Encourage small goals over time, which may eventually lead to the termination stage.

Figure 6.7 Research in Practice Illustration: Empowerment Informing Theoretical Components.

ways that components of several health behavior theories may function to persuade behavior change.

In the literature review of our study, we provided an argument that explained why HRT would initially serve as a metatheory to the RHBM. The justification for this proposed integration was included and the results from the analysis demonstrated that the integration was appropriate, specifically when trying to more accurately target motorcyclists to change their at-risk behaviors. However, the broad application of harm reduction tenets was revealed during our research project as well. The results indicated that several of the same issues relative to the five tenets of HRT emerged throughout and across the interviews. Because of the consistency in these tenets emerging throughout the interviews, it is not surprising that they may be useful in guiding other health behavior theories as well.

In this chapter we have been discussing the importance of accurately depicting your participants' feedback. However, we also want to mention the importance of taking your reader audience into account when reporting your results. Depending on your readership, you may have to justify your results to a different degree, which circles us back to an issue of validity and reflexivity.

Accounting for Different Audiences

In this final section of the chapter, we note the importance of audience analysis when reporting your results. Accounting for your audience is one method of ensuring validity and reflexivity in your research project. When discussing the results of our research project, we have to continually account for the variety of audiences, including you, who may read our results. Accounting for your audience, allows you, as a researcher, to maintain a higher level of reflexivity. Gilgun (2010) suggested becoming reflexive in this area as a means to being more cognizant of presenting your interpretations and recommendations in language that your audience(s) can appreciate and utilize, which is one reason we chose to incorporate research project in practice illustrations throughout this book. Gilgun (2010) went on to state the importance of clearly communicating thoughts regarding participants' experiences and what actions we, and other people in society, can take to respond to the barriers shared by participants.

So, each time you utilize your data to write a research paper or journal article, this process of reflexivity is important to consider. Depending on your target audience, different vocabulary and recommendations are necessary. For example, in this book we are focusing on an enhanced use of harm reduction theory, as a metatheory, and its implications in qualitative health and safety research. However, in other publications that emphasize aspects of motorcycle safety, the areas we highlight from the data are different. If we were trying to appeal to motorcyclists, drivers of cars and trucks, or policymakers, our recommendations would vary as well. The ability to be reflexive with your data and communicate in a way that your audience can understand is crucial to the results of your research project impacting the field of research and/or your target audience. The results of your research should have some degree of human relevance. Regardless of the actual results of your project, it is important to argue for the relevance of the findings to people outside the scope of your research community. Hammersley (1992) argued that if that connection cannot be made, then social scientific research would have no value.

SUMMARY

In this chapter we discussed the importance of validity and reflexivity during qualitative research projects. Specifically, we defined three major types of validity including descriptive, interpretive, and theoretical validity. Following a discussion of these types of validity, we provided examples of verification strategies that we used to ensure rigor and maintain trueness to our data. Reflexivity was an important verification tool that we utilized throughout our research project. In addition, we incorporated how the role of metatheory enhanced researcher reflexivity and how harm reduction metatheory functioned as a reflexive tool in our project. It is our hope that the research project in practice illustrations provided concrete examples of ways you can practice validity and reflexivity in future qualitative research projects. Particularly, these examples can help you build in your verification strategies at the beginning of your research project, rather than as an afterthought, to help ensure a valid and reliable study.

REFERENCES

Alasuutari, P. (1996). Theorizing in qualitative research: A cultural studies perspective. *Qualitative Inquiry, 2,* 371–384.

Alvesson, M. (2009). *Postmodernsim and social research.* Buckingham, PA: Open University Press.

Alvesson, M., & Skoldberg, K. (2000). *Reflexive methodology.* London: Sage.

Auberbach, C. F., & Silverstein, L. B. (2003). *Qualitative data: An introduction to coding and analysis.* New York: New York University Press.

Berg, B. L. (2004). *Qualitative research methods for the social sciences* (5th Ed.). Boston: Allyn and Bacon.

Brown, L. M., (1994). Standing in the crossfire: A response to Tavris, Gremmen, Lykes, Davis, and Contratto. *Feminism and Psychology, 4,* 382–398.

Brown, L. M. & Gilligan, C. (1992). *Meeting at the crossroads: Women's psychology and girls' development.* Cambridge, MA: Harvard University Press.

Campbell, T. (1996). Technology, multimedia, and qualitative research in education. *Journal of Research on Computing in Education, 30*(9), 122–133.

Connors, G. J., Donovan, D. M., & DiClemente, C. C. (2001). *Selecting and planning interventions: Substance abuse treatment and the stages of change.* New York: The Guilford Press.

Edwards, M. G. (2010). *Organisational transformation for sustainability: An integral metatheory.* New York: Taylor & Francis Group.

Finaly, L. (2002). Negotiating the swamp: The opportunity and challenge of reflexivity in research practice. *Qualitative Research, 2(*2), 209–230.

Fishbein, M., & Ajzen, I. (1975). *Belief, attitude, intention, and behavior: An introduction to theory and research.* Reading, MA: Addison-Wesley.

Flick, U. (2002). *An introduction to qualitative research* (2nd Ed.). Thousand Oaks, CA: Sage.

Gilgun, J. F. (2010). Reflexivity and qualitative research. *Current Issues in Qualitative Research, 1*(2), 1–31. Retrieved from http://www.scribd.com/doc/35787948/Reflexivity-and-Qualitative-Research.

Glaser, B. G., & Strauss, A. (1967). *The discovery of grounded theory: strategies for qualitative research.* Chicago, IL: Aldine Publishing Company.

Guba, E. G., & Lincoln, Y. S. (1981). *Effective evaluation: Improving the usefulness of evaluation results through responsive and naturalistic approaches.* San Francisco, CA: Jossey-Bass.

Hammersley, M. (1987). Some notes on the terms 'validity' and 'reliability. *British Educational Research Journal, 13*(1), 73–81.

Hammersley, M., & Atkinson, P. (1983). *Ethnography: Principles in practice.* London: Tavistock.

Hammersley, M., & Atkinson, P. (1995). *Ethnography: Principles in practice* (2nd Ed.). London: Routledge.

Johnson, B. R. (1997). Examining the validity structure of qualitative research. *Education, 118*(2), 282–292.

Kerlinger, F. (1964). *Foundations of behavioural research.* New York, NY: Holt.

Lincoln, Y. S., & Guba, E. G. (1985). *Naturalistic inquiry.* Beverly Hills, CA: Sage.

Lindlof, T. R., & Taylor, B. C. (2002). *Qualitative communication research methods* (2nd Ed.). Thousand Oaks, CA: Sage Publications.

Logan, D. E., & Marlatt, G. A. (2010). Harm reduction therapy: A practice-friendly review of research. *Journal of Clinical Psychology, 66*(2), 201–214.

Lyotard, J. (1984). *The postmodern condition.* Minneapolis, MN: University of Minnesota Press.

Mauthner, N. S., & Doucet, A. (2003). Reflexive accounts and accounts of reflexivity in qualitative data analysis. *Sociology, 37*(3), 413–431.

Maxwell, J. A. (2005). *Qualitative research design. An interactive approach.* London: Sage Publications.

Maxwell, J. A. (1992). Understanding and validity in qualitative research. In A.M. Huberman & M.B. Miles (Eds.), *The qualitative researcher's companion* (pp. 37–64). Thousand Oaks, CA: Sage Publications (Reprinted from Harvard Educational Review. 1992, 62, 3; 279–300).

Morse, J. M., Barrett, M., Mayan, M., Olson, K., & Spiers, J. (2002). Verification strategies for establishing reliability and validity in qualitative research. *International Journal of Qualitative Methods, 1*(2), Article 2. Retrieved January 12, 2013 from http://www.ualberta.ca/~ijqm/.

Patton, M. Q. (2002). *Qualitative research and evaluation methods* (3rd Ed.). Thousand Oaks, CA: Sage.

Runciman, W. G. (1983). *A treatise on social theory: Vol 1.* The methodology of social theory. Cambridge: Cambridge University Press.

Seale, C. (1999). Quality in qualitative research. *Qualitative Inquiry, 5*(4), 465–478.

Silverman, D. (2005). *Doing qualitative research: A practical handbook* (2nd Ed.). London: Sage Publications.

Stenbacka, C. (2001). Qualitative research requires quality concepts of its own. *Management Decision, 39*(7), 551–555.

Thomson, S. B. (2011). Qualitative research validity. *JOAAG, 6*(1), 77–82. Retrieved from http://joaag.com/uploads/6_1_-7_Research_Method_Thomson.pdf.

Walsh, K. (2003). Qualitative research: Advancing the science and practice of hospitality. *Cornell Hotel and Restaurant Administration Quarterly, 44,* 2;66–74.

Weinstein, D., & Weinstein, M. A. (1992). The postmodern discourse of metatheory. In G. Ritzer (Ed.), *Metatheorizing* (pp. 135–150). Newbury Park, CA: Sage.

Winter, G. (2000). A comparative discussion in the notion of 'validity' in qualitative and quantitative research. *The Qualitative Report, 4.* Retrieved from http://www.nova.edu/ssss/QR/QR4–3/winter.html.

Yin, R. K. (1994). Discovering the future of the case study method in evaluation research. *Evaluation Practice, 15,* 283–290.

Chapter 7

Harm Reduction Championing Research Ethics

In the previous chapter we discussed the importance of being aware of and addressing issues of validity, including descriptive, interpretive, and theoretical validity. We referenced several verification strategies to help determine validity, including reflexivity as a pivotal strategy. We also highlighted the role of our proposed harm reduction metatheory to address issues of validity and reflexivity. In this chapter, we continue to discuss some concerns and challenges of qualitative interviewing and ways that incorporating harm reduction as a metatheory into your qualitative project may help address some of these challenges and strengthen the research process. Specifically, we discuss incorporating a metatheory into social scientific research as a way to help adhere to research ethics. We continue to draw upon our utilization of the tenets of harm reduction throughout our interviews with at-risk motorcyclists. Our reflections depict how harm reduction metatheory can be used to enhance ethics in interviewing methodology. The following objectives frame this chapter.

- Provide ethical principles to consider during in-depth interviews including autonomy, beneficence, power, and establishing rapport with participants
- Consider ways that integrating harm reduction metatheory can facilitate and extend the adherence to ethical principles during the interview
- Present ethical challenges specifically related to *HRT* and how extending HRT as a metatheory begins addressing these ethical concerns
- Highlight how integrating a metatheory into your methodology strengthens theory, reflexivity, and accentuates participants' voices, further enhancing research ethics

We start with a basic review of ethical principles researchers need to consider throughout their qualitative research projects, especially those projects that utilize in-depth interviews to collect data.

CONSIDERING AND EXTENDING QUALITATIVE HARM REDUCTION RESEARCH ETHICS

According to Hammersley (1999), there are four main areas operating within contemporary social science qualitative research: empiricism, ethicism, instrumentalism, and postmodernism. With a heavy emphasis on ethics in current research projects, it is necessary to encourage and have an ongoing dialogue about the importance of adhering to ethical guidelines while still carrying out your research project. Pertaining to the level of ethics within the areas of health and public health, Wodak (2007) defined *ethics* as "attempts to identify moral standards that regulate right and wrong conduct, including good habits that should be acquired, duties that should be followed, or the consequences of our behavior on ourselves and others" (p. 59). According to Edwards and Mauthner (2002), "Ethical decisions arise throughout the entire research process, from conceptualization and design, data gathering and analysis, and report" (p. 19), making ethics a topic we all need to be familiar with as qualitative researchers.

However, a common critique discussed within the qualitative research is the lack of ethical examples (Orb, Eisenhauer, & Wynaden, 2000). The absence of details in conversations about ethics has resulted in some novice and even veteran researchers being unprepared going into the field and gathering data (Batchelor & Briggs, 1994). Therefore, although we realize that presenting a chapter that can demonstrate exactly what you need to do to research ethically is nearly impossible (Josselson, 2007), we thought it important to dedicate considerable space in this book to address ethical dilemmas you may encounter during in-depth interviews including tips to respond to these challenges, particularly when using HRT as a guiding framework. Our hope is that, after reading about our experiences integrating HRT into our research project, your awareness of and attitude toward ethical research increases and enhances the rigor of your own research projects. We begin with a discussion of ethical frameworks commonly practiced within social scientific research.

Ethical Frameworks within Social Scientific Research

Broadly, Kvale (1996) discussed three ethical frameworks that often are used when conducting research in the social sciences. As you will read throughout this chapter, most qualitative research draws from all three frameworks to inform research projects. These three frameworks are presented below:

Ethical Frameworks in Qualitative Research (Kvale, 1996, p. 122)

1. *Duty ethics of principles*: research is driven by autonomy, honesty, justice, and respect and cannot be strayed from during a project.
2. *Utilitarian ethics of consequences (or consequentialism)*: emphasizes the consequences of an action and prioritizes the positive outcomes of research such as knowledge, satisfaction, or happiness.
3. *Virtue ethics of skills*: stresses a contextual or situational ethical position, emphasizing researchers' morals and ethics. Strength of researcher reflexivity is needed.

Generally, the ethical principle of "do no harm" to participants should always apply in social scientific research (Hopf, 2004) by taking whatever precautions necessary, including assuring participation is voluntary and confidentiality is maintained throughout and after the interview (Kvale, 1996). Even though ethical principles are kept in mind and adhered to during the practice of qualitative research, there are several ethical challenges researchers encounter that are specific to the in-depth interview. These challenges are discussed in the next section.

Ethical Challenges Specific to In-depth Interviewing

Ethical concerns specific to interviewing methodology have been introduced by several qualitative scholars as an important research element to be aware of. Allmark and colleagues (2009) conducted a literature review using a variety of databases and categorized 88 references that discussed ethical issues related to: (a) in-depth interviews though not specifically connected to a research study; (b) study-connected papers in which authors discussed the ethical issues that emerged from using in-depth interviews; and (c) empirical studies that focused on ethical issues related to in-depth interviews. The findings of this review suggest that ethical issues are important to be aware of and address during your study.

To illustrate, we first discuss how we addressed some of the common ethical issues researchers experience while conducting in-depth interviews. And second, we consider how applying harm reduction as a metatheory helped challenge common theoretical discourse, extending the notion of research ethics during our project. We begin with some common ethical challenges you can expect to encounter during a research study using in-depth interviews including informed consent, confidentiality, power, and establishing rapport. We frame these challenges within the three main ethical principles: autonomy, beneficence, and justice.

Autonomy and Informed Consent

When discussing *autonomy*, Capron (1989) asserted that respect for participants should be a principle of any qualitative research study. Capron went on to discuss *informed consent*, the process of balancing between over-informing and under-informing the participant (Kvale, 1996), as a way to recognize the rights of participants in the study and allow them to freely decide whether or not they want to continue with the interview. Similarly, Orb et al. (2000) stated that allowing participants to "exercise their rights as autonomous persons to voluntarily accept or refuse to participate in a study" is essential for protecting participants (p. 95). Therefore, informed consent should always be addressed before the interview starts and should be reconsidered throughout the interview as a way to ensure participant autonomy.

Informed consent provides participants with the purpose of the study, types of questions that will be asked, and how the data will be used (Sinding & Aronson, 2003) so participants can make an educated decision about their desire to participate in the study. Organizations that conduct research with people typically have an Institutional Review Board (IRB) that can provide you with the specific information you must inform your participants about in order to meet ethical requirements of collecting data from human subjects. Although requirements may vary slightly, some basic topics you are likely to discuss with participants before obtaining consent follow.

General Information Discussed During the Informed Consent Process

- Purpose of the research
- Specific interview procedures
- Duration of participation
- Risks of participation
- Compensation
- Confidentiality
- Voluntary nature of participation
- Contact information
- Signature to document informed consent

However, even if your respective IRB approves your informed consent document and overall method of obtaining consent, it still can be difficult to obtain informed consent from vulnerable populations (e.g., children, prisoners, or those with mental illness). Depending on those you are conducting research with, you may need to develop a more detailed script describing how the study results will be used or you may have to take additional precautions to maintain participant confidentiality, such as not recording the interview and instead taking detailed, written notes. Because our sample of motorcyclists were not a vulnerable population, and due to the nature of this often marginalized group, participants were eager to volunteer and talk about their motorcycling experiences.

Even after informed consent is obtained from participants, it is important to continually monitor their comfort in sharing information with you. Despite our accounts of motorcyclists' willingness to share details of their risky and safe driving behaviors, you may encounter participants who are less open about their personal behaviors. Because of the sensitive topics often discussed during in-depth interviews, several researchers (Byrne, 2001; Field & Morse, 1992; Kvale, 1996; Miller & Bell, 2002; Nunkoosing, 2005) suggest that in addition to obtaining informed consent, *process consent*, also known as continuous consent or continuous renegotiation, can be used throughout the interview. For example, if you wish to learn more about something a participant said, instead of saying, "Tell me more about that," regaining permission by asking, "Is it alright if we talk more about that?" allows the participant to opt out of the conversation and not feel obligated to continue discussing a difficult topic (Allmark et al., 2009; Sinding & Aronson, 2003). Although not without flaws, this technique of ongoing consent reconfirms that participants are comfortable and willing to continue, or not continue, talking about or revisiting the subject matter you wish to probe about in more detail.

While conducting our in-depth interviews with motorcyclists, we incorporated a process of continuous consent through our discussion at the beginning of each conversation to ensure that participants qualified for our study and the nature of harm reduction metatheory guiding the interviews. Several of the same topics emerged across sections of the interview, so we often found it necessary to return to and probe topics including participants' previous crashes, alcohol consumption behaviors, and speeding behaviors. When these topics emerged, participants were given the option to further discuss their experiences and behaviors. An example of this technique is provided in Research Project in Practice Illustration Figure 7.1.

As you read, we simply asked the participant if she was willing to divulge more information about her previous accident. She was given the opportunity to say yes or no and since she said yes, we continued discussing that accident and subsequently, how that experience altered her safety behaviors. This example may seem insignificant. However, the process of renegotiating consent, depicted in this illustration, communicates concern for the participant and her comfort throughout the interview. In addition, the participant is

Research in Practice Illustration
Obtaining Process Consent During an Interview

E: Yeah, I bet. Umm so at the beginning of the interview you said that you have been involved in a motorcycle accident?
P1: Yes.
E: Okay, can we talk more about that?
P1: Yes.
E: Okay, great. So, was another vehicle involved in the accident?
P1: No. This is when I was...this was ages ago. Well I've been in a lot of little ones but probably the major accident would have been...(8.0)...back in my 20's when I was in Arizona and it happened because in Arizona it's so hot and the cars tend to drip their oil on the asphalt. And that's why motorcycles ride in the right or the left tire lanes and not the center because that's where all fluids fall. And I was pulling up to the uhh...light...prior to it changing and I was in the center where I shouldn't have been and when I went to pull the brake the rear wheel just surpassed the front wheel. It was because I hit a little oil.

Figure 7.1 Research in Practice Illustration: Obtaining Process Consent During an Interview.

continually offered a comfortable, accurate voice throughout the interview, helping the interviewer adhere to the ethical principle of participant autonomy. This technique is particularly recommended when you are inquiring about a difficult subject during which participants may become emotional. For example, sometimes participants' participation in an interview can be therapeutic (Birch & Miller, 2000), and their mental and emotional capacity to talk about topics such as violence, grieving, and health issues including cancer or miscarriage, may be difficult to sustain for the duration of the interview. Renegotiating consent is one way to better ensure participants' comfort during these challenging conversations while maintaining a positive attitude toward ethical research. In the next section we discuss the ethical principle beneficence and confidentiality.

Beneficence and Confidentiality

Another ethical principle considered during the research process is *beneficence*, which, more simply is doing good and preventing harm. When maintaining beneficence, communicating issues of *confidentiality* with participants is necessary, meaning discussing how information provided during the interview will be kept private by primarily not revealing which participant provided the information. It is important to indicate that confidentiality cannot always be guaranteed (Allmark et al., 2009). Some researchers (Orb et al., 2000; Richards & Schwartz, 2002) recommend using pseudonyms or initials whenever possible to help maintain participant anonymity. You probably already noticed in the research project in practice illustrations throughout this book that we referred to participants in confidential variations such as "P2," "Participant 3," or "Interviewee 15." These identifiers not only maintained participants' confidentiality when reporting the results of the interviews, but also helped us organize the data during the transcription and coding phases.

Another method we used so participants would not be identifiable was blinding any references participants made to their residence or the general geographic area in which they lived (Richards & Schwartz, 2002). Again, you probably noticed this blinding process throughout the research project in practice illustrations we provided. Since our research pool included individuals throughout an entire state, this blinding process allowed participants' identity and location of residence to remain unrecognizable. However, if your research pool consists of a sample from a much smaller location, such as individuals recruited from a specific unit in a hospital, or teachers from schools in the same county, you may have to go through extra precautions to ensure their confidentiality. Or, participants may need to be told that it will be difficult to guarantee their privacy because others may be able to recognize their identities during dissemination of the study results. You need to discuss this possibility during the informed consent process. Another ethical principle commonly referenced is justice. This principle is discussed next, followed by power balance as a way to account for participant justice.

Justice and Power Balance

Justice refers to being equal and fair during the interview and not exploiting participants upon completion of the interviews (Orb et al., 2000). Similarly, when considering justice for your participants, if the group you are studying is a vulnerable population, special permission may be necessary before interviewing these individuals. When adhering to the principle of justice, researcher *power* over the participant is an ethical consideration that should be taken into account during in-depth interviews. Issues of power to consider may include the interviewers' role in directing the conversation, the possibility of the participant feeling misled by the interviewer's role and/or expertise (Allmark et al., 2009), and the ability of the researcher to decide which quotes to use in the final dissemination of results (Sandelowski, 1994).

For example, throughout our interviews with motorcyclists participants often viewed us as motorcycle safety experts and asked several questions about injury and fatality statistics and the impact that personal protective equipment (PPE) may have on an individuals' health outcomes upon being involved in a crash. We understood that some participants may have wanted to participate in the interview to obtain answers as well as share information, so we had to strike a careful balance between how much information we shared, to not dominate the conversation or influence their responses when we provided the information they requested. Consequently, even though we chose to use our position of power to continue with our interview questions when participants desired to learn about research concerning motorcycle safety, we returned to their queries at the end of the interview. Taking this approach, we could show respect for participants' concerns and provide them with closure without unduly influencing how they responded to subsequent interview questions. An example of this power balance is presented in Research Project in Practice Illustration Figure 7.2.

Although it may be difficult to glean from the transcript, Participant 6 was genuinely surprised that the helmet statistic was approximately 37%. Even after we were finished with the interview he continued to ask if the number was really that high. If we would have provided that information at the beginning of the interview when he asked, this participant's responses toward safety may have been slightly different throughout the interview, erring on the side of safer responses, especially since he did not wear a helmet and consistently operated his motorcycle at high speeds. However, we did not want to ignore his earlier query which is why we allowed space toward the end of the interview to provide the information the participant requested.

Research in Practice Illustration
Responding to Questions During Harm Reduction Motorcycling Interview: Maintaining an Equal Relationship with Participants without Compromising the Data

Introductory Excerpt from Interview 6

E: Okay. Do you ever see any motorcycle safety media like messages or materials?

P6: Sometimes you see bumper stickers. Uhh like, "loud pipes save lives" and stuff like that. Uhh…"be careful on the road motorcycles are around"…uhh mainly bumper stickers.

E: Okay does that ever cue your own safety behaviors?

P6: Ya I mean I think about it and ya know, I think about it but I don't think about it that much. I mean I know the potential outcome is dangerous ya know. But that's it. I haven't really seen any stats on how many people…how many lives could have been saved by wearing a helmet. If they have something like that then that would be good for a campaign. Do you know that stat?

E: I can definitely give you some information about motorcycle safety when we're done, since you might have other questions come up, too. If I don't know the answer, I'll send you some information.

Concluding Excerpt from Interview 6

E: Okay well great. Those are all of my questions unless you have any comments for me at all before we end the interview? I know you asked about helmet protection information earlier.

P6: Do you know that stat?

E: Well the most recent information I've read said that in around 37% of the accidents…wearing a helmet could have saved the motorcyclists' life or prevented fatal injuries.

P6: So around 37%?

E: Yea.

P6: Did you research that?

E: It's in some traffic safety facts from the National Highway Traffic Safety Administration. If you Google their organization, you can see a lot of traffic safety statistics.

P6: Wow.

Figure 7.2 Research in Practice Illustration: Responding to Questions During Harm Reduction Motorcycling Interview: Maintaining an Equal Relationship with Participants without Compromising the Data.

Providing participants time to ask questions and subsequently provide genuine reactions helps keep the power balance between the researcher and participant in check.

However, it can be difficult to reduce these power imbalances while simultaneously reinforcing participants' confidence and comfort throughout the interview. In response, suggestions for giving something back to participants can be used as a method to make participants feel more comfortable to seek more information upon completion of the interview. Therefore, giving something back to participants is recommended, which provides them an opportunity to acquire knowledge and learn about the topic (Armitage, 2005).

In our case, we provided participants with a Motorcycle Safety at Purdue (MS@P) campaign t-shirt that, not only promotes motorcycle safety with our logo and safety message, but states the campaign's website (i.e., www.ItInvolvesYou.com; front and back of t-shirt design are depicted in the following Research Project in Practice Illustration Figure 7.3). The campaign website provides an outlet for motorcyclists, drivers of cars and trucks, and family and friends of motorcyclists to obtain information about traffic safety. Although we do not know how many participants visited the MS@P website, it is possible their fellow motorcyclists noticed it on their t-shirt as well.

The next ethical challenge of qualitative research we discuss is establishing trust, or rapport, with participants before, during, and after the interview.

Establishing and Maintaining Rapport

Previously we discussed the importance of obtaining consent before proceeding with an interview. However, this process of consent does not necessarily influence the information shared during the interview. Rather, the nature of the information disclosed during the interview is highly dependent on the rapport, or trust, you build with each participant (Josselson, 2007). Consequently, the manner in which you inform participants about the study, discuss the ways you will maintain their confidentiality, and continue to make them feel equal and at ease throughout the interview, all contribute to the level of trust you eventually establish. In this section, we discuss general issues of rapport. However, keep in mind that all of the aforementioned ethical principles discussed are important elements to help build and maintain a trustworthy relationship with your participants.

Establishing *rapport*, also known as building trust, facilitates participants' comfort in sharing personal information. Rapport is established early in the interview and begins by the researcher clearly and honestly stating the purpose of conducting the research (Lindlof & Taylor, 2002; Rubin & Rubin, 2012). Generally, establishing rapport involves communicating trust and respect for participants and the information they share during the interview

**Research in Practice Illustration
MS@P T-shirt Distributed to
Interview Participants**

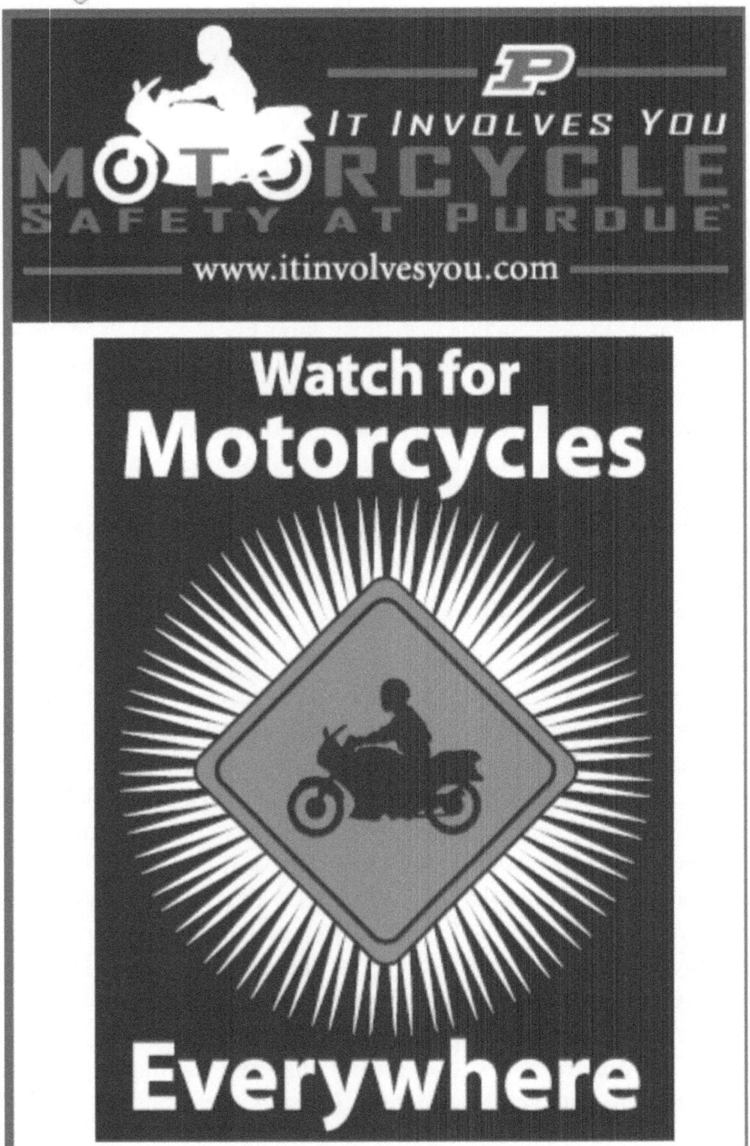
IT INVOLVES YOU
MOTORCYCLE
SAFETY AT PURDUE
www.itinvolvesyou.com
Watch for
Motorcycles
Everywhere

Figure 7.3 Research in Practice Illustration: MS@P T-shirt Distributed to Interview Participants.

(DiCicco-Bloom & Crabtree, 2006). Besides the verbal content shared during the interview, Josselson (2007) noted that participants also notice your subtle nonverbal cues including your ability to be "empathic, nonjudgmental, concerned, tolerant, and emotionally responsive as well as your ability to contain affect-laden material" (p. 539). Even the way we dress, how close we sit to participants, and how we initially present ourselves through the tone of our voice sends a perceived message to each person (Duncombe & Jessop, 2002). Therefore, your verbal and nonverbal communication cues affect participants' willingness to elaborate on their personal experiences.

Spradley (1979) described the stages of developing rapport as apprehension, exploration, cooperation, and participation. Spradley went on to say that the main purpose of establishing rapport is not necessarily and/or only to establish a relationship with the participant, but also to build a sense of respect toward each other. This respect often is implied through the emotional, rich dialogue that occurs during the interview. To help establish rapport and maintain a respectful relationship with participants, reciprocity, the two-way process of sharing and gathering information, should occur throughout the interview (Alvesson & Skoldberg, 2000; Booth & Booth, 1994).

Because of the continuous and in-depth level of information we share and respond to with each participant during an interview, continuous steps to maintain a positive ethical attitude are necessary. Duncombe and Jessop (2002) described rapport as a detached form of friendship. Although it is true that boundaries are necessary to limit the depth of emotions shared by researcher and participant, and a sense of overall ignorance is prescribed by some researchers (Glaser & Strauss, 1967) to achieve rapport with hesitant participants, we found that the application of harm reduction metatheory to engage participants helped facilitate a respectful, trustworthy relationship with the motorcyclists that we interviewed. Specifically, the tenets of harm reduction quite naturally guided a strong sense of researcher ethics, which we sensed among a majority of the motorcyclists we interviewed. In Chapter 4, we discussed how the development of the interview protocol and content shared during the interview was informed by harm reduction and facilitated a strong discussion. Below, we debrief this content and how the role of harm reduction metatheory helped us avoid ethical dilemmas that may be encountered during the process of establishing rapport before and throughout the interview.

Harm Reduction Metatheory Facilitating Rapport

Our research project in practice illustrations have referenced ways that integrating the metatheoretical perspective of HRT with another theory to guide interviews can help address the aforementioned challenges of interviewing while enhancing methodological rigor. The development of an interview guide and how you frame the interview questions toward participants is a pivotal approach to encouraging a balanced dialogue during which participants feel comfortable communicating with you about their behaviors and experiences. You probably noticed in Chapter 4, which discussed the methodology of our study, that the metatheoretical tenets of HRT helped us build trust with participants. In that chapter, we discussed how the use of metatheory informed the development of the interview guide. We stated that the openings of each interview section included harm reduction terminology in an effort to build participants' trust, increase their comfort in responding to questions, and encourage reflexivity during the interview (refer to Table 4.1: Column 1). We provided examples from the interview guide that depicted how each tenet aimed to facilitate a nonjudgmental, accepting attitude toward the participant (refer to research project in practice illustrations presented in Chapter 4).

However, besides guiding what we verbally communicated to motorcyclists who participated, the tenets of HRT also increased our ability to empathize and remain nonjudgmental throughout the interviews. In the research project in practice illustrations depicted in Chapter 4, you read the mental goals we established before each interview section, which were based on a tenet of HRT. Incorporating the metatheory to establish a framework for communicating with participants also served as a method to enhance our ethical attitude throughout the interviews since we were constantly exhibiting the principles of humanistic value and pragmatism. Being nonjudgmental and practical throughout the interviews helped us embrace a sense of empathy toward participants that, in some cases, may not be easy.

For example, we interviewed an individual who became a motorcyclist despite his father being killed in a motorcycle accident. According to this participant, "A drunk driver going 100 mph didn't stop at the light, just ran right through and rear-ended him" (Participant 2). Even though initially we may not have understood why this participant decided to become a motorcyclist himself, we expressed our appreciation for his willingness to share this experience with us and dialogue about the tensions that developed with his family as a result of him becoming a motorcyclist. Instead of immediately asking why he started motorcycling despite his father's accident, we proceeded with our interview questions and inquired about that accident where it fit within the interview, such as the section that discussed perceived severity and perceived susceptibility to crashes. As the interview progressed, the participant opened up about his father's accident and the ways it did and did not affect his safety behaviors. This natural progression makes sense, since oftentimes during an interview, as the relationship between the participant and the interviewer builds, participants start to open up and may even seek advice from the interviewer, or desire a personal response, based on the information they are providing (Josselson, 2007). Using the tenets of HRT, we were able to provide supportive, noncritical feedback, which in turn, aided trust. Josselson (2007) recommended providing a normalizing response as to make participants feel comfortable continuing with their narrative, despite any criticisms they may have received in the past. An example of this concept in action is provided in Research Project in Practice Illustration Figure 7.4.

Although this participant did not ask us for our opinion of his decision to ride a motorcycle, he indicated that others often questioned why he wanted to ride. In response, we felt it was a good point in the interview to quickly insert that other motorcyclists have a similar history and it is not uncommon. As our interview results demonstrated, motorcycling often is a family lineage, so a non-motorcyclist may not understand this decision. We wanted to communicate to the participant that we were not judging his decision to be a motorcyclist, despite his father's accident. In response, we continued to receive expanded narratives about this accident and the participants' personal path toward safer behaviors after he became a father.

We realize that the concept of using the overarching tenets of harm reduction to help establish trust may still be abstract. However, keep in mind that the tenets of harm reduction can be used to enhance and refresh your attitude toward ethical research, which in the process, helps establish a trustworthy relationship with participants. Now that we reviewed some common ethical situations you are likely to encounter during in-depth interviews, we slightly

Research in Practice Illustration
Harm Reduction as a Tool to Build Rapport

E: When you started practicing some safer behaviors, like wearing your helmet more and everything, was there any one event that sparked that particular change in behavior?
P2: Oh yeah. Having kids.
E: Having kids, okay.
P2: Like I said, my dad was killed on a motorcycle and umm a lot of people questioned why I ever got a bike. But, I grew up around them my whole life. Umm (5.0) I had dirt bikes since I was young. Umm and I knew that even though that was a fact, because I grew up around bikes, I didn't wanna be the…I wanted to sorta eliminate or diminish the possibility of my kids being without a father. So, that's when it changed…or at least when I thought about it.
E: Yeah. Well a lot of motorcyclists have had similar histories with riding. Many people may know someone who has been in an accident but it affects everyone differently.
P2: To be quite honest (5.0)...umm I was six when he was killed but I already was involved with motorcycles and it just continued and umm…my mom didn't want us to really be involved but we already had dirt bikes and we grew up in an area where there was nothing but woods by us so we were able to do those things. I think her opposition came if we wanted to motorcycle ride on the street. Umm…I didn't think about…I didn't think about that at all really. It was just natural to me. Umm again, people are killed in car accidents…does that mean you stop driving a vehicle? Umm…ya know motorcycles…I mean people are killed on bicycles. To enjoy life you're gonna do what comes natural. You're gonna do what you've been raised with. So ya know…those thoughts didn't come to mind at that point.

Figure 7.4 Research in Practice Illustration: Harm Reduction as a Tool to Build Rapport.

change the focus of our discussion. Consistent with our emphasis on research ethics, we consider it important to address the ethical barriers that HRT has encountered in previous research. Then, we discuss how extending HRT to a metatheory helped limit some of these common barriers. Finally, we conclude this section with broader implications of using metatheory in social science research as a means to challenge common discourses and thus, allow participants new opportunities to assist us in applying theories while further sharing their experiences.

THE DUALITY OF ETHICS IN HARM REDUCTION THEORY

Historically, the use of HRT and general harm reduction policies have been met with opposition. Although we believe the application of the tenets of HRT enhanced our sense of researcher ethics, these same tenets have contributed to HRT being misunderstood and condemned as encouraging illegal activities or spreading the wrong message to individuals and society (Sweanor, 2007). As previously discussed, since HRT accepts that people use drugs and HRT interventions may seem to encourage people to continue using illegal drugs, some argue that HRT interventions are a Trojan horse because they seem positive but actually are detrimental to society (DuPont, 2013; DuPont & Ford, 2000; Marlatt, 1998). Consequently, most of the ethical issues associated with conducting research with illicit drug users have been associated with harm reduction research, prompting ethical debates about its application in research and interventions with human subjects.

Despite those who are opposed to the general concepts of harm reduction, many practitioners, researchers, and policymakers support utilizing harm reduction approaches to minimize negative consequences of risky health behaviors while eventually lessening the occurrence of those risky behaviors. Even though we support applying HRT within these same situations, there still were ethical questions specific to this theory we had to consider throughout our research project with motorcyclists. We discuss some of the ethical issues we discovered embedded within HRT. During our discussion we challenge you to consider what ethical issues may arise as a result of a metatheoretical and/or theoretical framework you may choose to utilize during your qualitative research project.

Coinciding with the increased application of HRT to empirically study a variety of health behaviors, an increased engagement in ethics surrounding harm reduction research also has been called for (e.g., Fry et al., 2005; Golding, Dent, Nissim, & Stott, 2006; Paterson & Panessa, 2008). In this section, we discuss micro-level ethics concerning HRT, including the day-to-day issues that may be encountered during a harm reduction-related research project. Then, we focus on the macro level or broad issues that must be addressed to integrate a more ethical perspective in research that utilizes the tenets of HRT. After this discussion, we review how moving toward utilizing harm reduction as a metatheory may alleviate some of the ethical quandaries and backlash that may be encountered when conducting research that utilizes a harm reduction approach.

Harm Reduction Ethics at the Micro Level

You can expect to encounter the same ethical dilemmas during harm reduction research as in other social scientific research projects, including informed consent, confidentiality, safety, risks, and potential harms to participants (Fry & Hall, 2002). These basic interpersonal issues are termed *normative ethics*, *micro-level ethics*, or *ethics in practice*, which we have been discussing throughout this chapter. Some of the barriers to ethics in micro-level practice when conducting research that utilizes the tenets of harm reduction are listed in Table 7.1.

We will not explain each of these areas in detail since we already discussed the importance of gaining approval from respective institutions to study human subjects and involving participants throughout the research project in terms of developing rapport and appropriately disseminating results. However, one concern we did not have to contend with during our study but is commonly a concern within critical theory and particularly in harm reduction research, is vulnerable and/or marginalized populations (Punch, 1994). As we previously noted, harm reduction research is historically conducted with vulnerable populations, mainly drug users. However, according to Fisher (2004), although drug users are a vulnerable population, they often are not granted the same special protection as other groups including children, pregnant women, or prisoners. Because this vulnerable population often is not assured the same

Table 7.1 Barriers to Micro-Level Ethics Engagement in Harm Reduction Research

- Lack of understanding from institutional research ethics committees regarding harm reduction research.
  - Lack of institutional commitment to develop an ethical approach to complement harm reduction research, practice, and policy, and subsequently promote that approach to ethical research.
- Increased frequency of vulnerable populations within harm reduction research.
- Inadequate participant feedback during formative stages of research.
  - Vague utility of ethics as a formative tool for research and practice.
- Few applied concrete, ethical resources to help guide researchers during ethical dilemmas.
- Lack of appropriate dissemination of research findings to participants.

Source: Adapted from Fry et al., 2005; Irwin & Fry, 2007.

level of protection, ethical dilemmas, including confidentiality breaches, are common when conducting harm reduction research with drug users (Buchanan et al., 2002). Irwin and Frey (2007) argued that, as we continue to use harm reduction to engage new audiences (e.g., at-risk motorcyclists) and focus on new health issues, we will have to find better ways to maintain participants' confidentiality and protect them to the best of our ability during the research process.

We are optimistic that our research project can inform some of the common micro-ethical challenges that are encountered during harm reduction projects. As mentioned at the beginning of this chapter, although micro-level ethics frames the ways we conduct research, useful guidelines for how to respond to ethical dilemmas are lacking. However, several researchers (e.g., Guillemin & Gillman, 2004; McGraw, Zvonkovic, & Walker, 2000) offered reflexivity as a tool for guiding ethical actions during research projects.

Harm Reduction Metatheory Informing a Reflexive Approach to Research Ethics

McGraw et al. (2000) connected reflexivity and ethics when they described one feature of *researcher reflexivity* as, "A process whereby researchers place themselves and their practices under scrutiny, acknowledging the ethical dilemmas that permeate the research process and impinge on the creation of knowledge" (p. 68). Up to this point, we discussed reflexivity as a way to ensure rigor and produce knowledge throughout the research process. Also, in the previous chapter we discussed how reflexivity helped produce a more honest, noncritical dialogue with our participants. However, by being reflexive and, in a sense, more alert during the research process, Guillemin and Gillman (2004) argued that besides producing knowledge, we also can be more cognizant of ethical issues that can occur during the project. They stated that being reflexive is "acknowledging and being sensitized to the micro ethical dimensions for research practice and in doing so, being alert to and prepared for ways of dealing with the ethical tensions that arise" (p. 278). In addition, Irwin and Fry (2007) made the point that, as the use of harm reduction continues to expand into other health areas, settings, and interventions, the importance of researcher engagement and reflexivity will be important to help answer ethical questions that ensue. Being reflexive during interactions with participants makes the tasks of respecting the autonomy and confidentiality of participants easier, in turn, minimizing the risk to participants (Guillemin & Gillman, 2004). Although reflexivity is a broad tool for addressing ethical dilemmas, Guillemin and Gillman (2004) provided what and how a reflexive researcher should be able to predict, see, and respond to ethical dilemmas (Table 7.2).

Table 7.2 A Reflexive Approach to Research Ethics

- The researcher understands and acknowledges that ethics in research has different dimensions and that research practice is infused with micro ethics at all levels of everyday research practice. This acknowledgment encourages researchers to think about:
  - How they should enter into the research project;
  - How to prevent ethical dilemmas from occurring; and
  - How they would respond to such dilemmas, if dilemmas occur.
- The researcher understands and acknowledges the potential impact that both she/he and the research process may have on participants' lives. This acknowledgment reflects how the researcher:
  - Develops and words interview questions;
  - Frames questions toward the participant;
  - Orders and times the questions throughout the interview.

Source: Adapted from Guillemin & Gillman, 2004, p. 276–277.

By being reflexive throughout the interviews for our qualitative research project with motorcyclists, our ability to communicate with participants, and participants' feedback in relation to the metatheory and research questions were at the forefront. In tandem with this reflexive process, we also had to continually ask ourselves if the questions and interactions that occurred during each interview were ethically appropriate (Christians, 2001). To combat potential ethical dilemmas from occurring during the interviews, we maintained a reflexive approach while conceptualizing our interview guide. The order of the interview sections was a conscious decision in an effort to help our participants feel more comfortable and gradually elicit more in-depth information as the conversation progressed. Refer to Research Project in Practice Illustration Figure 7.5 for a description of our rationale behind the ordering of the interview sections as it pertains to the tenets of HRT and researcher ethics.

This systematic design of the interview protocol was a reflexive exercise to help anticipate and prevent negative reactions from participants. Had we designed the interview guide differently, it's possible that we may have had an adverse effect on participants' safety behaviors. For example, several of the motorcyclists that we interviewed indicated that they respond negatively to people and messages that are judgmental and critical. If we did not begin the interview guide probing about cues to action they find desirable, while maintaining a humanistic and pragmatic attitude, our support and appreciation for their feedback may not have been as evident. During the development of your interview guide, we encourage this same sense of reflexive mindfulness by being aware of how you frame and ask the questions, realizing that it could affect not only the responses from participants, but their behaviors after talking with you in the interview. Now that we discussed micro-level ethics

Research in Practice Illustration
Developing a Harm Reduction Interview Guide
Using Reflexive Mindfulness

Section 1: Humanistic Value

By beginning with the tenet humanistic value, we could begin the interview with a relaxed, non-critical mentality, to allow motorcyclists to feel supported, despite their risky behaviors while driving a motorcycle.

↓

Section 2: Pragmatism

Carrying this non-critical tone to the next section, utilizing pragmatism, we were able to state that we realize risky behaviors cannot realistically be changed all at once, or ever, based on the barriers present in an individuals' life at that time.

↓

Section 3: Immediacy/Goal Setting

Continuing forward with a non-critical and realistic perspective, we utilized the tenet immediacy and goal setting to probe participants about what they could change soon, if desired. Having just discussed realistic changes they could make, it made sense to move on to when they could make these changes and how.

↓

Section 4: Empowerment

Naturally, we progressed into the empowerment section of the interview, in which participants could continue discussing several options that are available for behavior change, and dialogue about which behaviors participants would choose.

↓

Section 5: Community Collaboration

Finally, after focusing on the individual throughout the interview, the discussion concluded with community collaboration. Participants were treated as subject matter experts, and their help was enlisted to tell us about who needs to be involved to make the roads safer for motorcyclists, who we need to target, and how we need to communicate with these target audiences.

Figure 7.5 Research in Practice Illustration: Developing a Harm Reduction Interview Guide Using Reflexive Mindfulness.

from a harm reduction standpoint, we move on to discuss harm reduction ethics at the macro level.

Harm Reduction Ethics at the Macro Level

In addition to the basic day-to-day research dilemmas, termed micro-level or normative ethics (Guillemin & Gillam, 2004; Rotgers, 2006), the application of HRT in research projects, mainly those pertaining to drug use and abuse interventions, has influenced broader issues and debates. On a macro level, some researchers believe harm reduction is a value-neutral approach to health and the population being studied (e.g., Erikson et al., 1997; Fry et al., 2005; Rumbold & Hamilton, 1998). These researchers suggested that harm reduction emphasizes its methods in order to bypass, or make no assumptions about, the moral status of drug use and the drug user(s), or whatever health behavior is being studied (Erickson et al., 1997). Strang and Fortsen (2004) stated it this way, "As long as it reduces harm, anything goes" (p. 102). In addition, Keane (2003) argued that harm reduction takes this value neutrality approach in order to achieve its prohibitionist policy objectives within certain environments.

Even though some researchers discuss HRT as a value-neutral stance, many also realize that HRT cannot be completely value neutral because the overall goal of reducing harm is a value statement in and of itself. For instance, Denning and Little (2011) explained the ethical framework of harm reduction as, "harm reduction principles have arisen in a secular framework that privileges the social contract that human beings have rights to make their own decisions, and that humans should take care of those who are less able to take care of themselves" (p. 299). In addition, Wodak (2007) provided an ethical argument in support of harm reduction when he said:

> Setting and achieving realistic but sub-optimal objectives is considered more effective than setting but failing to reach utopian goals. In other words, 80% of something is better than 100% of nothing. The essence of harm reduction is well expressed in the public health maxim to "never let the best be the enemy of the good" (p. 60).

On the other hand, some researchers are concerned that if ethics or values are "de-emphasized as second order issues next to empirical, clinical, and political considerations, their resulting absence from dialogue means we miss an opportunity to strengthen harm reduction further" (Fry et al., 2005, p. 450). Van Beek (2009) asserted that we must continually reemphasize that HRT is the first step on a continuum that promotes abstinence-based strategies. This emphasis would foster harm reduction both as a cure-based and care-based approach to health (Bruning, 1990). In addition, researchers have continued to reiterate that although HRT does include abstinence as an overall goal, many times abstinence is unrealistic and, in these situations, it is unethical to not provide other methods of reducing negative health consequences (Gunn, White, & Srinivasan, 1998). Therefore, by providing alternative solutions to abstinence, HRT may be providing a more ethical approach in terms of protecting vulnerable groups' long-term health. So, the question becomes how can we better engage ethics while emphasizing the values of HRT to researchers and practitioners?

Hathaway (2002) argued that playing down the overall values of HRT has hindered its advancement in health research. One of the main failures of HRT is that the guiding principles, or core values, are still undetermined (Hathaway, 2002). Similarly, Fry et al. (2005) stated that, before focusing too much on the empirical, political, and economic concerns that inform our formative research, we need to step back and answer the important macro-ethics question of harm reduction which is, "what are the core values of harm reduction?" (p. 452). For example, Keane (2003) indicated that, although HRT promotes humanistic value and rights, specific details of how this approach is applied in practice have not been clear or articulated in the literature. She noted that humanistic value often is listed as an important characteristic of harm reduction research but goes on to say in terms of drug users, "the specifics of what it means to respect the rights of drugs users, what a humane value system requires in terms of drug policy and how these values interact with the objective evaluation of harms and benefits tend not to be spelled out in detail" (p. 228). In addition, Aceijas (2012) suggested that, despite HRT's compliance with the main principles of bioethics in healthcare (e.g., autonomy, beneficence, and justice), the well-established tenets of HRT including pragmatism, goal prioritization, humanism, and a focus on harms and risks, have been weakly portrayed, illustrating a defeatist attitude toward risky health behaviors.

One reason the core values of harm reduction have not been identified is partly because of the diversity of harm reduction approaches. Many organizations, public health professionals, and policymakers practice harm reduction. Although this wide application may be considered a strength of HRT, it also has made it difficult to "conceptualize the core harm reduction values and beliefs around which even a basic level of debate and dialogue can be achieved" (Irwin & Fry, 2006, p. 76). The authors further argue that this has left the relationship between harm reduction and ethics as implied or taken for granted. By better articulating the core values of harm reduction and how these values can be applied in everyday harm reduction practice, a stronger model of ethics surrounding harm reduction can be developed. Because harm reduction ethics are abstract, a reorientation to ethics, in terms of guidelines, IRBs, and professional research, and a more formative, practice-based approach that can be applied in harm reduction research, practice, and ultimately policy, is necessary. Meeting this ethical challenge requires a discussion of the core values of harm reduction, and how to best integrate an ethical framework within HRT practice (Fry et al., 2005). Synthesizing about and perhaps operationalizing these core values of harm reduction, and addressing any ethical issues of these core values, may help advance the acceptance of the theory. More importantly, if a set of core values is available, then there may be motivation to hold researchers accountable in practice, resulting in an increased adherence to research ethics.

We identified some of these same issues during our formative research of HRT. It is common to encounter several tenets (i.e., core values) of HRT when reviewing previous interventions that utilize HRT applications. Early on in our HRT research, we determined that establishing consistent tenets to complement the application of HRT as a metatheory and to associate with HRT design, implementation, and evaluation was important not only to expand the use of HRT in the field of health communication, but also to consistently apply HRT interventions. By establishing the tenets of HRT to aid the consistent application of HRT among researchers, we also learned that an appreciation of researcher ethics may be enhanced as well. For example, according to Marlatt and Witkiewitz (2010), because appropriate HRT interventions often are tailored to the specific needs of an individual or community, a universal HRT intervention is not always practical. Because it is not realistic or appropriate to create a one-size-fits-all intervention to encourage behavior change, it is important for HRT to contain consistent tenets that can be adapted to fit specific individual problems and community issues.

To illustrate, think about receiving a cue to action, such as a persuasive health message about consuming more fruits and vegetables. Before initiating a change in your fruit and vegetable consumption behaviors, you are likely to think about and be faced with different challenges to this shift in behaviors than your friend or family member. You may not live close to a store that sells fresh produce and your friend may be unable to afford fresh produce. Similarly, you both may have different reasons for wanting to change your diet (e.g., weight loss, cost, taste preferences). In response, different messages and/or information may be needed to further influence your desirability and consequent action to start consuming healthier foods. Obviously, individuals are likely to have different situations and may need to change their environment or reassess their personal challenges and risks. It is possible that among the varying circumstances and resources individuals experience when deciding how to respond to a particular cue to action, the broad utility of HRT tenets can be specified to fit individual situations. So, although realistic, gradual messages that encourage substituting a banana for a cookie may work for one person while another message that emphasizes and discusses the plethora of healthy consumption options individuals have available may be empowering and influential for another person.

The results of our qualitative research project indicate that utilizing harm reduction as a metatheory may highlight the ethical values inherent in HRT. In our review and analysis of HRT, five central tenets emerged, including humanistic value, pragmatism, immediacy/goal setting, empowering the individual through an egalitarian relationship of choice, and evidence of collaboration with the community. The results of our research demonstrated that these five tenets have broad utility as a metatheoretical framework to guide other theories during qualitative research projects. However, in adapting and utilizing these five tenets of HRT, researchers' sense of ethics can be enhanced throughout a research project by promoting nonjudgmental communication, continually providing a voice to audiences and empowering decision-making, and involving audiences in more stages of the formative research process. Below, we provide examples using the HRT tenets empowerment and community collaboration.

Harm Reduction Metatheory Alleviating Macro-Level Ethical Concerns of Harm Reduction

When we sought to identify the core tenets of HRT, we had the goal of determining these tenets for their conceptualization and application of a metatheory. However, we did not consider the ethical implications that conceptualizing harm reduction as a metatheory would have on research and practice that applies a harm reduction approach. We showcase empowerment and community collaboration as examples, based on the results of our research project.

Empowerment. Empowerment is one tenet that we noticed emerging throughout our review of HRT interventions and we determined it had important utility as a metatheoretical tenet. The importance of empowering individuals often is emphasized in HRT practices, but generally empowerment has not been assessed in the implementation and outcomes of HRT interventions. Although empowerment can occur from short-term goal setting, creating and communicating choices that are available to individuals in terms of their behaviors also need to be emphasized. Keefe (1978) argued that harm reduction practitioners need to promote an egalitarian spirit of partnership between practitioner and client. The same argument can be applied in that qualitative researchers need to promote an egalitarian partnership between the researcher and participant. Empowerment may be the ethical bridge needed to facilitate this respectful relationship.

Specifically, during discussions of harm reduction interventions, some researchers have called for what they term "ethics engagement" or more generally "engaging others" as an ethical imperative during interventions (e.g., Fry et al., 2005; Golding, Dent, Nissim, & Stott, 2006; Paterson & Panessa, 2008). The results from our research project support that the HRT tenet empowerment can enhance engagement during health and safety interventions while simultaneously enhancing research ethics. More specifically, engagement can fit within the ethical principle autonomy. Paterson and Panessa (2008) stated, "Harm reduction interventions that are responsive to the ethical principle of autonomy provide opportunity for at-risk participants to provide input and feedback about the relevance and appropriateness of the design and implementation of the intervention" (p. 26). These researchers went on to argue that by engaging others, harm reduction interventions recognize individuals' rights and ability to make decisions about programs and policies that may affect them in the future. Therefore, if empowerment is systematically and consistently integrated into research projects, researchers may better be able to allow individuals autonomy throughout the interview, in addition to openly providing individuals the right to make informed decisions from a viable list of options upon receiving information relevant to their current stage in life (Halpern, Johnson, Miranda, & Wells, 2004). In this way, empowerment helps facilitate autonomy on the researchers' side of the interview while autonomy helps facilitate a sense of empowerment on the participants' side of the interview.

Therefore, by researchers emphasizing empowerment during qualitative interviews, participants may realize a more prominent voice not only in informing the researcher about viable choices for behavior change, but also informing the researcher about viable possibilities for communicating with other target audience members in the future. We took this approach during the section of the interviews guided by empowerment. Refer to Research Project in Practice Illustration Figure 7.6 for some questions that we asked during the interview.

In particular, you will notice that we inquired what choices participants felt were most important for themselves, based on their current status as a motorcyclist, and also what safety choices may be in the best interest of a novice motorcyclist. One theme we discussed in Chapter 5 that emerged from these questions was starting small to build confidence. Within this theme motorcyclists discussed one or both of the following scenarios. First, motorcyclists shared safety behaviors that they performed as a new motorcyclist to develop skills and build confidence. Or, motorcyclists shared safety behaviors they did not perform as a novice motorcyclist but wished they did to help build efficacy in risky situations. Regardless of whether or not the motorcyclists did or did not engage in these safety behaviors, all of the motorcyclists interviewed strongly advised that any new motorcyclist should perform specific safety behaviors in order to build confidence and develop their skills. These participants provided several options a new motorcyclist can choose to gain as much knowledge as possible before traveling on busy roads including finding a motorcycle that fits your body, taking time to familiarize yourself

Research in Practice Illustration
Empowerment Informing Ethical Interviewing

1. If you wanted to practice safer behaviors on the road but didn't know how:
   a. What behavior would you start with?
   b. What steps would you take to learn?
2. If a new motorcyclist approached you and wanted to practice safer behaviors on the road but didn't know how:
   a. What behavior would you tell him/her to start with? Why?
   b. What steps would you suggest they take to learn about this behavior? Why are these steps useful?

Figure 7.6 Research in Practice Illustration: Empowerment Informing Ethical Interviewing.

with the motorcycle, trial and error within your boundaries, engaging in rural riding, and taking a safety course.

A few research project in practice illustrations follow that demonstrate how empowerment informed our interview questions, guided the interview discourse, and resulted in motorcyclists providing a plethora of feedback, ultimately providing an opportunity to this marginalized group to openly share their views. Specifically, we share feedback from participants about the importance of empowering younger children to make safer decisions, before they become motorcyclists, and the assertion from participants that taking a safety course is vital for building confidence and being able to make more competent decisions while driving a motorcycle. The first illustration (Figure 7.7) showcases the value participants placed on empowering future motorcyclists.

Another area that we talked about during the empowerment section of the interview was encouraging motorcyclists to choose safer behaviors and/or steer new motorcyclists in a positive direction toward safety behavior. Participants often referenced ABATE as an empowering tool for new motorcyclists and that, upon taking a safety course, new motorcyclists would be able to make better decisions. As an example, refer to Research Project in Practice Illustration Figure 7.8.

When applied as a metatheoretical base to support the application of the Reconceptualized Health Belief Model (RHBM), another HRT tenet, community collaboration gave motorcyclists an opportunity to dialogue about who needs to be involved in creating and disseminating motorcycle safety harm reduction initiatives. By invoking this HRT tenet the motorcyclists interviewed were involved in the formative research process of developing a motorcycle safety research and audience analysis plan. Formative research is

Research in Practice Illustration
Empowerment Enhancing Researcher Ethics during Interviews:
Giving Participants an Accurate Voice

Empowering Future Motorcyclists

E: Do you think anything is missing from any of the materials that promote safety that you've seen?

P27: I dunno I think the best thing that's going on in motorcycle safety is starting in bicycling and that's the helmets on the bicycle level. And you see it in uh, uh snowboarding and so I think that, well just like drugs. I think we're starting it really, really early…all of it…sex…all of it. The earlier you get the kids indoctrinated in the right way, the more that's gonna pass on. Like seatbelts ya know when we're, we're taught to put those on when we're 15 in driver's ed and I never turn the key without having a seatbelt on. It's just something that I did and I'm really, I use that as an example of all of those things. Ya know you just make it a habit young. That's why I think that bicycle helmet safety is what, where it would begin, that message. So I'd say that messages start there.

E: Okay.

P27: Telling a 50 year old to put on a motorcycle helmet's kinda long…long too late, I think.

Figure 7.7 Research in Practice Illustration: Empowerment Enhancing Researcher Ethics during Interviews: Giving Participants an Accurate Voice.

Research in Practice Illustration
Empowerment Enhancing Researcher Ethics during Interviews:
Giving Participants Voice

Using a Safety Course to Elicit Safety Choices

Example 1

E: Okay and then if a brand new motorcyclist came up to you, they just a got a bike and they're gonna start riding, but they didn't know a lot about safety precautions, what are some steps that you would tell them to take to learn more?

P34: (4.0) Well they have safety…oh what's the name of it…ABATE…or something like that that's a bicycle school. I never took it but I would strongly recommend it to others. And then ya know I would have them ride with somebody who's experienced so they learn the pace and learn how to take corners by watching somebody doing it as opposed to just going at it.

Example 2

E: So if you were a new rider and you did not know anything about motorcycle safety but you wanted to start practicing different behaviors umm, where would you start?

P7: A motorcycle safety class.

E: Okay.

P7: And that's what we made both our kids take and I took. Tommy didn't because he was a rider for years but the motorcycle safety class is…is conducted in [blinded city] and umm…it's a 7 day course or it's done for 8 hours a day over the weekend…two days. Ya know so it's a 16 hour course I would say. And it covers everything and it really is important. I would say anybody who's riding should take that class.

Figure 7.8 Research in Practice Illustration: Empowerment Enhancing Researcher Ethics during Interviews: Giving Participants Voice.

a process that has been lacking in other harm reduction initiatives and consequently these initiatives have been criticized for ignoring the authentic voice of the target audience.

Community Collaboration. Based on the results of our research project, using community collaboration as a metatheoretical tenet to guide interviews also may enhance research ethics during qualitative research projects. Creating environments conducive to individuals reducing harm is critical (World Health Organization [WHO], 1986). It is necessary to consider and involve the relevant community in all aspects of a health campaign or intervention, including those guided by theory. Cooperation with the community is essential to create enabling environments for individuals whether it is through policy or removing structural barriers impeding behavior change (Rhodes & Hendrich, 2010; WHO, 1986). The structural aspect of health and safety interventions involves seeking to remove contextual or environmental barriers to harm reduction while enabling the social and environmental conditions to help protect the individual from increased susceptibility to harm (Blankenship, Friedman, Dwarkin, & Mantell, 2006).

Through collaborating with the target audience and other key stakeholders, there can be greater assurance that community members' voices are heard and the necessary formative research is being conducted. Ethical frameworks for health interventions continue to emphasize the importance of autonomy, beneficence, and justice (Halpern et al., 2004). In response, these principles must be given thoughtful consideration during the development of health and safety interventions. In order to ensure that autonomy of the target population is created and sustained, Paterson and Panessa (2008) argued that researchers must request participants' voices during the development and implementation of an intervention, fostering a collaborative relationship throughout the process. In addition to empowerment helping solicit information from individuals, community collaboration can be used to help researchers maintain reflexivity and gain feedback from a variety of participants. According to Gurstein et al. (2003), "Conceptualizing young people as partners and decision makers in harm reduction interventions is founded on the belief that their engagement is critical for achieving optimal outcomes" (p. 24). Integrating ethics into a harm reduction approach requires collaboration from the grassroots (Fry et al., 2005), indicating the value of engaging target audience and community members in behavior change initiatives. Refer to Research Project in Practice Illustration Figure 7.9 for some interview questions guided by the HRT tenet of community collaboration. As you will read, the questions focused on engaging participants and treating them as experts, to glean pertinent information about developing campaign materials and messages to best target, inform, and persuade this audience of at-risk motorcyclists.

Additional Research in Practice Illustrations (7.10 and 7.11), demonstrate how using community collaboration helped us become more familiar with the extended target audience of at-risk motorcyclists and ways to best communicate with this group specifically and involve other groups and organizations whose help is needed to facilitate a safer environment for motorcyclists. Although we could include several issues that participants mentioned during the interviews, we focus on examples during which participants continued to list younger children as an audience that needs to be targeted and involved

Research in Practice Illustration
Community Collaboration Informing
Ethical Qualitative Interviewing

1. Why, if at all, is it important for a motorcycle safety campaign or intervention to collaborate with other individuals/groups to enhance safety messages and materials?
    a. Who should we collaborate with?
2. What do you think is missing from most motorcycle safety awareness materials that you see?
3. What exists in the environment that impedes your ability to practice motorcycle safety behaviors?
4. What improvements can be made to your current environment to facilitate safety behavior change?
5. What types of motorcyclists (e.g., gender, age, behaviors, etc.) do motorcycle safety initiatives need to target?

Figure 7.9 Research in Practice Illustration: Community Collaboration Informing Ethical Qualitative Interviewing.

in motorcycle safety initiatives and ABATE as a partner organization that must be included in persuasive materials that promote safety. We showcase these examples to illustrate the ways that the tenets of HRT can work in tandem throughout interviews to continually provide openings for participants to assert opinions that are of interest to them. These examples highlight that using the tenets of HRT as a metatheory continually serves to engage and involve participants. In addition, the outcome of these discussions with participants help guide specific initiatives for future motorcycle safety initiatives.

These examples provide a minimal view of the ways that participants were involved with and informed the formative research needed to develop safety messages focused on motorcycle safety behaviors. Paterson and Panessa (2008) asserted that, to maintain a strong sense of research ethics, engaging participants and continually giving them an accurate voice must be considered as a goal and not an end. These researchers continued, asserting that involving the audience in a respectful and collaborative way can increase the efficacy of such interventions. We see community collaboration as a powerful metatheoretical tenet that can provide a solid foundation for research ethics, serving as a tool to continually offer individuals a "real voice in the creation

Research in Practice Illustration
Community Collaboration Enhancing Research Ethics during Interviews: Involving Participants in Formative Research

More Formative Research Needed with Future Motorcyclists

Example 1

E: Okay. Alright um do you think there's any particular demographic that needs to be targeted because maybe they have riskier behaviors?

P35: Um I would say probably, if anything, younger children. Younger children that aren't really interested in it but who's had a family who is or who has participated in riding a motorcycle. Because I've actually noticed that a lot of my friends whose parents are riding motorcycles, their children are riding motorcycles. And it's just kind of, to me it's kinda like a family tradition, it gets passed down. So I think, I think that would probably be the largest one.

Example 2

P10: But umm…they talk about safety and stuff like that but yeah…I think a lot of the motorcycle places, clubs, and stuff are really…I think they should do more because there's too many people riding motorcycles that don't know what…and even in like the high school…you get these kids running around on these mopeds. They should have some kind of thing…summer class or something where the parents can take their kids down there and teach them the right way to ride. Because that's where it all starts, when you get a moped. And you, ya know, see these kids out…you're not supposed to ride double on a moped but you see it. And the parents aren't controlling their kids. So, I think they should have a summer safety class like at school for like mopeds and motorcycles and that kind of thing.

E: Okay.

P10: I think yeah (6.0)…the Township or somebody should do something. Because [blinded town] has a lot of kids on mopeds and they don't know how to ride.

Figure 7.10 Research in Practice Illustration: Community Collaboration Enhancing Research Ethics during Interviews: Involving Participants in Formative Research.

Research in Practice Illustration
Community Collaboration Enhancing Researcher Ethics during Interviews: Involving Participants in Formative Research

Identifying Strategic Partnerships to Enhance Message Credibility and Resonance

Example 1

P21: Oh yeah I mean there's, there's uhh…something's available already. I think just harping on the safety equipment isn't what people want to hear. I think it just sounds like your mom telling you motorcycles are dangerous. But like uhh, ABATE offers an advanced rider course and it's uhh…I know a guy that's a die-hard rider, he rides a Mecotto, and he takes the ABATE advanced rider course every year. Even though he's done it for the past whatever, because he believes that it sharpens his skills. So yea, yeah I think it's good that people want to participate in things like that.

E: Okay do you think there's anything missing from motorcycle awareness materials that should be added? So, anything else that we can emphasize besides harping on safety?

P21: Umm…the thing that I think is so important with my safety when I'm riding is me being super aware of other drivers. And you always see the stickers, "motorcycles are everywhere, ya know be conscious, be aware," or whatever. Umm I think that that should be in reverse also harped on a lot with riders to be ya know, "be aware of your surroundings," ya know. Just I dunno.

Example 2

E: Mmmhmm. Okay, great. The last section discusses how motorcycle safety can be improved in this area in terms of enhancing safety materials and resources. Do you think it's important for a campaign to collaborate with individuals and groups in [blinded county] to enhance safety messages?

P10: Yeah. Ya know ABATE…we belong to ABATE who held the classes when we went. And if they could get some more…I mean there are millions of people that are riding motorcycles. Ya know if they could get some kind of incentive going and get some more classes going and…We belong to a club in [blinded city] and ya know…they…we go riding with them once in a while. They go to dinner rides like on Tuesday night and they have safety classes like at their meetings they'll talk about safety and stuff like that. But I mean as far as riding they don't go out there and direct you because they're not qualified.

Figure 7.11 Research in Practice Illustration: Community Collaboration Enhancing Researcher Ethics during Interviews: Involving Participants in Formative Research.

of programs and policies designed to serve them" (Weiker, Edington, & Kipke, 1999, p. 215).

The following checklist summarizes some mental notes that we utilized throughout the interviews. These reminders, developed from a harm reduction approach, also helped us adhere to the ethical principles we've discussed throughout this chapter.

Checklist for Adhering to Ethical Principles during Interviews:

- Did you recruit a range of participants for your research study as a technique to conduct solid formative research?
- Are you maintaining a noncritical attitude toward participants (both nonverbally and verbally)?
- Are you providing participants opportunities to share their opinions, express available options to them, and discuss personal choices throughout the interview?
- Are you focusing on choices and/or behaviors that participants perceive are realistic to adopt?

Now that you've read about the ethical debates surrounding harm reduction, and some ways that applying the five identified tenets of HRT consistently during in-depth interviews can enhance attention to research ethics, we conclude this chapter by highlighting how incorporating harm reduction metatheory or applying an existing theory in a new way can enhance ethics in social scientific research.

HARM REDUCTION METATHEORY CHALLENGING RESEARCH ETHICS IN SOCIAL SCIENCE

Throughout this chapter we strived to discuss ethical issues surrounding qualitative research projects in as much detail as possible. However, the role of ethics in qualitative research traditionally has been defined in more narrow terms, such as confidentiality and informed consent (Payne, 2000). Although these discussions are important, according to Morrow (1994), "The larger ideological implications of research are for the most part excluded from the 'ethics' question in standard methodology texts in social sciences" (p. 235). Morrow went on to assert that the absence of this discussion is problematic in research ethics. Specifically, researcher assumptions, including social values and moral consequences are embedded within these projects, regardless of whether we realize these assumptions exist, or they are taken for granted (Payne, 2000). Muruyama (1993) contended that metatheories, along with other broad, social paradigms, impact researcher assumptions, presuppositions, and ultimately, ethics. Similarly, we found that extending harm reduction as a metatheory offered a unique paradigm for research methodology (Morrow, 1994) thus, affecting the ethical mindset and considerations throughout the project, resulting in novel outcomes from the target audience of motorcyclists. Specifically, we focus on how the use of a new metatheory allowed for enhanced research ethics by increasing reflexive practice and minimizing power bias. Finally, we discuss the implications this new research paradigm can have on the development of realistic health and safety messages, in response to providing participants an enhanced voice throughout the interviews.

First, extending HRT to serve as a metatheory allowed for a more "unpredictable" study to occur. According to Brown et al. (1995), utilizing the same theories and frameworks throughout research studies, can eventually cloud ethical integrity and political agendas thus, limiting guidelines for solid research practice. Continued use of these theories then, perpetuates the same discourses and can dominate research practice, which Brown et al. (1995) stated, becomes a "value-neutral manipulation of things, becoming an amoral manipulation of persons" (p. 960). So, in this research project, although the metatheory did not explicitly guide our ethics, it implicitly enriched the discourse produced from harm reduction-related studies and resulted in an expanded practice and application in the research area of health and safety interventions and motorcycle safety initiatives.

Simultaneously, operating from a unique metatheoretical standpoint, we were able to continue exercising our reflexivity, particularly from a critical perspective of "ongoing dialoguing" which is less commonly practiced in qualitative research (Hosking & Pluut, 2010, p. 59). *Ongoing dialoguing* is directly related to and operates in tandem with metatheoretical premises. Utilizing metatheory can allow for an expansion of future practices through more involvement from participants (i.e., human inquiry) (Gergen & Thatchenkery, 1996). As a result of this greater level of involvement, participants are offered ample opportunity to discuss the behaviors they practice in their daily lives which, Hosking and Pluut (2010) argued, helps researchers broaden the scope of ethics and reflexivity, by providing new space for participants to reflect and contribute fresh knowledge.

Similarly, Schubert (1995) argued that practicing reflexiveness within a new research paradigm can help researchers identify social and/or rhetorical barriers that have previously hindered our viewpoints of a particular social area, and then subsequently challenge those barriers, resulting in ethical alternatives to research. This argument supports the notion of changing the way HRT, a theory with strong rhetorical and ethical barriers, was applied in our research project. Extending HRT as a metatheory helped transcend these previous limitations harm reduction faced as a theory and allowed participants an open, noncritical environment to dialogue with us about not only their motorcycle safety behaviors, but behaviors of other motorcyclists and drivers of cars and trucks as well.

Although this form of reflexivity can be practiced in any research project, a new metatheoretical perspective, in which we, as researchers, were treading in unfamiliar territory, allowed for a more collaborative learning process (Cunliffe, 2002), inviting the researcher and participant to co-learn and co-construct the relevant issues surrounding harm reduction efforts in motorcycle and traffic safety. By promoting an enhanced sense of ethical awareness in this way, we could minimize the power gap that often exists in qualitative research projects,. Although we realize it not always is possible to conceptualize and implement a new theoretical framework, it is practical to continually question how particular theoretical constructs have been used in the past. How can you change or utilize these constructs in ways that offer participants an expanded voice?

For us, proposing a revised framework to guide a new empirical study helped keep our ethics "in check" by challenging any presuppositions and values associated with HRT, the RHBM, and motorcycle safety. The results of using a metatheory to guide a theory in our research project challenged the ritualized, redundant findings and recommendations of HRT research that we identified through the review of literature. For example, recent research in the realm of health campaign messages has frowned upon the use of fear appeals (e.g., Hastings, Stead, & Webb, 2004; Morgan, 2012). However, in our interviews the discourse heavily focused on the use of fear appeals to persuade behavior change, indicating that for this target audience fear appeals should be considered in the development of health messages as a strong cue to action.

In response, administering a new metatheoretical framework or altering the way a theory has been used in the past, has potential to advance social science research specific to interviewing methodology, communication theory, and research ethics. In Research Project in Practice Illustration Figure 7.12, we provide an example of how applying harm reduction as a metatheory helped strengthen the application of the RHBM, which further resulted in unique discourse from participants that can inform the development of future motorcycle safety health campaign messages. Incorporating the tenets of HRT as a metatheoretical framework allowed us to converse with motorcyclists about cues to action to initiate behavior change, perceived benefits of and barriers to changing safety behaviors, and participants' confidence to perform safer behaviors while driving a motorcycle. Overall, this new use of the five tenets of HRT changed how this theory has been used in the past and as a result, enhanced application of the RHBM to better understand why motorcyclists do or do not adhere to safety recommendations.

For example, the Health Belief Model (HBM) was used previously in research that focused on traffic safety and motorcycle safety behaviors. When using the HBM alone, studies found gaps in messaging and concluded that improvements were needed in safety messages (Peterson et al., 2004). However, other than stating that changes were needed, these studies did not provide recommendations for improving safety messages and making them more realistic. The results of our research project, however, indicated that integrating HRT tenets with the relevant components of a health behavior theory can inform motorcycle safety behaviors and subsequently aid the development of accurate, targeted safety messages to motorcyclists. Refer back to Figure 7.12 for specific examples that participants provided to make safety messages and general campaign materials more realistic and persuasive. In this research project in practice illustration we present an excerpt from our codebook that illustrates the themes that occurred in response to desirable motorcycle safety materials, lack of materials, and specific examples from participants.

As you probably gleaned from this illustration, participants engaged in using the harm reduction tenets as well. They focused heavily on noncritical, yet realistic messages for motorcyclists, messages that empower motorcyclists

Research in Practice Illustration
Harm Reduction Metatheory and the Reconceptualized HBM Guiding Persuasive Motorcycle Safety Messages

Code: Disseminating realistic messages into local communities		
Theme 1: Targeting and using the family	**Definition:** Motorcyclists described supportive family members and children as a reason for changing their personal safety choices.	*Example:* *"Like I said, my dad was killed on a motorcycle and um…a lot of people questioned why I ever got a bike. I grew up around them my whole life. Um I had dirt bikes since I was young. Um and I knew that even though that was the fact I didn't wanna be the…I wanted to sorta eliminate or diminish the possibility of my kids being without a father. So, that's when it changed…or at least when I thought about it."* (Interview 2)
Theme 2: Using ABATE	**Definition:** Motorcyclists communicated that utilizing ABATE to support and promote safety messages was crucial because of their credibility.	*Example:* *"I do but I don't really pay attention to them. Like mostly what I paid attention to was ABATE like when we were in there they were always talking about things they knew I should watch out for and the messages were in there like…I think they were talking about it like you should re-take ABATE every so often they were saying or another because like rules change and stuff like that so that like…just the messages are kinda the same but ABATE is what teaches you everything about the messages."* (Interview 23)
Theme 3: Nonjudgmental so messages are received	**Definition:** Motorcyclists noted that they tune-out critical, judgmental messages and are more receptive to the nonjudgmental messages.	*Example:* *"…It depends on how it's presented. Ya know like after I got done riding and someone said, "Hey I saw you doing this" or "I, I seen that you stopped too suddenly when we were riding as a group and you need to, need to have more of a space between us." Yeah positive reinforcement as opposed to blah blah ya know."* (Interview 26)
Code: Sustain perceived susceptibility and increase perceived severity		
Theme 1: Be real, be graphic	**Definition:** Motorcyclists discussed the need to make media messages more realistic as a method to increase perceived severity, including showing graphic images of accidents.	*Example:* *"One thing I was expecting that I did not get there was kinda the scare tactic, showing actual accidents and like people after the accidents and like just the consequences and just like okay here's this accident, with a helmet and here's this accident without a helmet….just….cause visuals are big. If you can actually see that I think that would be a big thing."* (Interview 8)
Theme 2: Changing media formats	**Definition:** Since motorcyclists often only see or hear about parts of an accident, they often guess the details of the accident. Changing messages from more of a poster format to a commercial format would allow the entire event to be seen.	*Example:* *"Well maybe just videos demonstrating…(4.0) just like certain videos demonstrating um (3.0) what could happen in the result of like a motorcycle crash.* "(Interview 32)

Figure 7.12 Research in Practice Illustration: Harm Reduction Metatheory and the Reconceptualized HBM Guiding Persuasive Motorcycle Safety Messages.

Theme 1: Be real, be graphic	**Definition:** Motorcyclists discussed the need to make media messages more realistic as a method to increase perceived severity, including showing graphic images of accidents.	*Example:* *"One thing I was expecting that I did not get there was kinda the scare tactic, showing actual accidents and like people after the accidents and like just the consequences and just like okay here's this accident, with a helmet and here's this accident without a helmet....just....cause visuals are big. If you can actually see that I think that would be a big thing."* (Interview 8)
Theme 2: Changing media formats	**Definition:** Since motorcyclists often only see or hear about parts of an accident, they often guess the details of the accident. Changing messages from more of a poster format to a commercial format would allow the entire event to be seen.	*Example:* *"Well maybe just videos demonstrating...(4.0) just like certain videos demonstrating um (3.0) what could happen in the result of like a motorcycle crash.* "(Interview 32)
Theme 3: Setting easier, short-term goals to start with	**Definition:** Motorcyclists indicated that they quickly change behavior but do not sustain it. Promoting easier goals to sustain may increase longevity of safety practices.	*Example:* *"Like when I found out some of that happened I wore a helmet the next day when I rode my motorcycle."* (Interview 22)
Code: Minimize the barriers, maximize the benefits to empower change		
Theme 1: For the love of the motorcycle	**Definition:** Motorcyclists indicated that, in order to preserve the life of their motorcycle they wanted to be safer.	*Example:* *"Just being more aware of the things and the safety...I love my bike, I look at it every day but I don't ride when it comes to safety issues...I know the dangers of riding and others." (Interview 1)*
Theme 2: Focusing on youth and following them through adulthood	**Definition:** Motorcyclists indicated that to change the current motorcycle safety culture, change needs to start with adolescents and progress until they are adults, to begin changing the embedded culture.	*Example:* *"I think the best thing that's going on in motorcycle safety is starting in bicycling and that's the helmets in the bicycle level. And you see it in uh, uh snowboarding and so I think that, just like drugs, I think it's...we're starting it really, really early...all of it...sex...all of it. The earlier you get the kids indoctrinated in the right way, the more that's gonna pass on." (Interview 27)*
Theme 3: The choice IS yours, make the safer one	**Definition:** Motorcyclists communicated the importance of freedom of choice when it comes to motorcycle safety. Messages should promote the aspect of choice, but better communicate the benefits of safer choices.	*Example:* *"I think people should wear seatbelts if they want to wear seatbelts. People should wear helmets if they want to wear helmets. Guaranteed that the numbers do state that you're gonna, you're gonna survive better in most cases if you do...but I mean it's still your personal choice." (Interview 15)*

Figure 7.12 ***Cont.***

to make smarter, safer decisions and the importance of involving others in the development and dissemination of safety messages. Based on this feedback, it is possible that motorcyclists, and other target audiences, have specific feedback about ways to improve health and safety behaviors but, due to previous approaches to research that were restricted to the way a theory has always been used to guide studies in the past, these audiences were not provided openings to insert their voice. Integrating a new metatheory or theory is one approach to research ethics that can provide participants an enhanced voice that can often be silenced without the researchers' knowledge. In our case, integrating harm reduction tenets to inform the RHBM and motorcycle safety revealed new information about the target audience and their risky behaviors.

SUMMARY

Previously we discussed the ways that incorporating the tenets of HRT as a metatheoretical framework allowed us to converse with motorcyclists about cues to action to initiate behavior change, perceived benefits of and barriers to changing safety behaviors, and participants' confidence to perform safer behaviors while driving a motorcycle. Overall, the five tenets of HRT enhanced application of the RHBM to better understand why motorcyclists do or do not adhere to safety recommendations. However, the use of these five tenets, in tandem with the RHBM, also elucidated a greater sense of research ethics, by promoting autonomy, beneficence, justice, and establishing rapport. In addition, beginning to establish the same five core tenets of HRT may also help overcome some ethical dilemmas specific to harm reduction-related research in addition to promoting an egalitarian relationship between participant and researcher, and enhancing the formative research necessary in campaign development.

It is likely that, in the realm of philosophical, social scientific research, further inquiry about ethical considerations during in-depth interviews will consistently be necessary, due to the ever-changing research environments we encounter in the field. However, it is important to continue challenging our understanding of research ethics to have a positive impact on methodological research (Allmark et al., 2009). We believe incorporating a metatheory into qualitative research projects is a new approach to help challenge and strengthen research ethics and the ethical integrity of research projects. We provided numerous examples throughout this chapter to showcase how our use of harm reduction metatheory enhanced principles of ethical research, research reflexivity, and allowed openings for at-risk motorcyclists to insert their enhanced, accurate voice. Although no ethical framework or theory is able to solve all problems in a given research area (Sherwin, 1999), we conclude that the development and use of harm reduction metatheory has potential to strengthen the current state of qualitative social scientific research.

REFERENCES

Aceijas, C. (2012). The ethics in substitution treatment and harm reduction: An analytical review. *Public Health Reviews*, *34:* epub ahead of print.

Allmark, P., Boote, J., Chambers, E., Clarke, A., McDonnell, A., Thompson, A., & Tod, A. M. (2009). *Research Ethics Review, 5*(2), 48–54.

Batchelor, J. A., & Briggs, C. M. (1994). Subject, project or self? Thoughts on ethical dilemmas for social and medical researchers. *Social Science & Medicine, 39*(7), 949–954.

Birch, M., & Miller, T. (2000). Inviting intimacy: The interview as therapeutic opportunity. *International Journal of Social Research Methodology, 3*(3), 189–202.

Blankenship, K. M., Friedman, S. R., Dworkin, S., & Mantell, J. E. (2006). Structural interventions: Concepts, challenges, and opportunities for research. *Journal of Urban Health, 83,* 59–72.

Buchanan, D., Khoshnood, K., Stopka, T., Shaw, S., Santicles, C., & Singer, M. (2002). Ethical dilemmas created by the criminalization of status behaviors: Case examples from ethnographic field research with injection drug users. *Health Education and Behavior, 29*(1), 29–41.

Buning, E. (1990). The role of harm reduction programs in curbing the spread of HIV by drug injectors. In J. Strang & G.V. Stimson (Eds.), *AIDS and drug misuse* (pp. 153–161). London: Routledge.

Byrne, M. (2001). The concept of informed consent in qualitative research. *AORN Journal, 74*(3), 401–403.

Capron, A. M. (1989). Human experimentation. In R. M. Veatch (Ed.), *Medical ethics* (pp. 125–172). Boston, MA: Jones & Bartlett.

Christians, C. G. (2011). Ethics and politics in qualitative research In N.K. Denzin & Y.S. Lincoln (eds.), *The SAGE handbook of qualitative research* (pp. 61–80). Los Angeles: Sage.

Christians, C. (2000). Ethics and politics in qualitative research. In N. Denzin & Y. Lincoln (Eds.), *Handbook of qualitative research* (2nd Ed., pp. 133–155). Thousand Oaks, CA: Sage.

Cunliffe, A. L. (2002). Critical pedagogy: Reflexive dialogical practice in management learning. *Management Learning, 33*(1), 35–61.

Denning, P., & Little, J. (2011). *Practicing harm reduction psychotherapy: An alternative approach to addictions* (2nd Ed.). New York, NY: Guilford Publications Inc.

DiCicco-Bloom, B., & Crabtree, B. F. (2006). The qualitative research interview. *Medical Education, 40,* 314–321.

Duncombe, J., & Jessop, J. (2002). 'Doing rapport' and the ethics of 'faking friendship.' In M. Mauther, M. Birch, J. Jessop, & T. Miller (Eds.), *Ethics of qualitative research* (pp. 107–122). Thousand Oaks, CA: Sage.

DuPont, R. L., (2013). *The selfish brain: Learning from addiction* (2nd Ed.). Center City, MN: Hazeldon.

DuPont, R. L. & Ford, B. (2000). *The selfish brain: Learning from addiction.* Center City, MN: Hazeldon Publishing.

Erickson, P. G., Riley, D. M., Cheung, Y. W., & O'Hare, P. A. (1997). *Harm reduction: A new direction for drug policies and programs.* Toronto: University of Toronto Press.

Field, P. A., & Morse, J. M. (1992). *Nursing research: The application of qualitative approaches.* London: Chapman & Hall.

Fisher, C. B. (2004). Ethics in drug abuse and related HIV risk research. *Applied Development Science, 8*(2), 91–103.

Fry, C. L., Treloar, C., & Maher, L. (2005). Ethical challenges and responses in harm reduction research: Promoting applied communitarian ethics. *Drug and Alcohol Review, 24*(5), 449–459.

Fry, C. L., & Hall, W. (2002). An ethical framework for drug epidemiology: Identifying the issues. *Bulletin on Narcotics, 54,* 131–142.

Gergen, K. J., & Thatchenkery, T. J. (1996). Organization science as social construction: Postmodern potentials. *The Journal of Applied Behavioral Science, 32*(4), 356–377.

Golding, K. S., Dent, H. R., Nissim, R., & Stott, L. (2006). *Thinking psychologically about children who are looked after and adopted.* New York, NY: John Wiley & Sons.

Guillemin, M., & Gillam, L. (2004). Ethics, reflexivity, and 'ethically important moments in research'. *Qualitative Inquiry, 10,* 261–280.

Gunn, N., White, C., Srinivasa, R. (1998). Primary care as harm reduction for injection drug users. *Journal of the American Medical Association, 280,* 1191–1195.

Gurnstein, P., Lovato, C., & Ross, S. (2003). Youth participation in planning: Strategies for social action. *Canadian Journal of Urban Research, 12*(2), 249–274.

Halpern, J., Johnson, M. D., Miranda, J., & Wells, K. B. (2004). The partners in care approach to ethics outcomes in quality improvement programs for depression. *Psychiatric Services, 55*(5), 532–539.

Hastings, G., Stead, M., & Webb, J. (2004). Fear appeals in social marketing: Strategic and ethical reasons for concern. *Psychology and Marketing, 21*(11), 961–986.

Hathaway, A. D. (2002). From harm reduction to human rights: Bringing liberalism back into drug reform debates. *Drug and Alcohol Review, 21,* 397–404.

Hammersley, M. (1999). Some reflections on the current state of qualitative research. *Research Intelligence, 70,* 16–18.

Hopf, C. (2004). Research ethics and qualitative research. In U. Flick, E. von Kardorff & I. Steinke (Eds.), *A companion to qualitative research* (pp. 334–339). London: Sage.

Hosking, D. M., & Pluut, B. (2010). Re(constructing) reflexivity: A relational constructionist approach. *The Qualitative Report, 15*(1), 59–75.

Hunt, N. (2004). Public health or human rights: What comes first? *International Journal of Drug Policy, 15*(4), 231–237.

Irwin, K. S., & Fry, C. L. (2007). Strengthening drug policy and practice through ethics engagement: An old challenge for a new harm reduction. *International Journal of Drug Policy, 18,* 75–83.

Josselson, R. (2007). The ethical attitude in narrative research: Principles and practicalities. In D. J. Clandinin, *Handbook of narrative inquiry* (pp. 537–566). Thousand Oaks, CA: Sage.

Kvale, S. (1996). *Interviews: An introduction to qualitative research interviewing.* Thousand Oaks, CA: Sage.

Keane, H. (2003). Critiques of harm reduction, morality, and the promise of human rights. *International Journal of Drug Policy, 14*(3), 227–232.

Keefe, T. (1978). The economic context of empathy. *Social Work, 11,* 460–465.

Mauthner, M., Birch, M., Jessop, J., & Miller, T. (2002). *Ethics in qualitative research.* Thousand Oaks, CA: Sage.

Marlatt, G. A. (1998). *Harm reduction: Pragmatic strategies for managing high-risk behaviors.* New York: The Guilford Press.

McGraw, L., Zvonkovic, A., & Walker, A. (2000). Studying postmodern families: A feminist analysis of ethical tensions in work and family research. *Journal of Marriage and the Family, 62*(1), 68–77.

Miller, T., & Bell, L. (2002). Consenting to what? Issues of access, gate-keeping, and 'informed' consent. In M. Mauther, M. Birch, J. Jessop, & T. Miller (Eds.), *Ethics of qualitative research* (pp. 53–69). Thousand Oaks, CA: Sage.

Morgan, S. (2012). When health messages cause harm. Retrieved on February 17, 2012 from http://www.purdue.edu/newsroom/general/2012/story-print-deploy-layout_1_17433_17433.html.

Morrow, R. A. (1994). *Critical theory and methodology.* Thousand Oaks, CA: Sage.

Muruyama, M. (1993). Mindscapes, individuals and culture in management. *Journal of Management Inquiry, 2*(2), 140–155.

Munhall, P. L. (1988). Ethical considerations in qualitative research. *Western Journal of Nursing Research, 10*(2), 150–162.

Nunkoosing, K. (2005). The problems with interviews. *Qualitative Health Research, 15*(5), 698.

Orb, A., Eisenhauer, L., & Wynaden, D. (2001). Ethics in qualitative research. *Journal of Nursing Scholarship, 33*(1), 93–96.

Paterson, B. L., & Panessa C. (2008). Engagement as an ethical imperative in harm reduction involving at-risk youth. *International Journal of Drug Policy, 19,* 24–32.

Payne, S. L. (2000). Challenges for research ethics and moral knowledge construction the applied social sciences. *Journal of Business Ethics, 26,* 307–318.

Punch, M. (1994). Politics and ethics in qualitative research. In N.K. Denzin and Y.S. Lincoln (Eds.), *Handbook of qualitative research* (pp. 83–97). Newbery Park, CA: Sage.

Rhodes, T., & Hedrich, D. (2010). Harm reduction and the mainstream. In T. Rhodes & D. Hedrich (10th Ed.), *European Monitoring Centre for Drugs and Drug Addiction Monographs: Harm reduction evidence, impacts, and challenges* (pp. 19–33). Luxembourg: Publications Office of the European Union.

Richards, H. M., & Schwartz, L. J. (2002). Ethics of qualitative research: Are there special issues for health services research? *Family Practice, 19*(2), 135–139.

Sandelowski, M. (1994). The use of quotes in qualitative research. *Research in Nursing Health, 17*(6), 479–482.

Schubert, J. D. (1995). From a politics of transgression toward an ethics of reflexivity. *American Behavioral Scientist, 38*(7), 1003–1017.

Sherwin, S. (1999). Feminism and bioethics. In S.M. Wolf (Eds.), *Feminism and bioethics: Beyond reproduction* (pp. 47–66). New York, NY: Oxford University Press.

Sinding, C., & Aronson, J. (2003). Exposing failures, unsettling accommodations: Tensions in interview practice. *Qualitative Research, 3*(1), 95–117.

Strang, J., & Fortson, R. (2004). Supervised fixing rooms, supervised injectable maintenance clinics- understanding the difference [Commentary]. *BMJ, 328,* 102.

Sweanor, D. (2007). Harm reduction with David Sweanor. Retrieved January 30, 2010,from http://www.eudoxa.se/content/archives/2007/06/harm_reduction_7.html.

Van Beek, I. (2009). Harm reduction- an ethical imperative. *Addiction, 104,* 342–343.

Weiker, R. L., Edington, R., & Kipke, M. D., (1999). A collaborative evaluation of a needle-exchange program for youth. *Health Education Behavior, 26*(2), 213–224.

Wodak, A. (2007). Ethics and drug policy. *Psychiatry, 6*(2), 59–62.

World Health Organization, Health and Welfare Canada, Canadian Public Health Association (1986). Ottawa Charter for Health Promotion, WHO, Copenhagen.

Summary

Future Directions for Harm Reduction Metatheory

In this book, we extended beyond researchers' suggestions to integrate multiple theories into the design and practical outcomes of qualitative research projects, such as health campaigns and interventions (Nigg, Allegrante, & Ory, 2002; Noar, Benac, & Harris, 2007). Instead, we argued for the metatheoretical integration of *HRT* into the design of qualitative research projects. Throughout this book we demonstrated our process of considering and metatheorizing about harm reduction, how using harm reduction metatheory can guide qualitative research methodology and enhance the ways we traditionally apply health behavior theories, and how the constructs of health behavior theories can be enhanced when guided by harm reduction metatheory. To encourage further thinking about harm reduction metatheory, the following summary provides implications for future research considering harm reduction metatheory and suggestions for future research involving HRT as a metatheoretical framework.

RESPONDING TO THE ONGOING CONTROVERSY SURROUNDING HARM REDUCTION IN FUTURE RESEARCH

It is hoped that the research in practice illustrations about a motorcycle safety project presented throughout this book will advance the tenets and use of harm reduction metatheory. However, even though we extended the use and tenets of HRT, it is possible that HRT will remain stymied by its application toward the issue of illicit drugs and not overcome the social stigma surrounding harm reduction. Therefore, future research should employ harm reduction metatheory while addressing more controversial health problems. Possibilities to consider for future research follow.

Previous research suggests that harm reduction self-efficacy varies based on the type of high-risk situation being studied (Phillips, 2005). Therefore, it is important to acknowledge that if a topic other than motorcycle safety was explored in our research project, different themes might have emerged from the data. Motorcyclists identified several barriers that inhibit their safety behaviors while driving a motorcycle. It is likely that by using the tenets of harm reduction to guide a different health behavior theory surrounding a different health or safety issue, unique codes and themes would emerge that provide insights into the at-risk audience being studied. The results of our project indicate the importance of in-depth research with the target audience, whether that audience is motorcyclists who practice risky behaviors while driving their motorcycle or college students who binge drink on the weekends. In other words, we encourage future research that employs harm reduction as a metatheory to address both controversial and noncontroversial health issues.

Research projects surrounding harm reduction have historically focused on alcohol and other drug abuse. However, as illustrated toward the beginning of this book, the focus on these health issues impedes the reputation of HRT in applied health and safety research. In response, we addressed a less controversial health issue, motorcycle safety. However, to further harm reduction as a metatheoretical framework, future research also should address controversial issues, such as needle exchange programs or other drug abuse prevention programs to determine if similar results are rendered. For example, motorcyclists seldomly needed to discuss illegal behaviors they participated in while driving a motorcycle. Because there is no helmet law in Indiana, they did not have to worry about abiding by this law. The only unlawful behaviors motorcyclists mentioned were exceeding the speed limit and/or consuming alcohol beyond the legal BAC limit. However, revealing these behaviors is much different than an individual discussing their methamphetamine, heroin, cocaine, or other drug use, since possessing these drugs is a felony. Therefore, although integrating harm reduction tenets helped motorcyclists discuss their perceived safety behaviors, applying these same tenets may not render consistent results when drug users or other individuals engaging in illegal and/or socially-stigmatized behaviors are the target audience. Future research with a variety of at-risk populations likely will yield further insights.

In addition, besides considering health problems that are publically visible, future research should address self-harming behaviors that most often are hidden, such as eating disorders and intentionally cutting oneself. It is possible that at-risk populations that can hide their risky behaviors more easily may respond differently when probed with the five tenets of harm reduction. Incorporating the metatheoretical tenets of HRT to guide conversations with a variety of at-risk target audiences may reveal additional information that contributes to the development of new messages and interventions for these populations.

CONCLUSION

Previous research indicated that formal evaluation within the field of scientific inquiry has been absent in the development of metatheory (Edwards, 2010). Therefore, additional research applying harm reduction as a metatheoretical framework will initiate future iterations of harm reduction as a metatheory. Throughout this book we respond to the calls from other researchers to address the lack of empirically-tested harm reduction research. The results of our research project provide support for applying the tenets of HRT as a metatheoretical framework for enhancing the application of current health behavior theories within health and safety interventions. It is hoped that the continued integration of HRT as a metatheory with health behavior theories encourages harm reduction-oriented communication with at-risk populations. This communication approach will provide realistic, noncritical information that respects and guides individuals toward making their own decisions and choices on their path to becoming healthier and safer.

We hope our process of harm reduction metatheoretical integration helps advance your own harm reduction research, whether through conceptualizing a new metatheoretical orientation, improving upon current health behavior theories, or enhancing the ways you communicate with participants during data collection and dissemination of results. As we move forward in our personal research we define *Harm Reduction Metatheory* as a framework that consists of conscious and unconscious assumptions that emphasize realistic, nonjudgmental communication strategies to uncover and address barriers to immediate behavior change in guiding theoretical, empirical and practical work with at-risk, target audiences. Perhaps this framework can inform your own research. Ultimately, we hope this book and our research in practice illustrations provided encouragement that harm reduction does not have to be a taboo theory that is too difficult to grasp and apply. In addition, we hope our use of harm reduction metatheory illustrated that it is possible to more explicitly, rather than implicitly, integrate metatheory into our everyday research practice.

REFERENCES

Edwards, M. G. (2010). *Organisational transformation for sustainability: An integral metatheory*. New York: Taylor & Francis Group.

Nigg, C. R., Allegrante, J. P., & Ory, M. (2002). Behavior Change Consortium (Eds.). *Health Education Research, 17*, 493–679.

Noar, S. M., Benac, C. N., & Harris, M. S. (2007). Does tailoring matter? Meta-analytic review of tailored print health behavior change interventions. *Psychological Bulletin, 133*(4), 673–693.

Phillips, K. T. (2005). *Applying the relapse model to harm reduction: The development and evaluation of the harm reduction self-efficacy questionnaire.* Unpublished doctoral dissertation. Bowling Green State University, Toledo: Ohio.

Appendix A

Table A.1 Results for Humanistic Value Informing Motorcycle Safety Cues to Action

Code: It's a family thing		
Theme 1: Family member influential in motorcycling decision	**Definition:** The motorcyclist discusses a family member who rides/rode a motorcycle as the predominant reason for beginning to ride a motorcycle.	*Example:* *"Um actually my whole family rides motorcycles . . . that's, that's how I got brought into it. Um my dad, he's been riding forever and um my mom, she used to ride but she got a whole bunch of tendonitis from her job so that's how I ended up with the motor . . . with the Sportster. Um and then I took the uh Rider's Edge put on by Harley Davidson which is like a uh driver's ed course for motorcycles. So riding, being on two wheels throughout my whole family has just kind of been a lineage."* (Interview 35)
Theme 2: Inherited family member's tangible and intangible behaviors	**Definition:** The motorcyclist conveys that personal safety choices were heavily influenced by similar choices made by a family member who also rides a motorcycle.	*Example:* *"It's easy . . . my father, he rode. And he said that, if you're riding down the road going 50, 60 miles an hour and you get hit in the middle of the forehead with a june bug . . . you'll be, you'll wish that you had a helmet. Because for one, not only can that hurt, but it's gonna stun you and you could easily lose control of the bike. So that, those two experiences-my father's advice and then also the experience with the bumblebee encourages me to ride with uh appropriate gear."* (Interview 29)

Table A.1 Results for Humanistic Value Informing Motorcycle Safety Cues to Action (*cont.*)

Code: Fellow motorcyclists' influence		
Theme 1: Keeping the motorcyclist grounded	**Definition:** The motorcyclist identifies other motorcyclists who are part of a personal riding network as influential in practicing safer behaviors, or the motorcyclist identifies with being the role model to the personal riding network.	*Example:* *"Like normally he's always the one making sure . . . he's like really cautious when he drives like . . . he will do like 20 in a 30, like he's just so cautious. He's normally the one that like, well I'll lead but I'll have to make sure that he's with me and everything so he kinda helps settle me down and stuff like that."* (Interview 23)
Theme 2: Keeping up with group mentality	**Definition:** The motorcyclist discusses the role of group peer pressure in engaging in risky behaviors while riding a motorcycle; although some motorcyclists continue to give in to the peer pressure others avoid group riding.	*Example:* *"So initially when I'm flying down . . . well with the wheelie up like guys are doing because you know you have to do that or you're not a guy. You're just a punk, you're scared, you don't wanna be a chicken. It's just a whole mentality . . . you know I mean it sounds stupid and I'm telling you right now . . . me telling you about it . . . I feel like, "dang he's stupid, what would he do that for?" But at the same time ya know . . . ya know . . . you have to do it. I know it sounds stupid. It's like a fraternity. You have to do it because you wanna . . . you wanna be in the group."* (Interview 3)
Theme 3: Same riding styles, safe and risky	**Definition:** The motorcyclist describes the group in which they ride as practicing the same behaviors together, regardless of whether the behaviors are safe or risky.	*Example:* *"But just riding around town and out in the country, I like the no helmet thing. And that's, that's the way my buddies are . . . all the same thing."* (Interview 28)
Theme 4: Their choice, their fault, not my problem	**Definition:** The motorcyclist emphasizes the notion of choice when referring to motorcycle safety, that other motorcyclists know the risks of riding, and it is not their role to say something to other motorcyclists.	*Example:* *"Well my opinion is it should be your right to wear a helmet or not wear a helmet. And that's uh, that's all I can say about this. It's, it's not an issue that uh I believe or would be totally against it . . . . if you wore a helmet I wouldn't tell you shouldn't wear a helmet and I expect you won't to tell me I should be wearing a helmet. So it's the culture and the freedom of choice."* (Interview 19)

Code: Non-motorcyclists' influence		
Theme 1: Only if you follow her rules	**Definition:** The male motorcyclist indicates that his female partner is fine with his decision to ride a motorcycle as long as he wears a helmet or other safety gear.	*Example:* *". . . but when I go up to Chicago I have to have my helmet because she will kick my ass. . . . She'll break up with me so no, nah, that's it. The road rash she would just laugh at me, that's my own problem. Being a vegetable, that would be her problem."* (Interview 30)
Theme 2: Reluctantly go along with it	**Definition:** The motorcyclist indicates that non-motorcyclists are consistently worried about what will happen during a ride and always caution the motorcyclist to be safe.	*Example:* *"My wife goes along with it. Uh my kids go along with it and uh like my brothers have bikes, my son has a motorcycle, so we're, we're fine with it but I think in the back of everybody's mind there's always that doubt that maybe on one given day something bad will happen. So that's why, like my mom, when we, we were young kids she didn't want us to have motorcycles."* (Interview 28)
Theme 3: Wouldn't do it, don't support it	**Definition:** The motorcyclist states that relationships with non-motorcyclist family members are threatened because they do not support the decision to ride.	*Example:* *"And that spring I bought a 1971 Triumph Bonneville 650 . . . it was a . . . well that's what I bought. And my mother told me, she said, "You can have this but once you get rid of this, don't bring anymore around here." So I sold that motorcycle . . . I bought a Harley Davidson (haha). And my mother says, "You have to go" (Haha). So . . . I had to leave the house ya know, I had to move out and uh that was my mother's perception."* (Interview 25)
Theme 4: Exchange risky behaviors for children	**Definition:** The motorcyclist indicates that riskier choices were made while riding a motorcycle before having children and after having children, safer behaviors began.	*Example:* *"I have a family. Granted I have life insurance . . . some people think . . . but I wanna be here for them so I'm not gonna go out there and just be a rebel without a cause. And that's . . . I mean if I were single and didn't have a family there's a chance I probably wouldn't wear a helmet . . . more times. But knowing what I have to come home to . . . it makes you think differently."* (Interview 34)

Table A.1 Results for Humanistic Value Informing Motorcycle Safety Cues to Action (*cont.*)

Theme 5: Passenger cueing safety	**Definition:** The motorcyclist describes the differences in personal safety behaviors when a passenger is on the back of the motorcycle, including wearing safety gear and adhering to traffic laws.	*Example:* *"Well especially when you have a passenger because you're not only responsible for yourself, you're responsible for a passenger. I remember ya know, Jeannie's been on the bike with me plenty of times and you don't, you don't take the same risks you do."* (Interview 26)
Code: A motorcycle fatality, or close call		
Theme 1: Pulling out the gear	**Definition:** The motorcyclist references friends' accidents as the primary reinforcement to wear safety gear while riding.	*Example:* *"I think that other friends getting into accidents makes me think more about wearing your safety gear more. Uh I mean if somebody goes down and they say, "man, my head bounced off the concrete so hard, if I hadn't had my helmet on . . ." ya know. So that makes me think about it . . . more than the other stuff."* (Interview 21)
Theme 2: Driving more defensively	**Definition:** The motorcyclist uses the accidents of fellow motorcyclists to learn how to drive more defensively, safely, and make smarter decisions while riding.	*Example:* *"There have been times when I've been at a stop light stopped and I am constantly looking in my rearview mirrors or looking behind me to make sure that the car behind me is gonna stop . . . cause that's what happened to my dad. A drunk driver going 100 mph didn't stop at the light . . . ran right through. Umm so I think when I'm at a stop light and there's . . . there could be cars around but there's no body immediately behind me I start looking back to make sure everything's going to be okay."* (Interview 2)
Code: Where's the message		
Theme 1: Lack of information for drivers of cars and trucks	**Definition:** The motorcyclist discusses that a problem hindering safety is the prevalence of media that targets the motorcyclist, but that messages to inform drivers to be aware of motorcyclists are not prevalent.	*Example:* *"Um there's always more that could be said about motorcycle safety I think, just because of the fact that . . . nine times out of ten it's not the motorcyclist's fault when there's an accident, it is the other person's fault because they don't see the motorcyclist. So . . . there could never, in my opinion, be enough information out there for people."* (Interview 33)

Theme 2: Everyone in need of safety reminders	**Definition:** The motorcyclist thinks that there are small reminders that exist to caution everyone about motorcycle safety, such as bumper stickers and commercials, but there should be a lot more.	*Example:* *"I think that uh . . . uh I think it's really good because it hopefully like a non-biker who's in a car, who sees one of those bumper stickers will read it and it might just make them a little more aware ya know that there are bikes on the road and you do need to be more aware."* (Interview 18)
Theme 3: Don't drink and ride	**Definition:** The motorcyclist specifically references and offers feedback on the "don't drink and ride" campaign that targets motorcyclists as the primary messages prevalent in the media.	*Example:* *"Um the only commercials that I can really think that have been directed about motorcycles were like . . . um . . . drunk driving commercials and they'll have . . . they have the one where like they open a car door and all the alcohol spills out um and then there's one where they open the helmet visor and it, um floods out of there. So that's the only time I can really remember seeing a commercial directed toward motorcyclists."* (Interview 31)
Theme 4: Safety promoted via local clubs and events	**Definition:** The motorcyclist references local clubs or organizations, including motorcycle dealerships, clubs, and rides, as a medium that promotes safety.	*Example:* *"I work at Middle Steel so they have safety classes out there and once in a while they give one about motorcycle safety, especially in the spring when everybody's got their bikes out and stuff like that and we've had shows where we bring our bikes to the mill and they ask us about safety and they make sure we have all of the safety equipment on and everything."* (Interview 10)
Theme 5: ABATE teaching the media messages	**Definition:** The motorcyclist specifically references ABATE as the primary enforcer of motorcycle safety through their classes and bumper stickers.	*Example:* *"Like mostly what I paid attention to was ABATE like when we were in there they were always talking about things they knew I should watch out for and the messages were in there like . . . I think they were talking about it like you should re-take ABATE every so often they were saying or another because like rules change and stuff like that so that like . . . just the messages are kinda the same but ABATE is what teaches you everything about the messages."* (Interview 23)

Table A.1 Results for Humanistic Value Informing Motorcycle Safety Cues to Action (*cont.*)

Theme 6: Let's be real with it	**Definition:** The motorcyclist discusses making media messages more realistic as a method to change behavior including utilizing statistics and showing graphic images of accidents.	*Example:* *"One thing I was expecting that I did not get there was kinda the scare tactic, showing actual accidents and like people after the accidents and like just the consequences and just like okay here's this accident, with a helmet and here's this accident without a helmet . . . . just . . . . cause visuals are big. If you can actually see that I think that would be a big thing."* (Interview 8)
Code: Helmet mandates		
Theme 1: Helmet laws forcing safety	**Definition:** The motorcyclist shares opinions about Indiana's no helmet law and the impact (if any) it has on personal safety behaviors.	*Example:* *"I choose very wisely when I go through those states. I have chosen routes where I am going around states that have those laws because it's not as safe as they think it is. But I will if I have to."* (Interview 12)
Theme 2: Family rules enforcing safety	**Definition:** The motorcyclist discusses that the reason he/she wears a helmet is because of personal rules enforced by a family member.	*Example:* *"Um (haha) there was absolutely no way I could get on the bike without it . . . my parents just wouldn't . . . I was 17 when I started riding so they just would not allow it. Uh I was fine with it. Um now I like to wear my helmet because it's really cool looking."* (Interview 31)

Appendix B

Table A.2 Results for Pragmatism Informing Motorcycle Safety Perceived Benefits and Barriers

Code: Yeah I own it, doesn't mean I wear it		
Theme 1: Weather	**Definition:** The motorcyclist identifies weather, both hot and cold, as a contributor to the safety gear worn on a particular day.	*Example:* *"You have to think that, if you're going out for a ride . . . ya know it's hot and you can't leather up everyday cause in Lafayette it's like ya know 100 degrees and if you're in full leather . . . no. You'll sit there and sweat through your leather."* (Interview 17)
Theme 2: Uncomfortable	**Definition:** The motorcyclist is more comfortable riding without safety gear and believes riding is more convenient without safety gear as well.	*Example:* *"I think it has to be a conscious effort . . . a conscious decision. Because it is . . . it feels so much better to not have a helmet on. I mean the wind and, and the . . . you have to get used to a helmet, especially on a hot day. And the same with the leather jacket . . . you have to get used to wearing all the gear. The heavy boots, we ride in heavy boots. And it's . . . it's hot and it's uncomfortable when you stop and walk around. So yeah it has to be a conscious decision, you have to want to do it."* (Interview 7)

Table A.2 Results for Pragmatism Informing Motorcycle Safety Perceived Benefits and Barriers (*cont.*)

Theme 3: Who I'm with that day	**Definition:** describes the importance of living up to the mystique of being a motorcyclist and riding in groups, and not wearing safety gear is a part of that expectation	*Example:* *". . . a part of peer pressure is living up to the mystique of riding motorcycles. And they think that a helmet doesn't fit into the live to ride, ride to live sort of mentality and so yeah. Because I've spoken to my sister repeatedly, I've said, "listen, you need to wear a helmet ya know, why don't you wear a helmet?" and um and that's how I got on the subject with her that she said, "well none of my friends do."* (Interview 29)
Theme 4: The cool factor	**Definition:** The motorcyclist indicates that safety gear is not cool or fashionable enough to wear while riding a motorcycle, making safety gear less desirable.	*Example:* *". . . you can't tell me that it's not about style, that it's not about looking cool on the motorcycle. Nobody would, nobody would ride a, a clown colored motorcycle unless you're . . . well you know what I'm saying. No one would ride an ugly piece of crap motorcycle and really not give a crap what people think. So yea I'd say the barriers are style and looking cool ya know. I mean it doesn't look as cool to wear all the safety gear."* (Interview 21)
Theme 5: Freedom on the road	**Definition:** The motorcyclist experiences a sense of freedom without safety gear.	*Example:* *"But it just, it just goes against the spirit of riding a bike. Ya know like why wouldn't you just ride a fast car? Ya know it's for that openness and that takes away some of it."* (Interview 27)
Theme 6: It's more dangerous	**Definition:** The motorcyclist thinks that wearing safety gear is more dangerous due to dulling senses and reaction time, and can cause greater injuries if in an accident.	*Example:* *"Helmets, a lot of times, they hinder your view. And a lot of times the helmets will break your neck rather than just bang your head up, ya know."* (Interview 16)
Theme 7: Well, I wear something	**Definition:** The motorcyclist indicates that although a full set of safety gear is rare, a helmet is worn a majority of the time.	*Example:* *"Well I always wear something over my eyes. So if I don't have my helmet on then I would have eye protection."* (Interview 4)

Code: Age as initial barrier, later influencing change		
Theme 1: Getting older, getting wiser	**Definition:** The motorcyclist describes risky behaviors practiced when younger and aging as the primary reason for changing safety behaviors as personal riding progressed.	*Example:* *"Well just as I said when you're younger you don't realize the . . . the potential for accidents when you're younger. As you get older then you become to realize when you ride a motorcycle that you're really putting yourself at a big risk, a bigger risk of having an accident because there's no protection on a motorcycle. Where uh so you really have to slow down and watch. And ya know you just, you don't think, when you're younger you just don't think anything's gonna happen. And as you get older and wiser and uh you get a little bit safer."* (Interview 25)
Theme 2: Young and invincible	**Definition:** The motorcyclist indicates feelings of invincibility as a young motorcyclist as the main contributor behind engaging in risky riding.	*Example:* *"I practiced a lot of risky behaviors when I was really young. But after uh, after I turned 20 my risky behaviors declined exponentially. . . . When you're young you're always invincible. Come on think about it, how old are you?"* (Interview 15)
Theme 3: Detached from harm	**Definition:** The motorcyclist indicates that the younger you are, the more likely you are to try anything on a motorcycle.	*Example:* *"No because I think human nature is that you think it's never gonna happen to you. Um ya know I feel as though when I ride I'm doing it very safely, whether or not I am, I don't know! (haha)."* (Interview 34)
Theme 4: Can't afford to be safe yet	**Definition:** The motorcyclist indicates that the cost of safety gear is a barrier to being safer while riding.	*Example:* *"A lot of the newer safety gear is actually very expensive now. So I think obtaining new safety gear is probably not quite out of my control but it would be much more difficult than just avoiding an unfamiliar road."* (Interview 35)
Code: Taking a chance		
Theme 1: Only if you follow her rules	**Definition:** The male motorcyclist indicates that his female partner is fine with his decision to ride a motorcycle as long as he wears a helmet or other safety gear.	*Example:* *". . . but when I go up to Chicago I have to have my helmet because she will kick my ass. . . . She'll break up with me so no, nah, that's it. The road rash she would just laugh at me, that's my own problem. Being a vegetable, that would be her problem."* (Interview 30)

Table A.2 Results for Pragmatism Informing Motorcycle Safety Perceived Benefits and Barriers (*cont.*)

Theme 2: Reluctantly go along with it	**Definition:** The motorcyclist indicates that non-motorcyclists are consistently worried about what will happen during a ride and always caution the motorcyclist to be safe.	*Example:* *"My wife goes along with it. Uh my kids go along with it and uh like my brothers have bikes, my son has a motorcycle, so we're, we're fine with it but I think in the back of everybody's mind there's always that doubt that maybe on one given day something bad will happen. So that's why, like my mom, when we, we were young kids she didn't want us to have motorcycles."* (Interview 28)
Theme 3: Wouldn't do it, don't support it	**Definition:** The motorcyclist states that relationships with non-motorcyclist family members are threatened because they do not support the decision to ride.	*Example:* *"And that spring I bought a 1971 Triumph Bonneville 650 . . . it was a . . . well that's what I bought. And my mother told me, she said, "You can have this but once you get rid of this, don't bring anymore around here." So I sold that motorcycle . . . I bought a Harley Davidson (haha). And my mother says, "You have to go" (Haha). So . . . I had to leave the house ya know, I had to move out and uh that was my mother's perception."* (Interview 25)
Theme 4: Exchange risky behaviors for children	**Definition:** The motorcyclist indicates that riskier choices were made while riding a motorcycle before having children and after having children, safer behaviors began.	*Example:* *"I have a family. Granted I have life insurance . . . some people think . . . but I wanna be here for them so I'm not gonna go out there and just be a rebel without a cause. And that's . . . I mean if I were single and didn't have a family there's a chance I probably wouldn't wear a helmet . . . more times. But knowing what I have to come home to . . . it makes you think differently."* (Interview 34)
Theme 5: Passenger cueing safety	**Definition:** The motorcyclist describes the differences in personal safety behaviors when a passenger is on the back of the motorcycle, including wearing safety gear and adhering to traffic laws.	*Example:* *"Well especially when you have a passenger because you're not only responsible for yourself, you're responsible for a passenger. I remember ya know, Jeannie's been on the bike with me plenty of times and you don't, you don't take the same risks you do."* (Interview 26)

Code: A motorcycle fatality, or close call		
Theme 1: Pulling out the gear	**Definition:** The motorcyclist references friends' accidents as the primary reinforcement to wear safety gear while riding.	*Example:* *"I think that other friends getting into accidents makes me think more about wearing your safety gear more. Uh I mean if somebody goes down and they say, "man, my head bounced off the concrete so hard, if I hadn't had my helmet on . . . " ya know. So that makes me think about it . . . more than the other stuff."* (Interview 21)
Theme 2: Driving more defensively	**Definition:** The motorcyclist uses the accidents of fellow motorcyclists to learn how to drive more defensively, safely, and make smarter decisions while riding.	*Example:* *"There have been times when I've been at a stop light stopped and I am constantly looking in my rearview mirrors or looking behind me to make sure that the car behind me is gonna stop . . . cause that's what happened to my dad. A drunk driver going 100 mph didn't stop at the light . . . ran right through. Umm so I think when I'm at a stop light and there's . . . there could be cars around but there's no body immediately behind me I start looking back to make sure everything's going to be okay."* (Interview 2)

Code: Where's the message		
Theme 1: Lack of information for drivers of cars and trucks	**Definition:** The motorcyclist discusses that a problem hindering safety is the prevalence of media that targets the motorcyclist, but that messages to inform drivers to be aware of motorcyclists are not prevalent.	*Example:* *"Um there's always more that could be said about motorcycle safety I think, just because of the fact that . . . nine times out of ten it's not the motorcyclist's fault when there's an accident, it is the other person's fault because they don't see the motorcyclist. So . . . there could never, in my opinion, be enough information out there for people."* (Interview 33)
Theme 2: Everyone in need of safety reminders	**Definition:** The motorcyclist thinks that there are small reminders that exist to caution everyone about motorcycle safety, such as bumper stickers and commercials, but there should be a lot more.	*Example:* *"I think that uh . . . uh I think it's really good because it hopefully like a non-biker who's in a car, who sees one of those bumper stickers will read it and it might just make them a little more aware ya know that there are bikes on the road and you do need to be more aware."* (Interview 18)

Table A.2 Results for Pragmatism Informing Motorcycle Safety Perceived Benefits and Barriers (*cont.*)

Theme 3: Don't drink and ride	**Definition:** The motorcyclist specifically references and offers feedback on the "don't drink and ride" campaign that targets motorcyclists as the primary messages prevalent in the media.	*Example:* *"Um the only commercials that I can really think that have been directed about motorcycles were like . . . um . . . drunk driving commercials and they'll have . . . they have the one where like they open a car door and all the alcohol spills out um and then there's one where they open the helmet visor and it, um floods out of there. So that's the only time I can really remember seeing a commercial directed toward motorcyclists."* (Interview 31)
Theme 4: Safety promoted via local clubs and events	**Definition:** The motorcyclist references local clubs or organizations, including motorcycle dealerships, clubs, and rides, as a medium that promotes safety.	*Example:* *"I work at Middle Steel so they have safety classes out there and once in a while they give one about motorcycle safety, especially in the spring when everybody's got their bikes out and stuff like that and we've had shows where we bring our bikes to the mill and they ask us about safety and they make sure we have all of the safety equipment on and everything."* (Interview 10)
Theme 5: ABATE teaching the media messages	**Definition:** The motorcyclist specifically references ABATE as the primary enforcer of motorcycle safety through their classes and bumper stickers.	*Example:* *"Like mostly what I paid attention to was ABATE like when we were in there they were always talking about things they knew I should watch out for and the messages were in there like . . . I think they were talking about it like you should re-take ABATE every so often they were saying or another because like rules change and stuff like that so that like . . . just the messages are kinda the same but ABATE is what teaches you everything about the messages."* (Interview 23)
Theme 6: Let's be real with it	**Definition:** The motorcyclist discusses making media messages more realistic as a method to change behavior including utilizing statistics and showing graphic images of accidents.	*Example:* *"One thing I was expecting that I did not get there was kinda the scare tactic, showing actual accidents and like people after the accidents and like just the consequences and just like okay here's this accident, with a helmet and here's this accident without a helmet . . . . just . . . . cause visuals are big. If you can actually see that I think that would be a big thing."* (Interview 8)

Code: Helmet mandates		
Theme 1: Helmet laws forcing safety	**Definition:** The motorcyclist shares opinions about Indiana's no helmet law and the impact (if any) it has on personal safety behaviors.	*Example:* *"I choose very wisely when I go through those states. I have chosen routes where I am going around states that have those laws because it's not as safe as they think it is. But I will if I have to."* (Interview 12)
Theme 2: Family rules enforcing safety	**Definition:** The motorcyclist discusses that the reason he/she wears a helmet is because of personal rules enforced by a family member.	*Example:* *"Um (haha) there was absolutely no way I could get on the bike without it . . . my parents just wouldn't . . . I was 17 when I started riding so they just would not allow it. Uh I was fine with it. Um now I like to wear my helmet because it's really cool looking."* (Interview 31)

Code: Taking a chance		
Theme 1: Speeding	**Definition:** The motorcyclist describes speeding as a risky behavior during personal rides.	*Example:* *"As much as you could get away with, yeah. I like, I like to drive fast anyway so yeah, always. It'd be nothing to be double . . . ya know if it was 50 it'd be a 100. Cause bikes, ya know most bikes can do 120 in yards ya know. I'm not saying that, I don't condone that, that's just a fact. . . . Why would you own the bike if you didn't?"* (Interview 27)
Theme 2: Corner carving	**Definition:** The motorcyclist describes taking turns very tight and quick as a risky behavior during personal rides.	*Example:* *"Umm . . . (4.0) . . . uh even though Harley's aren't corner carvers I like to . . . I get on a turn and I like to lean into it. And I like to accelerate through a turn. It just gives you that fun feeling."* (Interview 21)
Theme 3: Drinking and riding (then or now)	**Definition:** The motorcyclist describes drinking heavily and then riding as a previous or current risky behavior during personal rides.	*Example:* *"Every time I'm out. Every time you're on a bike you stop at a bar. Whether it be one beer or ten. That's risky when you involve alcohol . . . that's risky. Slows your reaction."* (Interview 12)

Table A.2 Results for Pragmatism Informing Motorcycle Safety Perceived Benefits and Barriers (*cont.*)

Theme 4: Riding in bad conditions	**Definition:** The motorcyclist decides to ride despite dangerous weather conditions.	*Example:* *"I will ride in the winter ya know after it's snowed and it's been melted and dry for like three weeks but the wind chill is like 10 degrees. I'll bundle up and ride then but I guess that might be one of the more risky things I've done."* (Interview 29)
Code: Complacent		
Theme 1: There's not anything to change	**Definition:** The motorcyclist feels confident with personal skills and feels there are no safety behaviors to change.	*Example:* *"I went through a stiff of a couple years where I actually didn't wear my helmet and all that other stuff and I got back into it so I've pretty much made what changes I need to make."* (Interview 9)
Theme 2: Don't want to change	**Definition:** The motorcyclist describes a specific safety behavior that could be changed but takes no specific action to change current safety behaviors.	*Example:* *"I'd like to try a little more on safe behaviors but I don't think I will. It's one of those things where I should do it but I'm not going to. I'm not going to get around to it. It's just one of those things where it's right there . . . it's just right now I don't wanna grab it. It's the . . . I can do it . . . I just don't wanna."* (Interview 5)
Code: Driving defensively as key to being and feeling safe		
Theme 1: Know and stay within boundaries	**Definition:** The motorcyclist indicates that to maintain safety motorcyclists must establish personal boundaries and continue riding within those boundaries and personal abilities.	*Example:* *"Establishing boundaries as, as a rider, what you can and can't do. And (3.0) and sticking to those boundaries because if you don't you're putting your own life in jeopardy."* (Interview 33)
Theme 2: Aware of surroundings 100% of time	**Definition:** The motorcyclist indicates that to maintain safety motorcyclists must always be aware of their surroundings, such as environment and other drivers.	*Example:* *"Being an assertive, defensive driver, being aware of your surroundings at all times, trying to . . . trying to anticipate other drivers' actions."* (Interview 21)

Theme 3: Equip yourself and motorcycle with extras	**Definition:** The motorcyclist describes methods to furnish a motorcycle and the body to stay safer while riding on the road.	*Example:* *"On my bike, for example, I put air horns on it. Because a little horn on a motorcycle doesn't bring anybody's attention, but when you hear this then people are like, whoa what's that?!"* (Interview 1)
Theme 4: No (alcohol) influence	**Definition:** The motorcyclist indicates that one of the best ways to be safe on the road is to maintain awareness by only riding a motorcycle when sober.	*Example:* *"Motorcycle safety for me would be one, not to be under the influence of anything, obviously. I mean obviously you're a better rider when you're not under the influence of alcohol or drugs."* (Interview 3)
Theme 5: At the mercy of the car/truck's behaviors	**Definition:** The motorcyclist conveys that regardless of how safe motorcyclists are on the road, vehicles can make an error and the motorcyclist will lose based on the difference in vehicle size.	*Example:* *"Yeah somebody can pull out in front of me just as easily as they could back then. So no, no I don't. I feel pretty much, have been and always will be at the mercy of the other drivers. I just gotta watch out."* (Interview 24)
Code: Personal safety		
Theme 1: Check the bike	**Definition:** The motorcyclist describes various ways to check and upkeep a motorcycle to avoid a mishap while riding.	*Example:* *"Uh I check the equipment, check the tires, check the lights, um make sure everything's good to go. You really should do that every ride but I don't do it every ride. But I do, every other ride I'd say. And uh so yeah, checking the equipment is a big thing, your turn signals and things like that and if they don't function and you think you're functioning, you turn in front of somebody . . . well I had my turn signal on. Well you, it didn't work so that's kinda a big thing too."* (Interview 28)
Theme 2: Stay aware of surroundings	**Definition:** The motorcyclist indicates that staying aware of all types of surroundings and predicting other behaviors is necessary.	*Example:* *"Um I always, I think the biggest one is always scanning . . . don't . . . I try not to just kind of like just stare out into space and just kinda try to ride in a straight line. Like I always try to scan and see what's in front of me and beside me."* (Interview 35)

Table A.2 Results for Pragmatism Informing Motorcycle Safety Perceived Benefits and Barriers (*cont.*)

Theme 3: Helmet	**Definition:** The motorcyclist reports that a choice made to maintain personal safety is wearing a helmet.	*Example:* *"Uh wearing a helmet is a choice so I always do that."* (Interview 24)
Theme 4: Follow the laws	**Definition:** The motorcyclist indicates that when basic traffic laws are adhered to motorcyclists are doing all they can to maintain personal safety on the road.	*Example:* *"Um (3.0) and then just adhering to traffic laws the same way you would any other vehicle."* (Interview 31)
Theme 5: Being able to say no to the ride	**Definition:** The motorcyclist indicates that an important aspect of maintaining personal safety is being able to assess the surroundings and alertness and if applicable, not ride that day.	*Example:* *"There are times I guess when in heavy traffic . . . like I just made . . . a lot of times ride my motorcycle to veterinary meetings and I had one this week where I had to go around 465 in Indianapolis during rush hour and I consciously chose to drive the car because I didn't want to be in that situation on a motorcycle. So I do elect not to take it sometimes when I'm in a situation that's not ideal."* (Interview 24)
Code: Benefits of safe motorcycling		
Theme 1: Internal confidence	**Definition:** The motorcyclist attributes safer behaviors with being a more confident motorcyclist.	*Example:* *"Feeling more confident when riding. Um . . . (4.0) . . . I think that's really just about it, just feeling more confident while riding."* (Interview 33)
Theme 2: Quality of life, and the ride continues	**Definition:** The motorcyclist indicates that a key benefit of being safer on a motorcycle is the ability to continue riding happy and healthy.	*Example:* *"Well obviously I'm alive! Yeah and it's just a very enjoyable sport. I look at it as um a great way to spend a Saturday afternoon ya know. I just really enjoy it."* (Interview 7)

Theme 3: Costs of riding influences safety	**Definition:** The motorcyclist indicates that a benefit to maintaining safer behaviors is maintaining the life span of a motorcycle.	*Example:* *". . . if you're safer on your motorcycle then, then the maintenance upkeep of the motorcycle and your gear isn't nearly as what it could be. Uh ya know if you're real reckless and you could, you could be burning something up in the engine, you could be burning something up in the transmission, or you could actually be constantly just dropping the bike or something and then . . . in the end it all adds up pretty quick."* (Interview 35)
Theme 4: Invisible	**Definition:** The motorcyclist does not acknowledge any benefits of being safe on a motorcycle because being safe equates to uneventful rides.	*Example:* *"You don't see the benefits of it because it, ya know you don't, you don't think about it. If you don't get in an accident you're going well, this is kinda boring but you don't think of, well I'm being safe therefore I'm not in a wreck. So I think it's something you don't see but it's, it's just part of the game ya know."* (Interview 28)

Appendix C

Table A.3 Results for Immediacy/Goal Setting Informing Motorcycle Safety Perceived Susceptibility and Perceived Severity

Code: Speed as both safety and risk		
Theme 1: Unexpected can happen quicker	**Definition:** The motorcyclist describes speeding as a risky behavior based on having less time to react to an unexpected barrier on the road.	*Example:* *". . . if you're speeding at all there's a lot of times you can hit bumps in the road and they can, they can definitely surprise you when you hit them and everything, especially if you're not expecting them and when you're speeding you just gotta make sure you're not coming up on someone too quickly. Or you gotta watch out for things that could like really catch you or your bike off guard and that could definitely cause you to crash."* (Interview 23)
Theme 2: Natural reflex for the motorcyclist and the motorcycle	**Definition:** The motorcyclist describes speeding as a natural behavior when riding a motorcycle.	*Example:* *"You just feel it. It's great you just feel it, you just ride. You don't care about what that speedometer says. You feel the road . . . you feel it. You ride where you feel comfortable, whether it be 80, 90, 100."* (Interview 12)

Table A.3 Results for Immediacy/Goal Setting Informing Motorcycle Safety Perceived Susceptibility and Perceived Severity (*cont.*)

Theme 3: Highway yes, local road no	**Definition:** The motorcyclist describes speeding on a highway as a safety precaution to keep up with traffic and risky on local roads due to unexpected traffic stops and vehicles pulling out.	*Example:* *"Especially on uh local highways and things because of all the side roads and things that come into . . . you take like uh say highway 6, going out east. There's all those little roads that come in and you're runnin' 70 miles per hour and somebody pulls out in front of that and you got your hands full. So yeah I'd say more, the risk gets greater as you get down to the smaller roads and things. Main highways . . . you could go 85 on 80/94 and you'd be staying up with traffic! It's almost safer to run with the traffic than it is to try to hold the speed limit ya know."* (Interview 28)
Theme 4: Breaking the law	**Definition:** The motorcyclist indicates that speeding is safe until being 15 mph over the speed limit because then you can be charged for reckless driving.	*Example:* *"Well I would say one of them is watching your speed and not necessarily because someone could take you out but also . . . because ya know you can get pulled over ya know and then ya know it's . . . police . . . they make a big deal about speeding . . ."* (Interview 3)
Code: Alcohol embedded in the motorcycling culture		
Theme 1: Yes it impairs my skills, but it's just part of it	**Definition:** The motorcyclist conveys that consuming alcohol negatively impacts personal ability to ride a motorcycle safely but continues to participate in the behavior because it is expected in the motorcycling culture.	*Example:* *"So we shoot up there on Wednesdays and ya know we're up there . . . well . . . what's everyone doing up there? They're getting' shit feathered . . . oh I'm sorry . . . they're drinkin', they're eatin wings, ya know what I mean . . . they're hanging out. There's live bands there, everybody's drinking ya know, so . . . (4.0) . . . no it's not cool to drink obviously when you're on your motorcycle. But at the same time, it's the whole culture . . . that's what you're supposed to do. So if I'm drinking water people are like, "are you runnin' a marathon dude, or what? Where's the beer at?". I'm dead serious . . . dead serious. You see people hammering back shots."* (Interview 3)

Theme 2: Poker runs as enabling activity	**Definition:** The motorcyclist indicates that poker runs encourage motorcyclists to drink a lot of alcohol while on a ride.	*Example:* *"I've been on a few of those poker runs and . . . first couple I did . . . I went to every bar, drank a couple beers and as the day wore on I noticed I was getting a little bit . . . not doing too well on the bike ya know. So I said I can't do it and I've never had anyone on the back and done that so. But I think somebody needs to address that . . . the poker run thing where you drink. They outta start saying hey let's go, let's have a poker run but let's go over and have lunch and then we'll go to another place and we'll do . . . everybody will drink a bottle of water and then we'll go to the next place and then when we get back to our destination then we can drink beer ya know. And that, that . . . there's a wreck on those about every time they have one ya know."* (Interview 28)
Theme 3: The conscious drinker	**Definition:** The motorcyclist expresses that drinking and riding is not risky because personal tolerance and experience drinking is exceptional.	*Example:* *"Well I, I shouldn't say that I don't drink and drive, I've got a limit of two beers. If I'm ridin' that bike . . . well most of the time anymore when I'm ridin' that bike it's one beer. Anybody that's hammered and gets on a bike, that's wrong. Ya know I did that when I was younger."* (Interview 19)
Theme 4: Confronting the drunk motorcyclist	**Definition:** The motorcyclist describes the internal thought process before confronting fellow motorcyclists about their drinking behaviors while riding.	*Example:* *"I think you let them make that choice to a point. I'd say ya know if somebody is obviously intoxicated then yeah . . . I have wrestled friends for their keys before . . . tried to not, well ya know, arrange them rides or whatever. Um but yeah, but just ya know somebody comes in and has a 6-pack . . . they're a grown-up, they can decide. If they're not inebriated then they can make their own decisions."* (Interview 21)

Table A.3 Results for Immediacy/Goal Setting Informing Motorcycle Safety Perceived Susceptibility and Perceived Severity (*cont.*)

Code: Risk of accidents		
Theme 1: Always thinking about the possibility	**Definition:** The motorcyclist indicates that the possibility of having an accident is on their mind the entire ride.	*Example:* *"Every time I get on the bike it's the first thing I think about. It's like, "okay, I can get killed on this". And it affects me . . . it does. But . . . the . . . (5.0) . . . the way we ride and where we go . . . makes me feel okay. I overcome that and I want to do it so much . . . I enjoy it so much that . . . I mean it's the same risk I feel . . . I don't feel it in the car but I know in the car I could get killed just as easily."* (Interview 7)
Theme 2: If thought about it I wouldn't ride	**Definition:** The motorcyclist indicates that he/she would not continue riding if the thought of accidents permeated his/her thoughts while riding.	*Example:* *"It crosses my mind but it's not something I dwell on. I mean if I dwelt on it and really thought about it then I probably wouldn't ride. But ya know I mean like I said earlier I've got a family and I wanna make sure I get home to them."* (Interview 34)
Theme 3: It eventually happens to everyone	**Definition:** The motorcyclist indicates that every motorcyclist will have an accident while riding at some point.	*Example:* *"There are only two types of riders . . . those that have gone down and those that will go down . . . you eventually have to have an accident."* (Interview 1)
Theme 4: Not any more dangerous than everyday life	**Definition:** The motorcyclist describes motorcycling as risky as any other activity encountered in everyday life.	*Example:* *"You just have to be aware of your surroundings. It's not any more dangerous than anything else. You can fall down your basement stairs and break your neck."* (Interview 21)
Code: More experience, less susceptibility		
Theme 1: Feeling safer with every mile of experience	**Definition:** The motorcyclist indicates that the more miles driven, the more confidence exhibited on a motorcycle.	*Example:* *"I've got more miles under my belt so and, and I picked up some more uh tricks and I understand my motorcycles better so yeah I feel more confident."* (Interview 29)

Theme 2: Acquainted with the motorcycle and how it handles	**Definition:** The motorcyclist describes the process of learning the motorcycle as a contributing factor to lowering the chances of being in an accident.	*Example:* *"I would say like my reactions got better like um it was not just pertaining to my bike but just riding in general. Um also with my bike though I got to know the nuances of it like the rear brake and things like that. Um . . . and then I, having experienced enough different situations to kind of know how to react to newer ones on the fly."* (Interview 31)
Theme 3: Learning to go with your gut	**Definition:** The motorcyclist notes that with more experience it is easier to sense a dangerous situation.	*Example:* *"There's uh been some roads especially early in the season I've gotten like bad feelings before like, "maybe I shouldn't hit this corner at 60 mph," ya know. Although I have in the past and I'll come up on it and the whole corner is covered in gravel and I'm like, see . . . it's a good thing I chose not to do that."* (Interview 21)
Code: Consequences		
Theme 1: Road rash	**Definition:** The motorcyclist primarily associates an accident with road rash, scraping, and grinding all over a body.	*Example:* *"I guess with me . . . (7.0) . . . road rash would be the thing that I would think about. Just . . . I dunno . . . if . . . if I'm riding and I glance at the pavement I'm like, "oh if I fell off here it'd kinda scrape me up."* (Interview 8)
Theme 2: Head	**Definition:** The motorcyclist primarily associates an accident with a permanent head or neck injury.	*Example:* *"Brain injury or brain damage because the head's probably gonna be the first thing to hit the ground if you go flying forward off the bike. Or broken bones if you fall off the side. So, or probably a concussion as well so yeah."* (Interview 32)
Theme 3: Death	**Definition:** The motorcyclist primarily associates an accident with immediate death.	*Example:* *". . . it's really like a frieken death machine. Because all it takes is somebody to cut out in front of you and then sphew. And then you're hamburger meat."* (Interview 3)
Code: Personal accident or close-call accident		
Theme 1: Got right back on	**Definition:** The motorcyclist describes getting back on a motorcycle as the primary reaction after a personal accident.	*Example:* *"I was raised on a horse farm. What do you do? You get back on the horse, right?"* (Interview 15)

Table A.3 Results for Immediacy/Goal Setting Informing Motorcycle Safety Perceived Susceptibility and Perceived Severity (*cont.*)

Theme 2: Wake-up call	**Definition:** The motorcyclist indicates becoming more aware of personal vulnerability and safety behaviors while riding a motorcycle in response to an accident or close-call accident.	*Example:* *"I realized that you couldn't be defensive enough. You could never anticipate that in a million years and yet, it, it happened and that's not an accident, that's just ya know like insanity, like it's hard to describe. . . . And that was as close to an accident as you could have. But Natalie was just an infant, maybe a month old, and she would've been."* (Interview 27)
Theme 3: Just gimme a second (or more)	**Definition:** The motorcyclist stopped riding a motorcycle for a temporary period of time in response to an accident or close-call accident	*Example:* *"But um that really scared me. I mean . . . my dad, he was ahead of me in the other lane and he saw it happening in his rearview mirror and he said he could see it in my helmet and the look on me was "holy crap!" there were other words used but . . . holy crap. I was like what am I going to do . . . and it scared me to the point where for a week I wouldn't get on the bike but after that I was like . . . it's inevitable that I'm gonna get on a bike . . . I'm gonna do it and let's get this over with."* (Interview 5)
Theme 4: Making it a single vehicle (motorcycle) accident	**Definition:** The motorcyclist describes the behaviors engaged in before, during, and after an accident to avoid colliding with another object.	*Example:* *"And . . . um (3.0) a car stopped suddenly in front of me and rather than hitting him I laid it down. So that's what, that's what happened. . . . I wasn't going to hit him that was my sole purpose. So I had to do whatever I could to not hit him. Um (5.0) I dunno I just knew I wasn't gonna hit him. It didn't even occur to me or . . . I didn't even process the thought of going around, or . . . cause I didn't even know what he was doing I just knew that he stopped suddenly and then by the time I had already decided that I wasn't gonna hit him, he turned. And at that point it was too late."* (Interview 33)
Theme 5: It wasn't my fault	**Definition:** The motorcyclist feels angry toward drivers of other vehicles who caused an accident or close-call accident.	*Example:* *"Well, I believe that I try not to take risks and I try to obey the law and try to be a safe rider. So that being said, most of the time I'm really pissed that somebody was being an idiot and potentially ending up hurting me so yeah, I'm usually angry."* (Interview 2)

Code: Seeing/hearing it happen		
Theme 1: Maybe it *could* happen to me	**Definition:** The motorcyclist indicates that seeing or hearing about an accident causes feelings of susceptibility to surface because the accident could have happened to anyone.	*Example:* *"Hey this can happen to me ya know? And you're taking a chance every time you go on the bike but you like to ride so you've gotta control what you're doing with that motorcycle?"*(Interview 10)
Theme 2: Log it in the mind	**Definition:** The motorcyclist indicates that after seeing or hearing about an accident, details of the accident are mentally noted in order to avoid making the same mistake(s).	*Example:* *". . . you kinda start thinking about ya know the discussion you had in the lunch room about what they say when they have to go do stuff for his son because he couldn't do this or this and uh . . . you get on the bike that day and kinda think on the way home, ya know, "what did that kid do that was wrong?"* (Interview 10)
Theme 3: Temporary change in behavior	**Definition:** The motorcyclist indicates that after seeing or hearing about an accident a change in safety behaviors naturally occurs but eventually the motorcyclist reverts back to previous behaviors.	*Example:* *"Well it changes your, changes your outlook for a short period of time. I mean in reality ya know you slow down and you're more cautious. But then that . . . ya know."* (Interview 25)
Theme 4: Thinking twice	**Definition:** After seeing or hearing about an accident the motorcyclist describes feelings of apprehension and questions whether or not riding a motorcycle is worth the risk.	*Example:* *"After that accident we both . . . ya know Tommy couldn't ride because he was laid up with a cast and I ya know . . . we did. It was hard getting back on again and getting back in the groove again . . . (5.0) And ya know, the thing with your cousin too . . . that was a hard, hard thing to go through. I mean . . . terrible, well you were there, to watch your best friend lose his son. It was just horrible. And (8.0) . . . ya know that kind of stuff starts adding up and you hear about more and more people."* (Interview 7)

Table A.3 Results for Immediacy/Goal Setting Informing Motorcycle Safety Perceived Susceptibility and Perceived Severity (*cont.*)

Theme 5: Better motorcyclist than that motorcyclist	**Definition:** The motorcyclist indicates that seeing or hearing about an accident has no impact on personal behaviors because the motorcyclist in the accident was not as skilled of a rider.	*Example:* *"Um not really cause everybody has their own different situation. You don't know if that person was drunk, that person was doing crazy stuff or that person was going really fast ya know. I just try to kinda ya know keep that under control and not get too stupid while I'm riding."* (Interview 29)
Code: Compromise		
Theme 1: Weather-related safety	**Definition:** The motorcyclist describes safety behaviors practiced only when particular weather conditions are present.	*Example:* *"Sometimes since I'm still not quite as experienced if I know it's like really windy . . . I don't like riding when it's really windy . . . um . . . if it's gonna be really really hot, I'll take the air conditioned car. Um, but I guess I don't, I won't ride as much as like Jeff, my fiancé, does because he's a bit more comfortable with different weather conditions and stuff like that. But, I'll try and ride as much as I can. I'm just a little bit more picky as to the conditions that I will ride in."* (Interview 8)
Theme 2: Extra precautions for long rides	**Definition:** The motorcyclist describes safety behaviors practiced only when riding for an extended period of time.	*Example:* *"Um . . . just . . . if it's just a short trip . . . I'll usually just wear tennis shoes. If it's a longer trip I'll probably put boots on. And may wear a leather jacket. But if it's just short usually just a t-shirt or whatever."* (Interview 34)

Appendix D

Table A.4 Results for Empowerment Informing Motorcycle Safety Self-efficacy

Code: Becoming a safer motorcyclist		
Theme 1: Now more than in the past	**Definition:** The motorcyclist describes personal safety choices made now that were not practiced as a novice rider.	*Example:* *"I would say it's the opposite, that I was less likely to use safety precautions before when I was an early rider. It was all about being cool, ya know (haha). Now it's totally different. I can't think of anything that I could do much safer. I read all the books . . . "* (Interview 7)
Theme 2: Making the motorcycle safer	**Definition:** The motorcyclist describes ways to make the motorcycle safer to ride including loud pipes, headlights, and sidebars in case of a crash.	*Example:* *"I don't think I've ever laid it down, so I don't know how I would react. But it has skid bars on it and things like that that won't let it tip completely over flat. It's like a safety thing where you go so far and once the tire comes off the ground it'll slide. So in my mind I think that's what would happen but I don't wanna really find out (haha) ya know what I mean."* (Interview 28)
Theme 3: Avoiding panic mode	**Definition:** The motorcyclist thinks that it is easier to maintain composure and react quicker when facing a close call.	*Example:* *"Like . . . there's a . . . I'm sure you know studying what you study but there's like a common panic thing they have when they're not experienced riders and in a panic situation they can't help it. Like ya know . . . your panic has to go to avoiding the accident. Like instead of just ya know "ahhh" and going head on into something ya know you try to take some . . . (3.0) course of action to get away from it ya know."* (Interview 21)

Table A.4 Results for Empowerment Informing Motorcycle Safety Self-efficacy (*cont.*)

Code: Starting small to build confidence		
Theme 1: Motorcycle that fits your body	**Definition:** The motorcyclist advises starting with a smaller (650 CC) motorcycle to build skills.	*Example:* *"I would definitely point them towards that and I would definitely tell them, don't choose a bike that's too big. Get a, because if you choose a bike with too much power or that's too big or too awkward or something and you're not used to it then you're going to get hurt, no doubt about it."* (Interview 35)
Theme 2: Take time to familiarize yourself with the motorcycle	**Definition:** The motorcyclist recommends practicing and learning how the motorcycle handles before taking it out on the open road.	*Example:* *"When you first start out you don't know what's gonna happen with the motorcycle. As you get better you learn your own bike. It's kind of personal to your own vehicle. You jump on somebody else's bike that you don't know you're probably gonna wreck it (haha). I'm just saying. You'll be a lot safer. I mean if you know what your bike can do, handling it and all that you should be alright. Should be, anyway."* (Interview 22)
Theme 3: Trial and error within your boundaries	**Definition:** The motorcyclist indicates that confidence comes from making mistakes and learning from those mistakes by setting new boundaries.	*Example:* *"Umm . . . (6.0) . . . I've taken corners a little too fast and kinda lucked out. Um . . . the only time I ever did drop it was . . . I was in a parking lot seeing how tight I could do stuff and I ended up sliding it. But it wasn't a big deal. I didn't get hurt or anything."* (Interview 9)
Theme 4: Rural riding/ Parking lot	**Definition:** The motorcyclist advices new motorcyclists to engage in rural riding or on parking lots before venturing out on highways.	*Example:* *"Drive slow, drive slow. I would tell them to drive slow and stay in the country. Ya know don't go in congested areas. Uh drive the country roads to learn the motorcycle, all of its ya know, turn signals, lights and brakes and shifting and uh I'd just say stay in the country till you get comfortable with it."* (Interview 25)
Theme 5: Take the course	**Definition:** The motorcyclist recommends taking a safety course as the primary way to learn skills and build confidence.	*Example:* *"That's all you need. You take an ABATE class and they go through everything."* (Interview 12)

Code: Shift in societal norms impacting youth's safety		
Theme 1: Used to motorcycle experience from previous riding	**Definition:** The motorcyclist describes the rules of dirt bike riding as a sensitizing experience to wearing safety gear.	*Example:* *"Um I would say probably because I'm more comfortable with a helmet and I imagine that if I just kinda went from nothing to having to wear a helmet it'd be quite uncomfortable. So I'm, I'm used to knowing what a helmet feels like [from dirt biking] and knowing what it should feel like and how it should fit and everything."* (Interview 35)
Theme 2: Emphasizing safety for youth	**Definition:** The motorcyclist conveys that a larger safety emphasis exists to help target youth behaviors on a motorcycle.	*Example:* *"I think we are headed that way as far as people accepting uh wearing safety protection. Um the old schooler's are probably not gonna go along with it but the younger generation seems like they're, they're pickin' up on it. So I think we're headed in the right direction as far as safety."* (Interview 28)
Code: It involves motorcyclists to change too		
Theme 1: Keeping your cool	**Definition:** The motorcyclist describes angry, hostile responses to other drivers almost causing an accident.	*Example:* *"Just turned right in front of us and I'm like, "are you fucking kidding me"? I'm like, "let me off this fucking bike now. I will knock on the bitch's window and fucking sock her". Seriously, that's bullshit, it pisses me off when people do that."* (Interview 14)
Theme 2: I'm the exception	**Definition:** The motorcyclist indicates that other motorcyclists need to change their behaviors on a motorcycle.	*Example:* *"If you do want to be a serious motorcycle rider you need to take responsibility to be safe and don't put, like riding in groups, don't put your friends in jeopardy. Don't be the first guy to pull out in front of a semi with 6 bikes behind ya and he might be way down the road for him to pull out but the guys behind ya . . . they're gonna try to stay with ya and they'll pull out."* (Interview 2)

Appendix E

Table A.5 Results for Community Collaboration Informing a Harm Reduction Approach to Motorcycle Safety

Code: Collaboration is essential		
Theme 1: To raise awareness	**Definition:** The motorcyclist offers that collaboration is essential to help raise community awareness about the presence of motorcycles.	*Example:* *"Um personally I don't think much motorcycle safety gets to the riding community. As much as it is put out I've seen a lot of advertisements and its . . . it gets to a point and then talk to some people about it and they don't know what you're talking about. It's . . . it needs to get farther."* (Interview 5)
Theme 2: Sharing the road sharing the responsibility	**Definition:** The motorcyclist offers that by collaborating with several groups to discuss motorcycle safety all groups can get the message.	*Example:* *"It's an important message to get out there. I think . . . even . . . I know it sounds funny but even those little yellow bumper stickers, ya know, "be aware, motorcycles are everywhere," that's important. I mean especially for young drivers in cars even, they have to understand that there's more than just their vehicle on the road. it's . . . . it's a respect thing between everybody on the road. Um . . . and just knowing, seeing okay, there are motorcycles out here, there are bicycles out here. It's just a reminder of what's out there."* (Interview 2)

Table A.5 Results for Community Collaboration Informing a Harm Reduction Approach to Motorcycle Safety (*cont.*)

Theme 3: To get into the motorcycling culture	**Definition:** The motorcyclist indicates that collaboration with several groups may help infiltrate the embedded safety choices of the motorcycling culture.	*Example:* *"I don't think it would change just because the culture doesn't change. I mean ya know we're talkin about cultures, especially a Harley rider culture. Ya know it's just . . . it's just the whole live to ride, ride to live thing."* (Interview 3)
Code: Who's got the power		
Theme 1: Motorcycle clubs, organizations, and dealers	**Definition:** The motorcyclist offers that establishing relationships with various types of motorcycling organizations is the best way to reach motorcyclists.	*Example:* *"You need to meet at least one of each and they can generally tell you because um, (5.0) . . . the whole underworld of it is when you have your lettering, your things . . . you have to go before these other groups and organizations to put an organization in a community. So they will know who the other organizations are. If you meet one you know who all the other groups are . . . to learn how to get into partnering and meeting with the presidents, vice presidents, etc. And um, just pitching that sale to them and what the importance is and why it's important."* (Interview 1)
Theme 2: American Bikers Aimed Toward Education (ABATE)	**Definition:** The motorcyclist conveys that motorcyclists are most trusting of the safety advice from ABATE.	*Example:* *"I think just harping on the safety equipment isn't what people want to hear. I think it just sounds like your mom telling you motorcycles are dangerous. But like uh, ABATE offers an advanced rider course and it's uh . . . I know a guy that's a die-hard rider, he rides a Mecotto, and he takes the ABATE advanced rider course every year. Even though he's done it for the past whatever, because he believes that it sharpens his skills."* (Interview 21)
Theme 3: Bureau of Motor Vehicles (BMV)	**Definition:** The motorcyclist offers that partnering with the BMV to educate drivers of cars and trucks about motorcycles is necessary for safety.	*Example:* *"And then I think the um bureau of motor vehicles could do more to solicit safety information."* (Interview 33)

Theme 4: Law enforcement	**Definition:** The motorcyclist indicates that law enforcement would be influential in initiating safety practices.	*Example:* *"Um I think maybe the biggest one would probably be the uh . . . like the state patrol on the motorcycles. I know they don't have very many of them anymore. I know a lot of them are not doing it anymore or just switching to actual uh cars. But I think uh actually getting with them and making a solid program with them would be a pretty good asset."* (Interview 35)
Theme 5: Local venues and rides to educate	**Definition:** The motorcyclist suggests making education available to motorcyclists at events they already attend.	*Example:* *"But it's about uh other local rides that you have. Uh ABATE is not there, it's not there when . . . you have a lot memorial rides for people that have died ya know and that's where they should bring to mind the fact that it's more than let's ride . . . let's think about what we're doing . . . someone just got killed. He was riding drunk. Why are you doing that on two wheels, that's stupid."* (Interview 15)
Code: Addressing the risky motorcyclist		
Theme 1: Younger (crotch rocket) motorcyclists	**Definition:** The motorcyclist expresses that younger motorcyclists are less experienced and more willing to try daring stunts on their crotch rockets, making them a necessary target audience.	*Example:* *"Certainly the younger crotch rocketed ones I mean those bikes are made to be crazy. There's only one reason to own those. So I would say yeah as a demographic the ones that are buying that, that's usually . . . I mean a real young kid can't buy one because they cost so much but that, that younger group."* (Interview 27)
Theme 2: Older (Harley) motorcyclists	**Definition:** The motorcyclist expresses that older motorcyclists have slower reaction times and are stubborn to change how they ride a Harley, making them a necessary target audience.	*Example:* *". . . as far as the older population goes um (5.0) yeah they are very set in their ways and everything but a lot of them um if you . . . ya know they're usually I think of older guys on big Harleys and number one they've been riding forever (5.0) in my mind they've been riding forever so they know what to expect. Their bikes cost an insane amount of money and they're gonna do everything possible not to mess up their bike. Um so it would be good to target them but it's just because as far as year in safety I don't think they use it as much."* (Interview 8)

Table A.5 Results for Community Collaboration Informing a Harm Reduction Approach to Motorcycle Safety (*cont.*)

Theme 3: Everybody	**Definition:** The motorcyclist expresses that all motorcyclists, regardless of experience and behaviors, should be targeted to be safer on a motorcycle.	*Example:* *"I think it just needs to be, it just needs to be more of it. And I don't think demographics has anything to do with it. I think the more, the more that the information is out there, the better of any demographic would be."* (Interview 33)
Code: Clean up		
Theme 1: Road hazards	**Definition:** The motorcyclist describes common road hazards and conditions that are more dangerous for motorcyclists than other vehicles.	*Example:* *"All the construction. Ya know it's where there's tore up pavement but they let you ride on it it's more difficult for the motorcyclists to be on there than the cars. Um the steel bridges (haha) especially when they're wet . . . forget it. You just like, you just feel it like man, I'm goin down. But other than that no. Just the ongoing construction, the uneven pavement, the grooved pavement . . . it's really difficult to get a motorcyclist through that. So you really have to be aware."* (Interview 30)
Theme 2: Weather-related hazards	**Definition:** The motorcyclist indicates that the shorter riding season contributes to extra hazards and negligence on the road.	*Example:* *"Um not really I mean . . . cause of the winters and the spring you got a lot of loose gravel and stuff on the roads and the intersections and stuff you have to watch for . . . the salt and the cinders and stuff."* (Interview 36)

Index

alcohol abuse, harm reduction, 40–44; high-risk drinking, 50
alcohol-abuse interventions, harm reduction: Alcohol Misuse Prevention Study, 42; Brief Alcohol Screening and Intervention for College Student, 43; Life Skills Training Program, 42; Moderation Management, 42; School Health and Alcohol Harm Reduction Project, 43
autonomy, 204

beneficence, 206–7

community collaboration, 23–25; as a metatheoretical tenet, 160–68; interview questions that probe, 113–14. *See also* central tenets of HRT
confidentiality, participant, 206–7
consent, participant: informed, 204–5; process, 205–6
convenience sampling, 123
conversational techniques, types of, 100

empowerment, 21–23: as a metatheoretical tenet, 152–60; interview questions that probe, 112–13. *See also* central tenets of HRT
ethics, 202; frameworks of in qualitative research, 203; macro-level, 218–29; micro-level, 215–16

goal setting, in public health, 16
Grounded Theory, 116; analysis using, 117

harm minimization, 7–8
harm reduction metatheory: definition of, 234; integrated model of, 83
Harm Reduction Theory, 16; applications of, 36–44; barriers to, 4–10; central tenets of, 17–25; definitions of, 1–12; history of, 2–3; macro-level ethics of, 218–29; micro-level ethics of, 215–18
Health Belief Model, 76. *See also* Reconceptualized Health Belief Model
health promotion, 12
HIV test counseling, 46; integrated harm reduction model of, 48
humanistic value, 18–19; as a metatheoretical tenet, 128–34; interview questions that probe,

107–8; *See also* central tenets of HRT

immediacy, 20–21; as a metatheoretical tenet, 143–52; interview questions that probe, 111–12. *See also* central tenets of HRT
interviewing: analysis of, 115; as contextualized conversations, 99; ethnographic explanations of, 99; in-depth, 98; ordinary conversations, 100; question types, 99; responsive, 100; semi-structured, 104–5

justice, participant, 207–9

member checking, 181–83
metatheory: definition of, 74; integrated model of harm reduction, 83; reflexive tool, 193–97
motivational interviewing, 14
motorcycling behaviors, risky, 124

National Institute on Alcohol Abuse and Alcoholism (NIAAA), 53; four tiers of effectiveness, 54
needle exchange programs (NEPs), 36. *See also* history of Harm Reduction Theory
New Model for Public Health, 2

ongoing dialoguing, 230

power, researcher, 207–9
pragmatism, 19–20; as a metatheoretical tenet, 134–43; interview questions that probe, 109–11. *See also* central tenets of HRT
Purdue University: campus community retail bar coalition, 54–56; safer party magnet, 56; 21st birthday card, 60
purposive sampling, 122; maximum variation, 123

qualitative data analysis: constant comparative method, 117; initial coding, 116; negative case analysis, 117; open coding, 116; theoretical (or axial) coding, 117; theory-driven code development, 115; theme, 115

rapport, 209–211; harm reduction metatheory facilitating, 211–14
Reconceptualized Health Belief Model, 77; cues to action, 76, 83–85; perceived barriers, 85; perceived benefits, 85; perceived severity, 86; perceived susceptibility, 86; risk appraisal, 87; self-efficacy, 88
reflexivity, 183, 190–193, 197; metatheoretical, 187–90; postmodern aspect of, 185–87. *See also* verification strategies
research questions, crafting, 101
researcher bias, 181
risk reduction, 8

sampling, qualitative, 122
saturation, 125
snowball sampling, 123
Social Ecological Model, 51–53

theoretical sampling, 122
theoretical saturation, 124
theory, definition of, 74
Theory of Reasoned Action/Planned Behavior, 79–80, 194–95;
tobacco abuse, harm reduction, 38–40; e-cigarettes, 38; snus, 39
Transtheoretical Model/Stages of Change Model, 80–82, 195–96
Trojan horse, 5–6

validity, 176; descriptive, 176–77; interpretive, 180–83; metatheoretical, 191–93; theoretical, 190; verification strategies of, 177–80, 183–87

About the Authors

Emily J. Haas, Ph.D. (Purdue University, 2012), is a Behavioral Research Scientist at the National Institute for Occupational Safety and Health (NIOSH) Office of Mine Safety and Health Research (OMSHR). Her research seeks to integrate harm reduction with health behavior theories in the development of campaigns and interventions for several audiences and health issues including sexual violence prevention, motorcycle safety, and mine safety and health. Her current research involves initiatives to reduce the prevalence of injury and disease among the mining population including: developing, implementing, and evaluating multilevel interventions for mineworkers with a present emphasis on improving worker empowerment in response to new mining technology and improving mine site leadership to facilitate safer behaviors among workers; extending and refining theories about factors influencing mineworkers' risk perception and subsequent safety-related behaviors as a result of new technology; and mineworkers' self-escape training and competency assessment. She received her Ph.D. from Purdue University and her M.A. and B.A. from the University of Dayton. Her research is published in journals including *International Journal of Motorcycle Studies, Safety and Health at Work, International Journal of Qualitative Methods, Journal of Higher Education Outreach and Engagement, American Journal of Health Behavior,* and *Cases in Public Health and Communication Marketing.*

Marifran Mattson is Professor and Head of the Brian Lamb School of Communication at Purdue University and the Advisor to the Motorcycle Safety at Purdue campaign. She is an author of *Health as Communication Nexus: A Service Learning Approach* and has been teaching health communication courses for more than nineteen years. She is a Purdue University Community of Service Learning Faculty Fellow and an Indiana Campus Compact Faculty Fellow. Her primary expertise is in social marketing and advocacy campaigns and she served in a year-long fellowship at Centers for Disease Control and Prevention. She is the founder and faculty advisor for the Motorcycle Safety at Purdue (MS@P; www.ItInvolvesYou.com) campaign. Her health communication research has been published in journals and book chapters across disciplines.

www.ingramcontent.com/pod-product-compliance
Ingram Content Group UK Ltd.
Pitfield, Milton Keynes, MK11 3LW, UK
UKHW012036150926
475560UK00001B/39

9 780739 18056